Veterinary Pharmacology

A Practical Guide for the Veterinary Nurse

For Elsevier:

. . . .

Commissioning Editor: Mary Seager/Rita Demetriou-Swanwick
Development Editor: Rebecca Nelemans
Editorial Assistant: Louisa Welch
Project Manager: Elouise Ball
Designer: Stewart Larking
Illustration Buyer: Gillian Richards
Illustrator: Peter Cox

Veterinary Pharmacology

A Practical Guide for the Veterinary Nurse

By Amanda Rock BVSc MRCVS

Veterinary Surgeon, The Veterinary Hospital,
Estover, Plymouth, UK
Lecturer in Veterinary Nursing,
Rosewarne College, Camborne, UK

With contributions by

Sally Bowden BSc (Hons) CertEd VN

Glen Cousquer BSc (Hons) BVM&S CertZooMed MRCVS

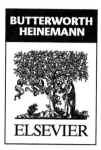

Edinburgh   London   New York   Oxford   Philadelphia   St Louis   Sydney   Toronto   2007

BUTTERWORTH
HEINEMANN

© 2007, Elsevier Limited. All rights reserved.

First published 2007

ISBN 978-0-7506-8862-8

British Library Cataloguing in Publication Data
A catalogue record for this book is available from the British Library

Library of Congress Cataloging in Publication Data
A catalog record for this book is available from the Library of Congress

 your source for books,
journals and multimedia
in the health sciences
www.elsevierhealth.com

Working together to grow
libraries in developing countries

www.elsevier.com | www.bookaid.org | www.sabre.org

ELSEVIER   BOOK AID   Sabre Foundation
              International

The
publisher's
policy is to use
**paper manufactured
from sustainable forests**

Printed and bound in the United Kingdom
Transferred to Digital Print 2011

Contents

Preface

Welcome to twenty-first century pharmacology!

This textbook focuses on the clinical application of pharmacology in veterinary medicine and surgery, and discusses currently used agents rather than those historically available. It is not intended to be a comprehensive formulary. Instead, representative agents from each group have been chosen to demonstrate the general mechanisms of action of the drugs rather than listing all those available. This will enable the reader to understand why a particular therapy is effective in treating a disease and encourages a problem-solving approach, which is the most effective way to learn about pharmacology and develop a working knowledge of the subject.

It is essential to have a basic knowledge of anatomy and physiology to understand how a drug acts on the body and how the body acts on the drug. Section two, therefore, concentrates on relevant body systems. This can be read as an introduction or can be referred back to whenever the need arises. The chemical science chapter and microbiology sections are aimed at those nurses wishing to gain a more detailed understanding of how medicines actually function.

At the start of each chapter the reader will find a list of the main learning aims and the objectives they should gain a knowledge of by studying the chapter. These have been based on the pharmacy certificate for veterinary nurses but incorporate all criteria for the level 2 and 3 veterinary nursing syllabus. The book is not a list of facts, however – more a discussion of the potential uses of drugs. For example, a reader could learn about all of the drugs used to treat allergic skin disease in one section rather than having to know the name of an agent to look it up.

Wherever possible, photographs accompany descriptions of the administration of drugs. Readers are thus encouraged to attempt new techniques, such as the administration of intramuscular injections into the gluteals rather than the leg muscles or the administration of a drug via nebulisation. The terminology used is explained in a comprehensive glossary and so the text is accessible to everyone with an interest in pharmacology – from animal nursing assistants through to veterinary students and surgeons alike. The practical pharmacy sections are of particular relevance to anyone working in a pharmacy manager type role.

Veterinary surgeons have a right to prescribe, but only a privilege to dispense medicines. This privilege is in danger of being taken away and given back to registered pharmacists if we as a profession do not start to manage our dispensaries more efficiently. The text highlights areas of good pharmacy practice we should be considering and gives tips on getting the most out of our therapies to achieve our ultimate aim – the alleviation or palliation of suffering in our patients.

Each chapter concludes with a variety of self-assessment questions to allow readers to ascertain their level of understanding and, in some cases, add to the knowledge already gained through studying the chapter. At the end of the text is a set of multiple choice questions, tailored specifically to the different levels of the veterinary nurse examinations.

This book can be used as a reference text whenever a clinical situation arises where drug knowledge is required. It is also intended as a piece of reading, designed to stimulate interest in the field of pharmacology. The author hopes that it will inspire nurses to take a more active role in the management of their patient's medications.

Amanda Rock,
2007

Introduction to Pharmacology

SECTION **1**

CHAPTER 1

The Role of the Veterinary Nurse in Drug Therapy

Amanda Rock and Sally Bowden

Learning aims and objectives

After studying this chapter you should be able to:

1. **Outline the importance of the veterinary nurse's role in ensuring accurate drug administration**
2. **List important aspects to consider when selecting a prescribed drug for administration**
3. **Name the 'five rights' of drug administration**
4. **Give some examples of side effects and various types of adverse reaction**
5. **Describe aspects of nursing care that may need alteration during drug therapy**
6. **Explain how to correctly discharge a patient requiring drug therapy at home**
7. **List factors affecting clients' understanding during patient discharge**
8. **Outline the importance of client' compliance**
9. **List methods by which veterinary nurses can improve client compliance.**

Introduction

The veterinary nurse (VN) plays an important role in all aspects of drug therapy. Veterinary practice has evolved and the days when the veterinary surgeon is constantly present to monitor every single patient under care have long gone. Equally, it is no longer common practice for veterinary surgeons to discharge every patient from the hospital, nor take all requests for repeat prescriptions. Thus, the VN's role has widened and increased in importance with regard to the welfare of patients both in and out of the hospital setting. This chapter explores all aspects of the VN's role in drug therapy and outlines the key components needed in order to practice safely and effectively. Where appropriate, other chapters in this book have been referenced to provide further detail.

Inpatient care

Medicines are commonly used to treat inpatients and VNs are well used to participating in the delivery of such treatment. However, when the practice is busy, it is easy to overlook the importance of one or more aspects of the drug therapy and for patients, this can lead to failure to recover, deterioration or complications in their condition.

It is not acceptable to assume that on-the-job training in the management of drug therapy is sufficient and there is no need for further learning or alteration in systems of delivery – whilst there are limited data available to demonstrate the rate of

3

drug errors made by VNs (Armitage et al 2005), there have been many studies regarding their veterinary counterparts. These all demonstrate significant errors made in all aspects of drug administration to inpatients. For example, Bruce & Wong (2002) recorded a 25.2% error rate and in the same year Taxis & Barber recorded a 49% error rate in a larger sample. VNs must ensure they are adopting best practice by actively reflecting on and reviewing their techniques and systems with regard to the key areas outlined below.

Selecting drugs

Once the veterinary surgeon has prescribed the medication for a patient, the VN may be required to select the drug from the pharmacy shelf. There is a vast array of different drugs available, many with several different names. The majority of drugs have one generic name and one or more brand names. It is important to understand the difference between a generic name and a brand name:
- the generic name is usually derived from the drug's chemical structure and is not protected by copyright
- the brand names are the copyrighted names given by the Marketing Authorisation (license) holder for their own particular make of that drug
- for example, generic amoxicillin is marketed as Clamoxyl (Pfizer), Duphamox (Fort Dodge) and Betamox (Norbrook) amongst others; generic furosemide is marketed as Dimazon (Intervet), Frusecare (Animalcare) and Frusedale (Arnolds) amongst others.

VNs should be aware of the generic names for all commonly used drugs, as different veterinary practices may stock different brands of the same

drug. Equally, it is important to know where to obtain information about drug names if necessary. Common sources of reference include the Animal Medicines Data Sheet Compendium (2005) and The Small Animal Formulary (Tennant 2005).

Drugs should be selected carefully and all practice staff should get into a habit of routinely checking their selection. A system of double-checking with another member of staff or via a computerised system should be employed. The important aspects to consider when selecting drugs for administration are detailed in Table 1.1.

Administration of drugs

There are several key points to consider when preparing for and administering drugs. Galbraith et al (1999) outline the 'five rights of drug administration', for human nurses, which are easily adapted for VNs, as Table 1.2 describes. For specific information relating to drug selection and administration, please refer to Chapter 3.

Observation and nursing of patients on drug therapy

Nurses are familiar with the recording of both subjective (the nurse's impression of the animal's condition such as bright, alert and responsive) and objective parameters (measurable indicators such as pulse rate and temperature). Patients receiving drug therapy may require additional observation because they are at risk of suffering from side effects and adverse reactions.
- A side effect is an expected, but unwanted, effect of normal drug therapy, usually related to its actions in parts of the body other than the area

Table 1.1 Important aspects to consider when selecting drugs for administration

Correct drug name	Note that some drugs have similar names, e.g. potassium chloride and potassium bromide, or phenobarbital, phenylbutazone and prednisolone
Correct strength	Most manufacturers make their packaging of the same drug a different colour for each strength, but not all do this. It is a good idea to write on similar packaging to help differentiate them, or keep them in containers of different colours (do not remove the drug from its original packaging; place the entire packet in an external container)
Stock rotation	A well-ordered pharmacy will only have one packet of each drug and strength open at any time. Do not open new packets unless it is necessary
Quality of product	Check the quality of the product – ensure it is not incorrectly stored, out of date or damaged and does not exhibit any unusual features such as difference in colour or viscosity (see Chapter 3 for further information)
Legal requirements	Remember to adhere to local rules, which comply with the Misuse of Drugs Act 1971 and Veterinary Medicines Regulations 2005, with regard to completion of a Controlled Drugs register and/or recording of batch numbers (see Chapter 2 for further information)

Table 1.2 The five rights of drug administration (adapted from Galbraith 1999)

Right drug	Ensure correct selection of drug from the pharmacy shelf. Correct interpretation of the veterinary surgeon's prescription is necessary – unfamiliar drugs should be checked using a suitable reference source, e.g. Animal Medicines Data Sheet Compendium. If the name of the drug is unclear, or the drug does not appear to match with the patient's condition, the prescribing veterinary surgeon should be consulted for confirmation of their instructions
Right dose	Ensure correct selection of drug from the pharmacy shelf. If drug calculations are required, VNs should double-check their calculations prior to drug administration. If the dose appears to be unusual for that particular size or species of patient, clarification should be sought from the prescribing veterinary surgeon (see Chapter 3 for further information)
Right patient	Ensure the correct patient has been identified. Some practices use paper collars to identify their patients; these and kennel name plates should be checked against the records prior to administration of drugs. Additionally, this is a good time to double check the drug is not contraindicated for the patient due to age, gender, status (e.g. pregnancy) or concurrent drug therapy. Some drugs stipulate 'special precautions' in certain circumstances and these should be double-checked too
Right route	Once the correct route has been identified, the correct administration technique must be used. For example, some drugs should only be given by slow intravenous injection, e.g. calcium borogluconate, metronidazole; not only must the VN identify the correct route but also inject the drug over time. Some orally administered drugs can only be administered with food, or must not be given at the same time as food. Some drugs can cause substantial damage to the patient if given via the incorrect route, or can be highly irritant, e.g. vincristine sulphate, which must be given intravenously – extravascular injection can cause serious tissue damage
Right time	This can sometimes be difficult, especially on a busy day in the practice. However, VNs must endeavour to administer drugs within the allotted time scale as blood plasma concentrations of drugs may dwindle below the therapeutic level if a dose is too late. This can lead to failure to recover

Box 1.1

Some examples of side effects of drug therapy

- muscular weakness from potassium loss with diuretic therapy
- breathlessness, restlessness and euphoria associated with steroid therapy
- depression associated with antihypertension drug therapy
- anorexia in patients on digoxin
- breakdown of oral mucosa in animals receiving cytotoxic drugs

being treated. Examples of side effects are shown in Box 1.1.
- An adverse reaction is an unexpected, harmful effect of drug therapy. It can be due to the drug, its administration or the patient. Adverse reactions are categorised into types, as shown in Table 1.3.

When observing a patient on drug therapy, it is also important to know which side effects and adverse reactions could occur and this requires a knowledge of specific medicines. For those less commonly used,

the VN can obtain this information from the product data sheet, so this should be kept to hand, near the patient (e.g. along with the patient's hospital record) so all nursing staff can gain easy access to it.

Suspected adverse reactions should always be reported to the veterinary surgeon immediately so that the patient can have any further treatment necessary. The Veterinary Medicines Directorate operates the Suspected Adverse Reaction Surveillance Scheme (SARSS), which provides report forms for completion in the event of a suspected adverse reaction. Further information regarding side effects and adverse reactions is found in Chapter 4. When considering the nursing care plan for individual patients, the need for additional frequency or type of observation should be taken into account. Table 1.4 outlines some additional observation and measurements which may be necessary.

Outpatient care

Discharging an inpatient

When anxiety levels are high, the ability to concentrate on detail is reduced. In such situations many clients do not listen carefully to discharge instructions. Studies show that most people can only retain

Table 1.3 Classification of adverse reactions

Reaction type	Description	Details	Examples
A	Augmented – enhanced drug effect	Predictable, dose-dependent, common, low mortality	Increased effect of drug due to hypoproteinaemic patient
B	Bizarre – allergic reactions	Unpredictable, not dose-related, high mortality	Urticaria, skin rashes, anaphylactic shock
C	Chronic – due to continuous therapy	Occurs when patients are on long-term therapy	Iatrogenic Cushing's from long-term prednisolone therapy
D	Delayed – occurring a long time after treatment	May not be apparent until several years after treatment	Teratogenicity of griseofulvin, carcinomas
E	End of treatment – occurring on withdrawal of therapy	Often caused by sudden withdrawal of a drug which should be slowly withdrawn	Seizure after phenytoin withdrawal, adrenocortical insufficiency after prednisolone therapy

three pieces of information from a consultation so it is clear that good communication skills are essential, even to impart the basics.

When discharging a patient, timing is everything – discuss the medications alone with the client before discharging the animal, which can serve as a distraction. Ensure the client can hear what you are saying easily – equipment, dogs barking, children in the room and the possibility of a deaf or hard-of-hearing client should all be considered. Ensure there is good lighting and wait for the client to put on their glasses. Written instructions can eliminate any ambiguity and ensure that clients have a written record to refer to.

Focus the learning by gleaning what information is essential and then what the clients want to know. It is best to begin with the client's questions and proceed from there, otherwise you may be explaining things they are not interested in knowing and they might not pay attention. By beginning with the client's needs, you give them some control over the learning process and increase the learning that takes place.

Check the details on the labels are clear, but do not assume all clients are literate – read all dose instructions out aloud. Explain any leaflets distributed with the medication. Assess the client's level of knowledge of the condition and break teaching down into stages if there is a lot to learn. For example, with diabetes mellitus cases arrange times to teach techniques when the client is familiar with the basic concepts and procedures. Box 1.2 shows the areas that should be discussed with clients at discharge.

Demonstration of medication techniques

Many clients will never have had to administer medication to their pet before. Whilst some will readily admit they need to be shown how to do this, some will be too embarrassed to confess to this and so it is a good idea to routinely demonstrate administration of medication to clients when discharging their pet, unless they specifically state they do not wish this.

It can be a challenge to administer a small amount of fluid to a kitten and wriggly dogs can prove impossible to get eye ointment into, even for the most experienced nurses. Therefore the client's manual dexterity, coordination of hand and eye and gentleness must be assessed before assuming competence in administering the medication. Repeated practice under supervision may be required and this should be offered when appropriate. Box 1.3 outlines some tips useful for effective demonstration to clients.

Client compliance

Client compliance is the extent to which the actions of the owner coincide with the instructions of the veterinary team with regard to care of an animal. It can be used to describe any aspect of treatment, but is most commonly referred to when discussing drug therapy and the likelihood that the owner will give prescribed medication correctly. Some human-centred nursing texts dislike the use of the word 'compliance', as it infers that people are being ordered to do as they are told, rather than following a course of treatment that has been negotiated and agreed. The terms 'adherence' and 'concordance' are preferred.

The importance of client compliance

Studies in human medicine show that patient non-compliance is a major cause of ineffective treatment. Studies undertaken in the veterinary field have also produced alarming results (Barter et al 1996,

Box 1.2

Areas that should be discussed with clients at discharge

Drug regime

- The client should be familiar with the name, dose, route of administration, desired action and storage of the medication
- When the medication should start and the length of the course
- Explain when the medication should take effect and when to seek advice if the effects are not seen
- How repeat prescriptions can be obtained if required
- How unused medications can be disposed of
- Cite possible side effects and ensure client is aware of the signs and symptoms of the reactions; also ensure the client knows when to report them and seek advice
- Discuss the general approach to management of other illnesses whilst on the medication, i.e. alert the veterinarian to the drug therapy and do not give other medications without seeking advice
- What to do if a medication is missed or vomited up
- Ensure the client is aware of any records they have been asked to complete

Exercise

- Often the promotion of exercise can reduce the need for drug therapy, i.e. analgesics for arthritis and any flexibility in dose should be discussed
- Some medications require exercise levels to be consistent, i.e. insulin

Diet and liquids

- The interrelationship between medications and food may be relevant, for example in diabetes mellitus, where the timing must coincide with the peak action of insulin
- Some medications must be given with food but some, like the antibiotic oxytetracycline, must not
- Patients on prescription or special diets might not be able to take their medications with any other foods and so nurses must ensure the tablets are not wrapped in meat or dairy products by clients desperate to administer the medication
- Some medications may cause nausea or vomiting and reduce appetite so management of inappetence and the provision of regular, small volumes of water might be relevant

Box 1.3

Tips useful for effective demonstration to clients

- Avoid creating a mirror image – sit alongside the client so they can see how you load a syringe, e.g. from the same angle as they will be expected to do it
- Teach the correct methods and do not demonstrate bad techniques
- Demonstrate a skill first, then describe it – if necessary, demonstrate again afterwards; avoid asking the client to absorb two sources of information at once
- Teach in stages and reiterate points of importance
- Demonstrate any other skills required to draw up or administer the medication, e.g. if syringes must be loaded
- Make use of 'props' such as soft toys or oranges for clients to practice with before handling their pet
- Once you have demonstrated, if possible ask the client to repeat the demonstration back to you to check their level of understanding – obviously, this applies to the technique only, to avoid overdosage!

Table 1.4 Additional observation and measurements for patients receiving drug therapy

Aspect of monitoring	Rationale	Nursing action
Patient alertness, body strength and ability to interact with nurse	More frequent checks are required to monitor patient correctly for adverse reactions	Increase frequency of checks – report any changes outside normal parameters. Provide additional mobility support if necessary. Provide appropriate physiotherapy if necessary
Temperature, pulse and respiratory rate measurement	More frequent checks are required to monitor patient correctly for adverse reactions	Increase frequency of checks – report any changes outside normal parameters
'Special precautions'	Some drug manufacturers advise special care be taken when using certain products in certain patients, e.g. clomipramine must be used with care in patients with cardiovascular dysfunction or epilepsy	Follow the advice given on the drug data sheet regarding 'special precautions'
Nutritional and fluid intake	Some drugs may require changes in food and water intake. Some can cause anorexia, inappetance, pica, polydipsia, etc.	Instigate changes in diet and fluid intake as necessary. Monitor calorie intake carefully in inappetent patients and provide assisted feeding if necessary. Measure fluid intake and ensure sufficient water is available in polydipsic patients
Elimination patterns	Some drugs may cause changes in elimination patterns, e.g. pollakiuria, polyuria, oliguria, stranguria, diarrhoea, haematochezia, melena, etc.	Report any changes. Provide additional opportunity for elimination. Obtain samples if necessary
Skin and mucous membranes	Petechial haemorrhage, rash, urticaria and ulceration can indicate an adverse reaction. Also, oral dryness and reduction in lacrimation are common side effects of some drugs	Report any changes outside normal parameters. Provide artificial tears and other lubrication when necessary
Urinalysis, faecal examination and blood sampling	These can be good indicators of the patient's tolerance to the drug	Ensure diagnostic quality samples are collected at appropriate times. Look for excessive protein and blood in urine and faeces. Hepatic and renal profiling may be useful
Therapeutic effect	The VN should know when to expect the drug to start having a therapeutic effect – if this does not happen it is important non-response is recognised	Report and record changes in the animal's condition. If an expected therapeutic effect does not occur, alert the veterinary surgeon immediately

Berendson & Knol 2002, Adams et al 2005). Ensuring client compliance will improve the health and welfare of the patient and the veterinary professional should facilitate this.

Factors affecting compliance

There are five main factors that affect client compliance – patient characteristics, treatment regime, the nature of the disease, the client themselves and their relationship with the veterinary team (Table 1.5).

The nurse's role in improving compliance

The veterinary nurse is ideally placed within the team to play a major role in increasing compliance and, in doing so, improving the wellbeing of patients. Box 1.4 outlines the various ways in which the VN can support the client.

Other methods of improving compliance, which involve manipulation of the prescription and therefore liaison with the veterinary surgeon, include:
- for short-term treatment, offering to medicate the patient if the owner is incapable, either by

Table 1.5 Factors affecting compliance

Factor	Description
Patient characteristics	The patient's temperament and lifestyle – animals who are aggressive or spend a lot of time away from the house may be less likely to receive regular treatment
Treatment regimen	The complexity of the treatment regimen – frequent dosing intervals and polypharmacy may reduce compliance
Disease nature	There is evidence in human studies that prophylactic treatment regimens and treatment regimens for chronic or terminal patients may be less likely to be adhered to
Client characteristics	Aged clients or those who have disabilities or illnesses may be less likely to comply to treatment regimens
Relationship with the veterinary team	A good relationship with the veterinary team will enhance the possibility the client will return for assistance if they encounter difficulty adhering to a treatment regimen

Box 1.4

Various ways in which the VN can support the client

- Educate the client – people are more likely to dose their animal if they understand why it is necessary, especially when the disease is asymptomatic, like hypertension
- Demonstrate how to give medication and encourage the owner to repeat the dosing technique whilst in the practice
- Offer medication aids such as reminders, pill givers
- Use written instructions and take advantage of commercially produced literature, videos, slides, models, charts, etc.
- Call the client one or two days following commencement of treatment to see how they are progressing
- Assure the client they can return to check progress or discuss treatment at any time
- Offer nurse consultations for patients diagnosed with long-term conditions, and/or consider a system of named nurses for chronically ill patients to encourage confidence
- Check repeat prescriptions are being ordered at the correct time intervals and query any discrepancies tactfully with the client
- Ask the client if they are able to manage the treatment programme easily when they call for a repeat prescription
- Ensure clients bring their pets back for routine blood testing if applicable, e.g. fructosamine and phenobarbitone serum levels
- If urinalysis is required, make sure the client is competent to collect a sample and understands storage requirements
- Check the drug is having the desired therapeutic effect when the client calls or visits the practice

daily trips to the surgery or hospitalisation for a period of time
- simplifying the drug regime – the more often a patient has to take a drug the less likely it is to receive it
- reducing unwanted side effects, e.g. steroids could be given in the evening to cats and in the morning to dogs to reduce restlessness.

The two case studies below can be used in role play training exercises.

CASE STUDY 1.1

A hypoproteinaemic dog with a hepatic tumour is medicated with morphine to control the pain. He suffers from regular atopic flare ups which respond to antihistamine therapy with chlorpheniramine (Piriton) plus an initial short course of prednisolone. What special precautions, additional observations and extra nursing care will be required due to the potential for enhanced CNS or respiratory depression which may occur with the concurrent administration of two CNS depressants?

The VN responsible for caring for this patient should consider the clinical management of the patient's condition. It is useful to formulate a plan as described below:

Preparation: Be aware of the patient's history and condition as well as all drug requirements, interactions and special precautions. Know how the patient has responded to any treatment so far and any potential complications that have arisen, e.g. difficult to dose orally. Know the aim of treatment – is it to cure or to manage the condition?

Implementation: Prepare clear, easy to follow instructions regarding drug administration and ensure plans are easily accessed by all nursing staff to guarantee continuity of care. Administer drugs according to plan, using the 'five rights' to make certain there are no errors. Alter observation and nursing care plans accordingly.

Evaluation: Observe the patient closely, according to the observation and nursing plan. Make any changes as necessary. Ensure all records are available for the veterinary surgeon during rounds in order for them to assess the patient's progress.

CASE STUDY 1.2

A cat has been diagnosed with hyperthyroidism and a urinary tract infection which she gets regularly due to stress. The following list of drugs needs to be administered:

- atenolol – a β-blocker to slow the heart and reduce the systemic hypertension (high blood pressure) caused by the hyperthyroidism (1 once a day for 1 week then a blood pressure check is required)
- methimazole (Felimazole) – a drug that interferes with the synthesis of thyroid hormone (1 twice a day for 3 weeks then a blood test is required)
- amitriptyline – a tricyclic antidepressant that is used to treat psychogenic disorders where there is a component of anxiety (0.5 ml once a day orally)
- amoxicillin/clavulanate (Synulox) – antibiotic (1 twice a day for 10 days).

The patient regularly takes cimetidine (Tagamet) syrup orally (0.5 ml twice a day) to control her stress-related gastritis and vomiting, but as it may increase the plasma levels of β-blockers the cimetidine should be stopped for the next few weeks.

The VN responsible for discharging this patient should consider the clinical management of the patient's condition once discharged. It is useful to formulate a plan as described below:

Preparation: Be aware of the patient's history and condition as well as all drug requirements, interactions and reactions. Know how the patient has responded to treatment as an inpatient and any potential complications that have arisen, e.g. difficult to dose orally. Know the aim of treatment – is it to cure or to manage the condition? How much information does the owner require in order to carry out the treatment correctly?

Implementation: Provide the client with the background detail regarding their pet's disease and drug therapy necessary for them to undertake the instructions correctly. This may involve several consultations, demonstrations, using written instructions, pill reminders and any other number of different techniques and aids.

Evaluation: Ensure the client is fully supported once the patient has been discharged by carrying out follow-up telephone calls. Make follow-up appointments for them as necessary and monitor progress using methods described in Box 1.4.

References and further reading

Adams V, Campbell J, Waldner C, Dowling P, Shmon C 2005 Evaluation of client compliance with short-term administration of antimicrobials to dogs. Journal of the American Veterinary Medical Association 226(4):567–574

Animal Medicines Data Sheet Compendium 2005 National Office of Animal Health, Middlesex, UK

Armitage E, Wetmore L, Chan D, Lindsey J 2005 Evaluation of compliance among nursing staff in administration of prescribed analgesic drugs to critically ill dogs and cats. Journal of the American Veterinary Medical Association 227(3):425–429

Barter L, Watson A, Maddison J 1996 Owner compliance with short term antimicrobial medication in dogs. Australian Veterinary Journal 74:277–280

Berendsen M, Knol B W 2002 Treatment compliance. Tijdschr Diergeneeskd 127(18):548–551

Bruce & Wong (2002), Taxis & Barber (2002) both cited at www.saferhealthcare.org.uk/IHI/Topics/MedicationPractice/WhatWeKnow/Whatweknowoverview.htm accessed 13.02.06

Galbraith A, Bullock S, Manias E, Hunt B, Richards A 1999 Fundamentals of pharmacology, 2nd edn. Addison-Wesley Longman, Harlow, p115–116

Tennant B (ed) 2005 Small Animal Formulary, 5th edn. British Small Animal Veterinary Association, Gloucester, UK

www.vmd.gov.uk/Publications/SARSS/sarss.pdf

Questions for Chapter 1

1. How could you differentiate between two strengths of the same drug on the pharmacy shelf, if the manufacturers' packaging was the same?

2. List the 'five rights' of drug administration.

3. What is the difference between a side effect and an adverse reaction?

4. To whom should suspected adverse reactions be reported?

5. List four aspects of monitoring and/or nursing care that may need to be altered due to drug therapy.

6. List six methods of providing information to a client.

7. Give four tips to providing an effective drug administration demonstration to a client.

8. List six ways in which the VN can improve client compliance.

For answers go to page 237

Pharmacy Law

Learning aims and objectives

After studying this chapter you should be able to:

1. **Understand the legislation relating to the use of drugs and medicines**
2. **Understand regulations applying to dangerous substances and consumer protection**
3. **Understand the role of professional organisations influencing pharmacy**
4. **Understand legislation affecting pharmacy.**

Veterinary drug legislation

Since 2001 the Competition Commission has been looking at medicines within veterinary practices. Its recommendations have been implemented through changes to the legislation and the RCVS Guide to Professional Conduct. Virtually all of the Competition Commission's recommendations affecting veterinary surgeons (but not the zero dispensing fee) have been implemented in the RCVS Guide to Professional Conduct and improve the transparency of medicine prices within veterinary practices. The law on veterinary medicines has been uncoupled from the Medicines Act 1968 and some revisions from a European directive have been incorporated. The resulting Veterinary Medicines Regulations 2005 came into force on October 30 of that year. The regulations apply the relevant provisions of European law and set out UK provisions in areas such as fees, distribution, appeals, advertising, inspection and enforcement of any veterinary medicinal product (VMP) as defined in Box 2.1. The VMR 2005 sets out the distribution categories for UK drugs as follows:

- Prescription Only Medicine – Veterinarian (POM-V)
- Prescription Only Medicine – Veterinarian, Pharmacist, Suitably Qualified Person (POM-VPS)
- Non-Food Animal – Veterinarian, Pharmacist, Suitably Qualified Person (NFA-VPS)
- Authorised Veterinary Medicine – General Sales List (AVM-GSL).

Box 2.1

VMPs

A Veterinary Medicinal Product is defined as:

a. any substance or combination of substances presented as having properties for treating or preventing disease in animals; or

b. any substance or combination of substances which may be used in, or administered to, animals with a view either to restoring, correcting or modifying physiological functions by exerting a pharmacological, immunological or metabolic action, or to making a medical diagnosis.

A VMP that has been classified as POM-V may only be dispensed by a vet or pharmacist and a clinical assessment must be made by the vet first. A product is included in this category when it:

- contains a new active ingredient not previously used in a veterinary medicine in the EU
- requires a strict limitation on its use for specific safety reasons
- requires the specialised knowledge of a veterinary surgeon for use/application
- has a narrow safety margin requiring above average care in its use
- is Government policy to demand professional control at a high level
- requires specific use, linked to a prior clinical assessment of the animals.

A POM-VPS drug can be prescribed by a Registered Qualified Person (RQP) which is defined as follows:

1. a registered veterinary surgeon
2. a registered pharmacist
3. a registered suitably qualified person (SQP).

SQPs will be registered with a body that has provided training to them and they will have had to have passed an examination and be present at each sale of the VMP. Although a clinical assessment of the animal is not a prerequisite, the prescribing RQP must be satisfied that the person administering the product has the competence to do so safely. All those supplying veterinary medicinal products will be required to abide by the Veterinary Medicines Regulations. Those supplying VMPs must also comply with labelling requirements, advise on safe administration, warnings and contraindications, and be satisfied that the person using the product is competent to use it safely and intends to use it for a purpose for which it is authorised.

AMTRA has been given the authority to run training courses in conjunction with some colleges to allow qualified and listed VNs to upgrade to become SQPs. The examination will consist of a 2-hour written assessment and training day courses are available. The modules will be designed to allow SQPs to supply for all animals or for all food-producing animals, horses, companion animals or particular species. The content will mainly focus on the changes to the legislation detailed below, but will also assess knowledge of the other pharmacy laws such as COSHH, RIDDOR and Health and Safety at Work. Packaging, labelling and dispensing will all be reviewed.

The Veterinary Medicines Regulations 2005 state that SQPs may prescribe and supply certain categories of veterinary medicines – mainly parasiticides and other medicines for the routine control of endemic disease. SQPs are able to prescribe and supply POM-VPS and NFA-VPS products for the species in which they have training.

It is still the case that veterinary surgeons have a right to prescribe and supply medicines such as POM-Vs and POM-VPSs as appropriate. Dispensing has always been a privilege rather than a right. Dispensing of those medicines by others was lawful prior to October 30, 2005 and in the view of the Royal College remains lawful under the new Veterinary Medicines Regulations. Listed VNs will be able to supply POM-VPS and NFA-VPS products in their own right if they become SQPs.

NFA-VPS drugs may be supplied by an RQP without a clinical assessment but with advice relating to any warnings or contraindications of use. AVM-GSL may be supplied by any retailer as there are no restrictions on its supply.

There were also changes made to the RCVS Guide to Professional Conduct, which took effect on November 3, 2005. The RCVS enforces these recommendations made by the Competition Commission. Any complaints are investigated by the Preliminary Investigation Committee and may be referred to the Disciplinary Committee. Key changes relate to providing information to clients about the availability of prescriptions and the prices of most of the commonly prescribed medicines:

- clients must be able to obtain prescriptions as appropriate
- clients must be informed of the price of any medicine to be prescribed or dispensed and the price must be made available to other parties who make reasonable requests
- itemised invoices must be made available to distinguish between fees charged for services and medicines and where possible itemised for individual products

- clients must be informed of the frequency of and charges for further examinations and repeat prescriptions
- new and existing clients must be provided with this information in writing
- there must be a sign in the waiting room (Box 2.2) detailing the current prices of the 10 veterinary medicinal products most commonly prescribed during a recent and typical 3-month period
- the exceptions to these requirements are when a delay in supply or administration would be unreasonable or where the medication is to be administered by injection and is only available in packs containing multiple doses.

Box 2.2

Client advice

Client advice as follows should be displayed on a large, prominently displayed sign in the waiting room:

- Prescriptions are available from this practice
- You may obtain relevant medicinal products from your veterinary surgeon *or* ask for a prescription and obtain these medicines from another veterinary surgery or a pharmacy
- Your veterinary surgeon may prescribe relevant veterinary medicinal products only following a clinical assessment of an animal under his or her care
- A prescription may not be appropriate if your animal is an inpatient or immediate treatment is necessary
- You will be informed, on request, of the price of any medicine that may be prescribed for your animal
- The general policy of this practice is to re-assess animals requiring repeat prescriptions or supplies of relevant veterinary medicinal products every X months, but this may vary with individual circumstances. The standard charge for a re-examination is £XX
- The current prices for the 10 relevant medicinal products most commonly prescribed during [a typical 3-month period] were:
  - [The 10 most commonly prescribed medicines and their prices listed]
- Further information on the prices of medicines is available on request

The RCVS also gives advice about communication with clients via the internet about animals that are under their care. The VMR do not define the phrase 'under his care' and the RCVS have interpreted it as meaning that:

a. the veterinary surgeon must have been given the responsibility for the health of the animal or herd by the owner or the owner's agent
b. that responsibility must be real and not nominal
c. the animal or herd must have been seen immediately before prescription or
d. recently enough or often enough for the veterinary surgeon to have personal knowledge of the condition of the animal or current health status of the herd or flock to make a diagnosis and prescribe
e. the veterinary surgeon must maintain clinical records of that herd/flock/individual.

What amounts to 'recently enough' must be a matter for the professional judgement of the veterinary surgeon according to the circumstances of each case.

The RCVS guide to professional conduct provides the advice shown in Box 2.3 on retail supplies. Legislation is constantly updated and takes into account reviews of and changes in both UK and European legislation. Up to date information can be obtained from reliable sources such as the RCVS and the VMD.

If there is no authorised medicinal product in the UK for a condition affecting a non-food producing animal, the vet may use the cascade system to relieve suffering. This means using a product authorised for use in another species, or for another condition in the same species. If no such product exists, then a product designed for human use may be used or one authorised in another member state. Only as a last resort should a home made preparation be used. The cascade should be followed in the order:

- a VMP authorised in the UK for use in another animal species, or for another condition in the same species; or
- if, and only if, there is no such product that is suitable, either a medicinal product authorised in the UK for human use or a VMP not authorised in the UK but authorised in another member state for use with any animal species (in the case of a food-producing animal, it must be a food-producing species); or
- if, and only if, there is no such product that is suitable, a VMP prepared by a pharmacist, a veterinary surgeon or a person holding a manufacture authorisation authorising the manufacture of that type of product.

See Chapter 3 for some applications of the cascade system in dispensing for exotics.

RCVS advice on retail supplies

A veterinary surgeon who supplies POM-V, POM-VPS or NFA-VPS veterinary medicinal products must:

a. always advise on the safe administration of the VMP

b. advise as necessary on any warnings or contraindications on the label or package leaflet; and

c. be satisfied that the person who will use the product is competent to use it safely, and intends to use it for a use for which it is authorised.

A veterinary surgeon that makes retail supplies of POM-V veterinary medicinal products on the prescription of another veterinary surgeon (i.e. for animals that are not under his or her care) should ensure that those to whom the medicines are supplied, or may be supplied, are informed that such supplies are made without a clinical assessment of the animal and that the animal is not under his or her care.

A veterinary surgeon who is associated with retail supplies of POM-VPS, NFA-VPS or AVM-GSL VMP (or makes such supplies), should ensure that those to whom the medicines are supplied, or may be supplied, are informed of:

a. the name and qualification (veterinary surgeon, pharmacist or SQP) of any prescriber

b. the name and qualification (veterinary surgeon, pharmacist or SQP) of the supplier

c. the nature of the duty of care for the animals.

Veterinary surgeons may prescribe POM-VPS VMP in circumstances where there has been no prior clinical assessment of the animals and the animals are not under his or her care. In these circumstances veterinary surgeons should prescribe responsibly and with due regard to the health and welfare of the animals.

Prescriptions and recording of medicines

The Veterinary Medicines Guidance Notes outlines how a prescription should be written. The following information should be included:

- the name and address of the prescriber
- the particulars which substantiate that the prescriber is a veterinary surgeon, e.g. MRCVS

- the name and address of the person to whom the product is supplied
- a description of the animal(s) it is prescribed for
- the date.

The prescription should be written in ink or another indelible format and should be signed or otherwise authenticated by the prescriber.

Records must be kept by keepers of food-producing animals outlining the purchase of all medicines and the identification of the animals treated. The manufacturer must also record all batches of VMPs and keep the records for 5 years. All prescriptions should be detailed and a copy kept for 5 years also. Wholesalers should keep their records for at least 3 years.

Dosage levels

Pharmacological studies are carried out on all new products to ascertain the safe dose range. The safety documentation always details the investigations undertaken in laboratory animals and all relevant information observed during clinical studies in the target animal. In order to reduce the number and suffering of the animals involved, new protocols for dose toxicity are continually being developed. Both single-dose toxicity studies and repeated-dose toxicity tests are carried out to reveal the acute toxic effects of the substance and time course for their onset and remission. These studies are normally carried out in at least two mammalian species and at least two routes of administration are studied. Evaluation of the toxic effects is based on observation of behaviour, growth, haematology and physiological tests – especially those relating to the excretory organs.

Safe and effective therapy can only be achieved with doses that produce optimal concentrations of a drug in the plasma and the tissues. Smaller doses will be ineffective and larger doses will not increase the benefits and may increase the toxicity. Between these two doses is the therapeutic dose range. Some drugs have a narrow range, such as digoxin, whilst others, like fenbendazole, have a wide safety margin.

Controlled drugs

We have a legal obligation to keep Schedule 2 drugs and some Schedule 3 agents locked away in a safe attached to the floor or wall of the building. This is because of the legislation in place to govern their safe usage, namely:

- The Misuse of Drugs Act 1971
- Misuse of Drugs Regulations 1985.

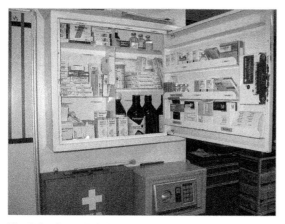

Fig. 2.1   Controlled drugs cabinet

Figure 2.1 shows a dangerous drugs cupboard with an electronic keypad below where the key is kept so that access is restricted to the vets in the practice who know the code. The record-keeping requirements for Schedule 2 drugs indicate that they must be entered in the register when purchased and also each time they are used within 24 hours – signed by the vet. The register must be a bound (not loose leaf) book and a separate register must be kept for each premises where controlled drugs are used. A separate part of the register must be used for each drug which must be specified at the head of each page. Entries must be indelible and in chronological order, without amendments. The register must be kept for 2 years from the last date of entry.

Schedule 2 controlled drugs must not be disposed of or destroyed except in the presence of a person authorised to do so by the Secretary of State. Examples are pethidine, morphine and fentanyl.

Schedule 3 includes buprenorphine, pentazocine, pentobarbital, phenobarbital and some minor stimulant drugs. These drugs are subject to prescription and requisition requirements but do not have to be recorded in a controlled drugs register. Temazepam, diethylpropion and buprenorphine must be kept locked away, but this does not apply to other Schedule 3 drugs.

Schedule 4 includes the anabolic substances and the benzodiazepines. They are exempt from most restrictions but due to an ethical obligation for safe use, many practices keep diazepam locked away.

Schedule 5 includes certain preparations of cocaine, codeine and morphine that contain less than a specified amount of the drug. They are exempt from all controlled drug requirements except for the need to keep relevant invoices for 2 years.

Veterinarians have no right to keep Schedule 1 drugs on the premises. The RCVS recommends that other drugs with the potential for abuse such as ketamine are stored in secure containers.

Other relevant legislation

Please refer to Chapter 3 for details of:
- The Health and Safety at Work Act 1974
- RIDDOR 1995
- COSHH 2002
- The Management of Health and Safety at Work Regulations 1999.

Questions for Chapter 2

What schedule are the following drugs in?

1. Diazepam
2. Phenobarbital
3. Methadone
4. Temazepam
5. Amfetamines

For answers go to page 238

Three

CHAPTER 3

Pharmacy Practice

With contribution from Glen Cousquer (Exotics pharmacology)

Learning aims and objectives

After studying this chapter you should be able to:

1. **Perform dosage calculations**
2. **List the forms drugs are available in**
3. **Compare the different routes of administration of medicines**
4. **List the relevant health and safety legislation**
5. **Describe the procedures for record keeping and stock control**
6. **State the requirements for packaging and labelling medicines.**

Dosage calculations

- *Solutions* are mixtures of substances that are not usually combined with each other. They consist of a solvent (the dissolving substance), and a solute (the dissolved substance).
- *Suspensions* are mixtures containing very large particles of solute. They settle out on standing and need to be shaken before administration as different parts of the mixture will not contain equal amounts of solute.

The amount of solute dissolved in the solvent is referred to as the concentration of the substance. Concentrations can be expressed as:

- parts
- weight per volume (w/v) for liquids
- volume per volume (v/v) for liquids
- weight per weight (w/w) for solids.

Most veterinary preparations are expressed as w/v. For example, diazepam is available as a 5 mg/ml solution for injection. Electrolyte solutions are often expressed in terms of milliequivalents per litre (mEq/L). IU stands for International Units and is used for the measurement of drugs and vitamins. Webster's Dictionary defines IU as: 'a quantity of a biologic (such as a vitamin) that produces a particular biological effect agreed upon as an international standard'. What this means is that IU is dependent on the potency of the substance, and each substance would have a different IU to milligram conversion. For example, 1000 IU of vitamin C would have a different weight than 1000 IU of vitamin A.

To work out how many ml of a drug a patient requires, just remember two things:

1. **Dose =** $\dfrac{\text{body weight} \times \text{dosage}}{\text{concentration of drug}}$

(i.e. divide what you need by what you have got).

2. **To get percentage solution into mg/ml, just multiply by 10.**

Example 1

A 20 kg dog requires a drug at 10 mg/kg. It is available in a 2% solution. How many ml does it need?

- Apply rule number 2: there are 20 mg/ml in this solution (2% × 10)
- Apply rule number 1:

$$dose = \frac{(20\ kg \times 10\ mg/kg)}{20\ mg/ml}$$

The units cancel themselves out, leaving you with the answer in ml – Dose = 10 ml.

Example 2

A cat weighs 11 pounds, and requires a drug, dose rate 1 mg/kg. The solution is 0.5%. How many ml does it need? To convert pounds to kilos, you divide by 2.2 (Box 3.1 shows some of the conversions).

- Cat weighs 11 ÷ 2.2 = 5 kg
- Solution contains: 0.5 × 10 = 5 mg/ml, so

$$dose = \frac{(5\ kg \times 1\ mg/kg)}{5\ mg/ml}$$

Dose = 1 ml.

Example 3

A dog weighs 25 kg and needs an agent with a concentration of 125 mg/ml. The dose rate is 0.5 mg/kg. How many ml are required?

- There is no need to work out the drug concentration because it is stated for you as 125 mg/ml:

$$dose = \frac{(25\ kg \times 0.5\ mg/kg)}{125\ mg/ml}$$

Dose = 0.1 ml.

When calculating dosages for most cancer chemotherapeutics, body surface area is correlated with the weight of the animal. Tables are available in most formularies for converting an animal's weight to surface area in square meters. In these cases the formula applied is:

Dose = mg/m² (from the drug's data sheet or a formulary) × m² (see conversion table).

Box 3.1

Conversion of pounds to kilograms

5 kg = 11 lb
10 kg = 22 lb
15 kg = 33 lb
20 kg = 44 lb
25 kg = 55 lb
30 kg = 66 lb

Forms of drugs and routes of administration

Oral administration

Materials required

- for oral administration of tablets – pilling gun
- for oral administration of liquids – syringe without a needle or a dosing syringe.

Technique

For oral administration of tablets to a *dog*. Ask an assistant to control and reassure the patient. Hold the top jaw with one hand and push your fingers into the premolar area to open the mouth. Insert the tablet into the mouth with the other hand and push it over the tongue to the back of the pharynx. The gag reflex closes off the airway and prevents the medicine from entering the trachea. Various methods of encouraging swallowing have been suggested, including blowing into the animal's nose and rubbing its throat.

For oral administration of tablets to a *cat*. Ask an assistant to restrain the cat with one hand on each front leg to prevent being scratched. Have the cat facing you. Place one hand on top of the head and place the thumb and third finger of that hand under the eye sockets. Point the nose of the cat towards the ceiling. This allows the jaw to be opened using the middle finger of the other hand. The tablet can now be inserted using either a pilling gun or your fingers. Covering the tablet with a palatable substance such as Katalax, butter or marmite may help with difficult patients.

For the majority of our patients, oral administration of medicines is the method of choice. Oral administration can be taken to include drugs that are specifically designed to dissolve under the tongue (sublingual) and those that can be absorbed through the mucous membranes of the cheek (particularly

Summary of oral medications

Oral solids

- tablets (powdered drugs compressed into discs)
- capsules (drug inside a gelatine container)
- granules

Oral liquids

- mixtures
- suspensions (insoluble drug in a liquid base)
- emulsions (drops of oil in water or water in oil)
- linctus

Potential problems

Gastrointestinal irritation, aspiration of medicine, person administering the drug being bitten, poor patient compliance due to unpleasant tasting medicines

useful to get sedatives like α-2 agonists into feral cats). Box 3.2 lists the oral medications.

Sublingual medications, either in tablet form, granules or aerosol spray, have little role in veterinary medicine due to the difficulties in preventing the animal from swallowing – although it is an excellent method of administering a drug to an anaesthetised or unconscious patient. First-pass metabolism is avoided as the drug does not need to be absorbed through the gut and taken to the liver before entering the circulation. Homeopathic granules are often best taken this way.

When administering oral liquids from a stock bottle a separate dropper should be used for each patient to avoid cross contamination.

Tablets may be enteric coated (Fig. 3.1) and therefore are designed not to be crushed or split else the drug is exposed to the acid in the stomach and not absorbed effectively.

Capsules likewise should not be opened in case their purpose is to protect the drug inside or to save the patient from tasting a bitter drug. Some capsules contain different sized granules and are designed to slowly release the medicine as the different granules dissolve. If a tablet or capsule sticks in the oesophagus it can cause inflammation and potentially ulceration and so they should be given with a bowl or syringe of water when possible. Often a drink of water before administering a tablet moistens the mucous membranes and helps the medicine go down.

When reconstituting powdered medicines, such as unstable antibiotics, it is important to mark the date of preparation on the bottle and store any unused medicine in the refrigerator unless the data sheets advise to the contrary. Another important point is to shake well before use.

Rectal administration

Rectal administration is practiced in veterinary medicine elsewhere in Europe and in human medicine. This is effective due to the large colonic surface area and the ability of the colon to absorb fluids and drugs from the gut lumen. Enema solutions can be administered using a Higginson's syringe (Fig. 3.2).

Injections

Materials required

Syringe containing the correct amount of drug, correct gauge and length needle, cotton wool swab soaked in surgical spirit.

Technique

1. Attach the needle firmly to the syringe by applying pressure and slightly twisting the needle onto the hub of the syringe.

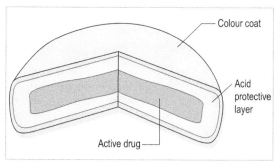

Fig. 3.1 Enteric coated tablets.

Colour coat

Acid protective layer

Active drug

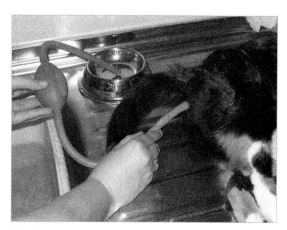

Fig. 3.2 Administration of an enema.

2. Swab the bottle's rubber diaphragm with surgical spirit before withdrawing the correct amount of drug.
3. Remove the needle's cap carefully and keep to one side. Insert the needle through the centre of the rubber diaphragm with the bottle inverted until the tip is visible inside the bottle. Over insertion may result in the needle drawing air into the syringe from inside the bottle. Withdraw the correct amount and then withdraw the needle.
4. Tapping the syringe with the needle uppermost will result in any air bubbles rising to the surface where they can be released by pushing slightly on the plunger. It is important not to create an aerosol of the drug. Live vaccines, e.g. the feline respiratory virus vaccine, can cause disease if inhaled. Replace the cap onto the needle unless the injection is to be given immediately.
5. Swab the area to be injected with surgical spirit and insert the needle into the appropriate site. Pull back on the plunger to ensure no blood is seen and that the needle tip is under the skin. This is identifiable by the plunger returning to its original position because of the negative pressure created by pulling back on the plunger. Depress the plunger to administer the drug.
6. Massage the area to encourage absorption of the drug and to minimise pain.
7. Correctly dispose of the administration equipment (see below).

Parenteral medications (avoiding the gut) can be injected into muscle, veins or under the skin and this method may be preferable due to a number of reasons including:
- the patient is unable to take the medication orally
- the drug is broken down in the gut, e.g. insulin
- the drug may not be absorbed in the gut, e.g. gentamicin
- the drug is metabolised extensively by the liver when taken orally and so little is available for use around the body, e.g. lidocaine
- fast onset of action is required
- very accurate dosing is required.

Plastic containers can sometimes interact with the drug and so glass containers remain the preferred method of drug presentation (this is one reason why drugs should not be left drawn up in syringes). Box 3.3 shows the types of containers used for injectable preparations.

The most suitable route of administration for a drug depends on the data sheet recommendation,

Box 3.3

Containers for injectable medicines
Glass ampoule (Fig. 3.3)
- Shake down solution from the neck
- Identify weakened area of neck marked with a dot or pre-scored line or use a file to make a scratch on the vial neck
- Snap off top using an ampoule sleeve to protect the fingers
Glass rubber-capped vial
- Remove protective disc from top
- Swab surface with an alcohol swab and allow to dry
- Can be used as a multidose container if the stability of the contents allows

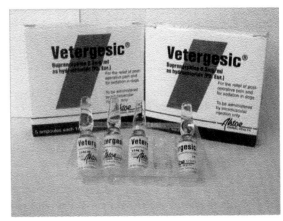

Fig. 3.3 Glass vials of buprenorphine. Courtesy of G. Cousquer.

the speed of onset required and patient compliance. Figure 3.4 shows the layers a needle passes through to administer a drug into the muscle. It is important to select an appropriate sized needle to ensure delivery of the drug to the correct place. The direct cutaneous artery is shown to highlight the importance of drawing back on the syringe to ensure the tip of the needle is not in the vessel.

The subcutaneous route is used for non-irritating, water-soluble substances such as insulin and vaccines. Oily solutions, aqueous suspensions and irritating drugs should be delivered intramuscularly.

Figures 3.5 and 3.6 show the preferred sites for administration of intramuscular injections. The thigh muscles are contained within a tight facial sheath and injection of large volumes can be painful. The back muscles and the gluteals (easily found by palpating the 'cat spay' landmarks) are not sheathed

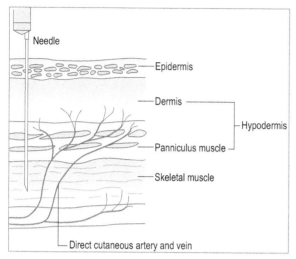

Fig. 3.4 Intramuscular injection.

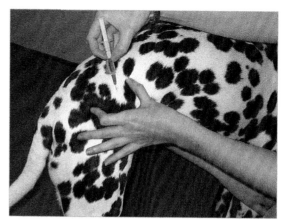

Fig. 3.6 Intramuscular injection into the gluteals muscle.

Potential complications of intravenous injections

- Tearing the vein with the needle causing a haematoma
- Necrosis of tissues surrounding the vein if an irritating drug escapes
- Phlebitis at the injection site if injections are repeated or prolonged
- Death or intoxication if the dose given is too high

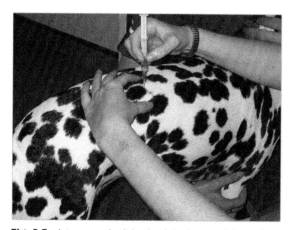

Fig. 3.5 Intramuscular injection into the epaxial muscles.

in this manner and patients tolerate injections much better. Another important point is to remember that needles are single-use and blunt quickly. A new needle should be used after withdrawal of drug from a rubber capped vial to minimise discomfort to the patient. Needles should be inserted quickly, the drug injected slowly and then the needle removed quickly to make the experience the least painful possible.

Box 3.4 shows the potential complications of intravenous injection. Other routes of injection include the following.

- Intra-arterial – used to administer radiopaque substances for selective contrast studies.
- Intra-articular – this involves injecting a drug directly into a joint. Corticosteroids are sometimes injected into joints to relieve inflammation. Care must be taken to ensure the

site is prepared aseptically and that a sterile technique is employed during the procedure. It is recommended that a sample of the joint fluid is collected prior to administration of any drug to allow culture and sensitivity and other diagnostic tests to be performed.

- Intraperitoneal – delivery of drugs into the abdominal cavity. Potential disadvantages include the variable onset and duration of action of drugs given by this route, the potential for puncture of abdominal organs and the formation of adhesions. Fluids and euthanasia drugs are occasionally given by this route.
- Intradermal – this involves injecting an agent into the skin. Part of the myxomatosis vaccine should be administered in this way.
- Epidural – injection into the spinal canal but outside of the dura mater (outer layer of the meninges).
- Intrathecal – this is administration of a drug into the subdural space (cerebrospinal fluid). If a drug has low lipid solubility it will not pass the

blood–brain barrier. Water-soluble antibiotics therefore are injected this way to treat meningitis to ensure the cerebrospinal fluid concentration is sufficient.

- Subconjunctival – injection under the conjunctival membrane. Antibiotics are sometimes administered in this way.
- Intracardiac – injection through the chest wall, directly into the heart chambers. It allows the drug to access the bloodstream quickly. Euthanasia and cardiac resuscitation drugs are occasionally administered this way.
- Intraosseous – injection of a substance directly into the bone marrow in the medulla of either the femur or the humerus. It is most often used to provide fluids to very small patients, those with damaged veins or those with very low blood pressure.

Topical administration

Percutaneous administration refers to the absorption of a drug through the skin or across mucous membranes. It is affected by drug concentration, contact time, thickness of skin and hydration of the tissues. It can also be increased by placing the drug into a vehicle such as dimethyl sulfoxide (DMSO). Fentanyl patches have become popular, especially in orthopaedic surgery, to deliver a controlled release of analgesia, to allow a reduction in anaesthetic and to provide good postoperative pain control. The patches release a prescribed medication through a semipermeable membrane for several hours to three weeks when applied to intact skin. These patches must not be cut down or allowed to get hot (e.g. when a patient lies on a heat pad) as the release of drug may be too rapid.

The respiratory mucosa may be medicated by the inhalation of aerosols or sprays (nebulae). Bronchodilators and corticosteroids are occasionally given this way.

Medication may also be applied to the mucosa of the oral cavity (sublingual), as suppositories to the rectal mucosa, the uterus, vagina, eyes and ears (aural).

Drug administration and dispensing in exotic patients

Exotic patients frequently present to veterinary practices for examination and treatment. Nursing staff hospitalising such patients must be familiar with and competent in the administration of medications to such patients. Where patients are returned to the owner for ongoing care at home, clear advice on

drug administration must be given. The wide range of species dealt with makes this a broad subject, as the route of administration must take into account important differences in anatomy, physiology, biology and behaviour. This discussion will limit itself to the subject of fluid therapy and drug administration in common birds, small mammals and reptiles and the key considerations nursing staff need to be aware of.

Drug administration for the avian patient

Fluid therapy can be provided by the oral, cloacal, subcutaneous, intravenous and intraosseous routes. Crop gavage, or crop tubing, is a technique that should be carefully learnt and practised regularly to ensure proficiency in this technique. The procedure should be performed quickly and smoothly in order to minimise stress to the patient and the risks of regurgitation. All equipment and materials should be prepared in advance to avoid unnecessary delays and stress. The patient should be gently but securely held by an assistant, leaving the operator's hands free to secure the head, pass the crop tube, palpate the crop to check its location and administer the fluids and any accompanying oral treatment(s).

Crop tubes are likely to require lubrication, especially in the dehydrated patient. Specially designed stainless steel crop tubes for birds with a large atraumatic end are available commercially; alternatively urinary catheters or lamb feeding tubes can be used. The tube should be introduced via the commissure of the beak and slid down the inside of the cheek and down the neck to enter the crop. The tube should be palpable on the left side of the neck, where the oesophagus tends to lie in most birds. Volumes of between 1% and 2.5% body weight can be administered into the crop. Following administration, the bird should be returned to a dark quiet box and all further stress avoided.

In sick, weak, severely dehydrated or otherwise compromised birds, oral fluid therapy may not be possible. In such situations a parenteral route should be chosen. Subcutaneous fluids can be given into the fold of skin immediately cranial to the thigh. Absorption rates from such sites will vary depending on the adequacy of perfusion of this area; perfusion is likely to be poor in a collapsed and dehydrated patient. Use of the enzyme hyaluronidase in fluids will promote fluid uptake from subcutaneous injection sites. Intravenous catheters can be placed in the basilic or medial tarsometatarsal veins. The latter is particularly useful in waterfowl. Maintenance of these catheters can prove difficult and the basilic vein is easily blown.

Intraosseous catheters are much better tolerated than intravenous catheters and their use is recommended. In birds the aerated bones, namely the humerus and femur, should be avoided as an injection of fluid into these bones is likely to enter the lung-airsac system. The preferred sites for placement of intraosseous catheters are the proximal and distal ulna, together with the proximal tibia. The skin should be aseptically prepared and a spinal needle, or similar, introduced at the appropriate site. The catheter should be bunged and protected from the patient. Water soluble preparations suitable for intravenous use can be administered via the intraosseous route.

Drugs that can not be given in this way can either be administered intramuscularly or via the subcutaneous route. Subcutaneous injections can be given in the loose skin of the axilla and groin. Small volumes can be injected under the skin overlying the tibiotarsus as this area is easily immobilised and cleaned when the bird's leg is extended. Intramuscular injections are best administered into the distal third of the pectoral musculature. Aseptic injection techniques should always be followed. The possibility of tissue damage should not be overlooked when administering i.m. injections and should be avoided in wild birds, where muscle damage may affect flying ability and fitness.

Drug administration in small mammals

The size of the patient should not be a reason to overlook the need for fluid therapy. Fluid losses can become very significant in small patients and efforts should always be made to minimise these (immaculate haemostasis, warming and humidification of inspiratory air, etc.). It is recommended that all small mammalian patients should receive fluids – this is particularly important when their fluid intake is reduced through illness, stress and debility. At the very least subcutaneous or intraperitoneal fluids should be provided. Fluids should always be warmed to body temperature. They should be injected in an atraumatic and aseptic manner.

The intraperitoneal route allows for the injection of significant volumes of fluids into a body cavity with a large surface area for absorption. This route is often better tolerated than the subcutaneous route. Consideration should be given to the abdominal anatomy and the key structures to be avoided. Palpation of the abdomen is appropriate to determine the size and fill of structures such as the spleen and the caecum. The cranial quadrants should be avoided where the liver and/or spleen are palpable. The caudal midline should be avoided where the bladder is full. The caudal left quadrant should be avoided where the caecum is full. This is likely to leave the right caudal quadrant as the most suitable site for an intraperitoneal injection. Volumes of 1–3 ml in mice, 2–4 ml in hamsters and gerbils, 10 ml in rats

and 25–50 ml in rabbits are appropriate. The use of indwelling intravenous catheters should be viewed as routine in ferrets and rabbits. With practice, the placement of fine gauge (e.g. 22, 24 and 27 gauge) catheters is readily mastered.

Use of the cephalic and saphenous veins is possible in both rabbits and ferrets. In the rabbit the marginal ear vein can also be used. The skin should be aseptically prepared and can be desensitised with local anaesthetic cream to facilitate catheter placement. In collapsed ferrets and rabbits with low blood pressure, as well as in young and small individuals, attempts to place an intravenous catheter may be unsuccessful. Use of intraosseous needles is appropriate in these situations. The proximal femur is easily accessed in both species and can also be used in guinea pigs, chinchillas and other small mammals. Placement of the catheter/needle is best performed under general anaesthesia. Medications can be provided via the oral, subcutaneous, intramuscular, intravenous and intraosseous routes, providing they are compatible with that route.

Syringe feeding of rabbits via a dosing syringe requires skill and patience. It is, however, an invaluable skill and one that all nurses should acquire for it will contribute to the nursing care and successful treatment of most sick patients. It is also a skill that needs to be clearly demonstrated and explained to owners who wish to continue supportive care at home. In smaller mammals, such as rats, intragastric drug administration is possible using a metal feeding needle (similar to the metal avian crop tubes). Tubes should always be measured up prior to insertion, by measuring the distance from the nares to the last rib. Subcutaneous injections can be administered into the loose skin of the neck and back in most species. Intramuscular injections are rarely indicated as most drugs can be administered via either the intravenous route (where a catheter has been placed) or via the subcutaneous route.

The limited muscle mass in small mammals is a limiting factor, especially in cachectic patients. The quadriceps musculature is probably the most accessible muscle mass but it is tightly enveloped in fascia and large injections are therefore likely to prove painful. In rats the maximum volume that can be injected into the quadriceps is approximately 0.2–0.3 ml. This falls to 0.1 ml in hamsters and gerbils and 0.03 ml in mice. Intravenous injections can be administered into the cephalic and saphenous veins in the rabbit and ferret, whilst in smaller mammals the lateral tail veins are likely to be appropriate. Intraosseous drug administration is also practical and is indicated in any patient where i.v. access is impractical. In small rodents a 24–26 gauge needle can be placed into the proximal femur, providing rapid access to the circulatory system.

Drug administration in reptiles

Fortunately most reptiles will take up fluids, both orally and via the cloaca, when placed in a bath. This avoids the need to handle and stress patients and will also promote defaecation and urination. Fluid presentation may have been inadequate and novice owners, of chameleons particularly, may require advice on how to provide a recognisable and hygienic source of water. Where the patient is too sick to rehydrate itself orally, fluid therapy should be provided via oesophageal gavage or via a suitable parenteral route. A blunt-ended gavage tube should be pre-measured to the level of the stomach prior to insertion. In chelonia the stomach is positioned level with the midpoint of the plastron. In snakes the distal oesophagus/stomach is situated approximately 33–50% of the snout-to-vent length from the mouth. Suggested maximum volumes are 5–15 ml/kg in chelonia, 10–20 ml/kg in lizards and 15–30 ml/kg in snakes.

The intravenous, intracoelomic and intraosseous routes are all suitable routes for parenteral fluid/ drug administration. The subcutaneous route is less useful in reptilian compared with mammalian patients due to the relative inelasticity of reptile skin. Significant leakage of injected material from subcutaneous injection sites can be seen and is obviously undesirable. The intracoelomic route is preferred to the subcutaneous route and is comparable to the intraperitoneal route in mammals. In chelonia, access to the coelom is obtained by injecting into the prefemoral fossa; an alternative 'epicoelomic' route is accessed by inserting a needle immediately caudal to the shoulder joint, just dorsal and parallel to the plastron. In lizards, intracoelomic injections are administered with the animal in lateral or ventral recumbency, by inserting the needle into the sub-lumbar fossa and advancing it cranially almost parallel to the body wall.

In snakes, injections should be made into the caudal quarter of the coelomic cavity, via the left flank, to avoid the extensive right air sac. The intramuscular route is probably the most practical and useful parenteral route. Suitable muscle masses include the epaxial muscles in lizards and snakes. In lizards and chelonia, the triceps brachii and quadriceps femoris can also be used. Intravenous access is possible via a number of sites including the jugular vein in chelonia, lizards and snakes, the ventral coccygeal vein in lizards and snakes and the dorsal tail vein in chelonia. Intraosseous catheterisation is extremely useful, both in chelonia and lizards. The most readily accessible site for needle placement in chelonia is the caudal plastrocarapacial pillar, accessed immediately cranial to the plastrocarapacial bridge area. In lizards, suitable sites include the distal humerus, distal femur and proximal tibia.

Drug dispensing in exotic patients

Drug therapy in avian and exotic veterinary medicine presents veterinary professionals with some interesting and challenging problems:
- the range of species dealt with is enormous
- very few drugs are licensed for use in exotic species
- treatment is, sadly, often initiated without a diagnosis
- small size may make accurate dosing difficult
- differences in metabolic rate may need to be taken into consideration
- targeted drug delivery to specific tissues may require specialist techniques and preparations
- important differences may exist between species:
  - drug pharmacokinetics
  - animal handling
  - route of administration
  - water consumption
  - drug side effects.

A good understanding of avian and exotic animal medicine is required in order for appropriate choices to be made. It is essential that general practitioners recognise their limitations and offer clients the option of referral where appropriate. Avian and exotic animal medicine is now a highly specialised discipline and the gap between the standard of care offered in general, as compared with specialist, practice will continue to widen. Specialist advice should therefore be sought wherever possible in order to ensure that clients are informed about the full range of options available to them.

It is no longer acceptable for every sick avian and exotic patient to be prescribed enrofloxacin (Baytril) without a diagnosis being made. This approach/ practice arose for two main reasons:
- interpretation of the prescribing cascade would appear to suggest that Baytril, as the only antibiotic licensed for use in avian and exotic patients, is the most appropriate choice
- failure to examine and investigate patients adequately will result in failure to arrive at an accurate diagnosis and failure to select a more appropriate treatment; the prescription and dispensing of Baytril in this manner can be viewed as irresponsible and will only result in the propagation of resistant strains of bacteria.

Selection of an appropriate medication for use in an avian or exotic patient will follow the prescribing cascade for non-food-producing animals. Certain companion animals may, in point of fact, be food-producing animals and this fact should not be overlooked. Rabbits, pigeons, quail, waterfowl and a number of other avian species are potentially food-producing animals as their meat, milk and/or eggs may be intended for human consumption. It is the prescribing veterinary surgeon's responsibility to establish that the patient is a non-food-producing animal.

Informed consent should be obtained from the owner of any exotic pet presenting to a veterinary surgeon. The consent form should clearly indicate that unlicensed medications are likely to be used in their animal and that this may carry risks. A separate section should establish whether there is any possibility that meat, eggs or milk from that animal is intended for human consumption. The form should clearly identify the animal (ID chip, closed leg ring, tattoo, ear tag, etc.) wherever possible.

If there is no medicine authorised in the UK for a condition affecting a non-food-producing species, the veterinary surgeon responsible for treating the animal(s) may, in order to mitigate unacceptable suffering, treat the animal(s) in accordance with the cascade system (see Chapter 2). Additionally, where an EU authorised veterinary medicinal product is unavailable, there exists the possibility to import an EU authorised human medicinal product or an authorised veterinary medicinal product from the rest of the world. At this stage the VMD should be contacted for advice on the most appropriate course of action. The VMD will issue an SIC for the importation of an EU Veterinary Medicinal Product, or an STC for an EU human medicinal product or any product (veterinary or human) from the rest of the world.

The lack of suitable authorised products in avian and exotic pets means that the prescribing cascade will frequently be referred to. The following three examples illustrate how a specific product can be chosen and reformulated where appropriate, for use in a specific indication in a specific species.

Example 1

A Blue Fronted Amazon parrot fed on an all-seed diet and presenting with pruritus, impaction of the salivary glands, hyperkeratosis of the oral cavity and periorbital swellings. These are all classical signs of hypovitaminosis A. In addition to correcting the diet, such a patient requires treatment with an injectble formulation of vitamin A. No injectable vitamin A preparation (veterinary or human) is, however, available in the UK. Treatment with an injectable formulation is indicated under the prescribing cascade because:

- a rapid response to treatment is required
- dietary supplementation is less reliable
- dietary changes are unlikely to be well accepted by the patient and a change to a complete balanced diet will only be possible over time.

A rapid improvement will also encourage owners to comply with the recommended changes as they are less likely to question the diagnosis and treatment in the face of successful treatment.

In this situation, application must be made to the VMD for an STC or SIC, allowing the importation of an alternative product. Injectable vitamin A is available from Romania and the United States. Both products are human medicinal products and will therefore require an STC.

Example 2

A rabbit presenting with purulent rhinitis and dacryocystitis is found to have a *Pasteurella* infection. Culture and sensitivity testing confirms the diagnosis and highlights resistance to tetracyclines and fluoroquinolones, but good sensitivity to gentamicin, chloramphenicol, penicillin and potentiated sulphonamides. Of the suggested antibiotics, only gentamicin (Tiacil, Virbac) has a UK licence for use in rabbits. Whilst topical treatment is appropriate, the patient is likely to benefit from systemic treatment. Both penicillin and potentiated sulphonamides are licensed for use in other animals and can, therefore, be considered. Procaine penicillin (e.g. Depocillin, Intervet) is a depot preparation that can be administered by the subcutaneous route on a once weekly basis for 3–6 weeks.

This practical option may make it a suitable choice. Consideration should be given, however, to the possibility that the drug, even though given parenterally, may provoke a severe (or even fatal) dysenterobiosis. In view of this, use of a potentiated sulphonamide may be preferable. Daily administration will necessitate daily injections with a suitable product licensed for use in other animals. If this is impractical, use of an oral preparation may be indicated. Oral preparations are available, e.g. sulfadimethoxine (CoxiPlus, Genitrix), for administration in the drinking water. An assessment may be made that medication via the drinking water is too inaccurate, in which case an alternative oral formulation must be used. Use of a human paediatric solution can be selected under the prescribing cascade because:

- it is available in a dilute form that can be more accurately dosed
- it is available in a palatable form that will be well accepted by the patient
- it is indicated on culture and sensitivity grounds
- it is deemed to be safer than alternative products.

Where the infection has invaded the bony tissues, the preparation and implantation of antibiotic impregnated beads is likely to be appropriate. In such cases reformulation of a gentamicin preparation to include it in suitably sized methylmethacrylate beads is appropriate.

Example 3

A goldfish presenting with a tumour requires surgery under general anaesthesia. An authorised product for the induction and maintenance of general anaesthesia, tricaine methanesulfonate (MS222, Pharmaq), is available in the UK. Where an alternative product is used, the veterinary surgeon should be able to justify the decision to do so on clinical grounds. Alternative anaesthetic regimens include the use of injectable medetomidine and ketamine or clove oil. The former could be justified where reversal of the anaesthetic agent is desirable. The latter can be used under the Small Animal Exemption Scheme for minority species. This scheme lists a number of products that have been used historically in a number of small species (e.g. permethrin in rabbits, carnidazole in pigeons) but where the market is too limited to warrant the expense of applying for a marketing authorisation. Products currently on the market can continue to be marketed until 2007, by which time they need to become specifically listed under the scheme.

Health and Safety

Health & Safety at Work Act 1974

Under this Act, employers are required to have a policy setting out how they ensure that risks to health and safety of employees, contractors and customers are kept as low as is reasonably practical. Where five or more people are employed, this policy must be set down in writing. Such a written policy must include:
- a statement of general policy
- delegated responsibilities for dealing with specific areas (e.g. equipment, substances, training, first aid, fire, reporting of accidents, etc.)
- general instructions to staff arising out of the significant findings of the risk assessments.

Such a document must aim to be concise, pointing the reader to more detailed guidance where necessary.

Management of Health & Safety at Work Regulations 1999

These regulations require employers and the self-employed to identify:
- the hazards arising from their work
- who could be affected by those hazards

- the measures to control the risk of those hazards causing harm.

The measures identified by the risk assessment will include the need to comply with other regulations (e.g. ionising radiations) as well as those to deal with specific hazards not covered by regulations (e.g. the hazardous behaviour of animals). They must, in order of priority, seek to:
- eliminate the hazard (e.g. substitute a disinfectant containing glutaraldehyde with a less hazardous one)
- physically control access to the hazard (e.g. prevent entry into areas where ionising radiations are being used)
- provide information, instruction, training and supervision to ensure people work in a safe manner (e.g. SOPs, safety signs, local rules, proper training)
- consider if personal protective equipment needs to be provided (e.g. face masks or goggles).

Where five or more people are employed these significant findings of the risk assessment must be recorded (often as an attachment to the health & safety policy). Risk assessments for the employment of young persons (under 18 years of age) are required.

A risk assessment assessing whether the practice premises does, or is liable to, contain asbestos, any risk arising therefrom, and action taken to manage the risk, may be required (Control of Asbestos at Work Regulations 2002). Employers have a legal duty to consult with their employees regarding health & safety. This should include:
- the regular circulation of the health & safety policy amongst staff, including the significant findings of risk assessments
- the regular circulation of the results of any monitoring of health & safety standards in the work place and action for their improvement.

Control of Substances Hazardous to Health Regulations 2002

The risk to health and safety from veterinary medicines and other substances has to be assessed under the Control of Substances Hazardous to Health Regulations 2002 (COSHH). There is wide variation in risk – many are low to medium risk but there are some substances in veterinary practice which pose a very serious risk to health. Implementing measures to control the exposure to low- or medium-risk substances can be adequately achieved when they are assessed by their therapeutic group/type/route of administration, etc. The practice can set out standard measures to control exposures to medicines such as:
- injectable anaesthetics
- pour-on anthelmintics

- steroidal compounds
- antibiotics.

Within these groups, practices must identify any specific medicines or substances that could have longer-term health risks, such as allergies (e.g. penicillin) or sensitivities (e.g. latex). Specific and detailed assessments and the resulting measures to control exposure must be made for high-risk substances such as:

- any hormones
- oil-based vaccines
- cytotoxic drugs
- glutaraldehyde disinfectants
- tilmicosin (Micotil).

It is recommended that practices request and keep COSHH sheets for all products used on their premises. These sheets should be obtained from the manufacturers whenever a new product is ordered. If, for example, an incident occurs at work following which a member of staff must attend Accident & Emergency, they can take with them full details of the product with which they have had contact.

Administering medicines

Improvements in drug presentations have meant increases in safe practice for nurses but have put increased demands on their technical skills, e.g. in the use of syringe drivers and pumps. The traditional role of the nurse does not include training in such areas and these electronically controlled delivery systems may require additional training if used.

Dispensing medication for clients to use at home

- Personal hygiene when administering oral medications to pets must be reinforced,

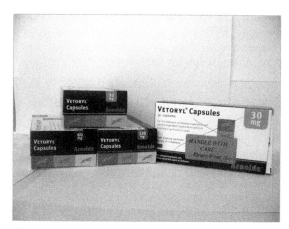

Fig. 3.7 'Handle with care' label.

especially if the patient has an infectious condition.

- Wear gloves for the handling of all medications where practical – and essential for those that are absorbed through the skin or being administered by clients with sensitivities or allergies. Figure 3.7 shows a hazardous drug labelled with instructions to wear gloves. Every bottle should be labelled both inside and on the outer packaging.
- Ensure the client is aware of any effects self-administration might cause and when to seek medical advice.

Disposal of administration equipment

Needles and other sharps should be carefully disposed of in the sharps bins, which are then collected for incineration. It is advisable that this is done immediately after use. The sharps must be collected in an approved container, which can be sealed and which has a handle. Unofficial containers, such as used tablet pots, are not acceptable. Syringes containing medicines should be disposed of into DOOP containers (see Disposal of unwanted medicines below). Empty syringes may not always require to be disposed of as special waste.

Disposal of contaminated body secretions and excretions

Specialist advice should be sought wherever there is a need to dispose of contaminated body waste (e.g. a chemotherapy patient's urine/faeces). Trace chemotherapy and other hazardous drugs should be disposed of by a regulated medical waste company through incineration. These recommendations are consistent with current knowledge of the toxicity of antineoplastic (cytotoxic, chemotherapeutics, anti-cancer) agents.

Record keeping and stock control

Ordering/requisitioning procedures

Most practices utilise an automated ordering system similar to ESCOS, which has a built-in stock level specific to your practice and transfers the order directly to the supplier. The Misuse of Drugs Regulations 2001 was amended in 2003 to allow computer-generated requisitions for controlled drugs but all Schedule 2 medicines require an original order with a vet's signature before they can be processed. Schedule 3 drugs require an MDA form.

Stock control

There must be an efficient stock control system to ensure a continuous supply of all products and removal of out-of-date medicines. An adequate supply of medicinal products and materials used in the treatment of patients must be readily available.

Depending on the workload of the practice, some agents may be used infrequently, which results in some drugs exceeding their shelf-life. Adequate stock control is therefore required. Many of the common injectable and oral agents require refrigeration; these agents should be kept away from animal or human food sources. Although cytotoxic drugs are not controlled by law, they can be abused with serious results – locked refrigeration is recommended. Drug residues have been found on the outside of manufacturers' packaging and on surfaces adjacent to stored, unused cytotoxic products. Thus from the time the drug arrives in the practice, the agent should be handled with gloves and should only be dispensed by trained personnel. It is also wise to store the agents in clear, plastic, zip-lock type bags.

To avoid surplus stock, some practices may charge the client for the entire amount of drug in a pack. If small amounts of medicines are only required for occasional use, the provision of a prescription is often more suitable.

Storage of medicines

It is recommended that all drugs are stored in accordance with manufacturers' recommendations, whether in the practice or in a vehicle. If it is stipulated that the drug be used within a specific time period, it must be labelled with the opening date. It is advisable that at least one member of staff must have completed an appropriate pharmacy course within the last 5 years to keep up to date with current recommendations. There are many specific storage requirements for drugs and it is always wise to consult the data sheets of any drug you unpack which you are unfamiliar with.

- Rimadyl (carprofen) should be stored in the refrigerator until opened and then kept at room temperature.
- Max/min thermometers should be used both in drug refrigerators (Fig. 3.8) and in the dispensary to ensure the environmental conditions do not fluctuate outside the recommended ranges.

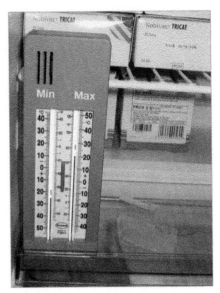

Fig. 3.8 Maximum/minimum thermometer.

- Light-sensitive drugs, such as injectable oxytetracycline, should not be drawn up and left in clear syringes for dispensing. The syringe should be placed in a brown envelope or bag until used.
- All environmental variables should be considered, including humidity and so it is unwise to store drugs near to the autoclave.
- Health and safety considerations include storing large containers on the ground and any potentially hazardous chemicals away from the general public.
- Affix a practice label to each item before it is placed in stock and write the date of first use on multidose vials to ensure the recommended period of use is not exceeded.
- Once stock has been dispensed it should not be accepted back into the dispensary because there may have been storage problems whilst the product was not under your care.

Disposal of unwanted medicines

Pharmaceutical products, veterinary compounds and Prescription Only Medicines (POMs) constitute 'special waste' and therefore out-of-date products must be disposed of in accordance with the Special Waste Regulations 1996 (as amended) and the Groundwater Regulations 1998.

- POMs which are prescribed for use in the 'home' and which enter the home for use by the animal owner are considered to be household waste and are exempt from the regulations.

- VMPs which are classified as P (no longer exists), PML (now POM-VPS or NFA-VPS), GSL and MFSX (now POM-V or VPS) are not defined as special waste and do not come within the scope of the regulations. But:
- Some of these VMPs will become special waste if they exhibit certain other properties such as particular physical/chemical, toxic or ecotoxic properties; more details are given in the Special Waste Regulations (1996).

Most pharmaceutical waste should be placed in the DOOP (disposal of old pharmaceuticals) bin, but Schedule 2 drugs which are no longer required should be stored and destroyed in the presence of a police officer from the drugs squad or a member of the home office who then countersigns the controlled drugs book. It is also a requirement that the drug is destroyed in a manner that renders it unavailable for further use. The easiest method is to inject it onto cat litter, which will absorb the agent. This then should be incinerated. The disposal instructions reflect the results of the required safety tests and take into account any potential risks to the environment, health of humans, animals and plants.

Pharmaceutical waste, being classed as special waste, has to be collected separately from other clinical waste. There are still some grey areas as to what is covered by pharmaceutical waste, but it includes the following:

- prescription-only medicines
- any part-full bottles or part-used ampoules
- out-of-date medicines
- discarded chemicals
- cytotoxic products.

This implies that empty syringes and pharmaceutical bottles, including vaccine vials, need not be placed into DOOP bins but it is advisable to seek specialist advice when setting practice policies.

Special waste must be collected and disposed of by a registered contractor. Responsibility for pharmaceutical waste remains with the veterinary surgeon (the producer) until it is disposed of correctly. Collection requires completion of a six-part form, which documents and traces the waste from producer through carrier to incineration. The waste contractor will often provide the documentation. In addition, pre-notification is needed, for each collection, to inform the local authority that the waste is being collected. Pharmaceutical waste must be treated separately by the carrier; if the carrier does not differentiate between pharmaceutical and other clinical waste, it is advisable to document this for your own benefit.

Accidental injection or ingestion

Cytotoxic drug tablets should not be split or crushed and capsules should never be opened and divided. Safe dosing schedules can be devised by increasing the dosing interval, sourcing alternative formulations or reverting to injecting the drug. Whenever possible, tablets and capsules should be dispensed without altering the manufacturer's packaging and an additional warning should be added to the label instructing owners not to crush or split the tablets.

An accident book is required by law and must meet the requirements of the Data Protection Act. It must record the following:

- date and time of accident or occurrence
- full name and address of the person involved and the injury or condition suffered
- where the accident or occurrence happened
- a brief description of the circumstances
- in the case of a reportable disease: the date of diagnosis, the occupation of the person concerned and the name or nature of the disease.

This information must be kept for at least 3 years and all staff must know where it is located.

Practices should have a procedure for the Reporting of Injuries, Diseases and Dangerous Occurrences as required by RIDDOR regulations 1995. Any injury, accident or work-related illness which keeps an employee off work or unable to do their normal job for more than three days must be reported to the Incident Contact Centre (ICC) within 10 days. The ICC is the single point of contact for all incidents in the UK. Incidents can be reported by Telephone 0845 3009923, Fax 0845 3009924, or by Post to ICC, Caerphilly Business Park, Caerphilly, CF83 3GG (HSE).

There should be a suitably stocked first-aid box, as required under the Health and Safety (First Aid) Regulations 1981, and a person or persons should have been appointed to take charge should someone fall ill or be injured, and to re-stock the first-aid box as required. There is no standard list of items to be included in the first-aid box, although there is a suggested minimum:

- a leaflet giving general guidance on first-aid
- 20 individually wrapped sterile adhesive dressings
- 2 sterile eye pads
- 4 individually wrapped triangular bandages
- 6 safety pins
- medium-sized individually wrapped sterile unmedicated wound dressings
- 2 large sterile individually wrapped unmedicated wound dressings
- 1 pair of disposable gloves.

Suspect adverse reactions

Adverse reactions in humans or animals to medicinal products should be reported promptly to the Veterinary Medicines Directorate and to the manufacturer (see Chapter 1 for more details).

Packaging and labelling of medicines

Packaging

Guidelines for dispensing are available in the current BSAVA Small Animal Formulary and the BVA Code of Practice on Medicines (2000). The Royal Pharmaceutical Society of Great Britain recommends that when repackaging medicines from bulk containers, they must be dispensed in appropriate containers, both for the product and the user.

- Tablets and capsules must be dispensed in crush-proof and moisture-proof containers.
- Solid dose and external preparations should be dispensed in a re-closable, child-proof container.
- There can be exceptions made if the medicine is in the manufacturer's original pack such as a blister pack. These should be dispensed in paper board cartons or wallets or paper envelopes.
- Discretion may be exercised in the use of child-proof containers for the elderly and infirm. Advice must be given to keep all medicines out of the reach of children.
- Paper envelopes and plastic bags are unacceptable as the sole form of packaging of veterinary medicines.
- Sachets should be dispensed in paper board cartons or wallets, or paper envelopes.
- Under The Medicines (Fluted Bottles) Regulations 1978, certain medicinal products for external use should be dispensed in fluted bottles so that they are recognisable by touch. This requirement does not apply to volumes in excess of 1.14 litres or to eye or ear drops supplied in plastic containers.

- Creams, dusting powders, granules, ointments, pessaries, powders, suppositories and semi-solids should be dispensed in wide-mouthed jars made of glass or plastic.
- The dispenser has a duty to ensure that the owner understands any instructions on the label and knows how to use the product safely.

Labelling

The Medicines (Labelling) Regulations 1976 recommends that the label must be mechanically printed or indelibly and legibly printed or written in accordance with statutory requirements. Biro, felt tip or ballpoint pen are acceptable; ink and pencil are not. The label must include the following:

- name of owner or keeper
- address where animal is kept
- name and address of veterinarian
- date of dispensing
- the words 'for animal treatment only' unless the package is too small
- the words 'keep out of the reach of children' or words to the same meaning
- the words 'for external use only' or 'not to be taken internally' for medicines that are for topical use, e.g. eye or ear formulations, lotions, liquid antiseptics
- ideally the label should not obscure the expiry date of the preparation or important printed information on the manufacturer's label or pack; small tubes may be dispensed in an appropriately labelled envelope
- product information leaflets should be dispensed where possible with the product.

Common prescribing abbreviations

Directions should preferably be in English without abbreviation. It is acceptable, however, to use some Latin abbreviations when dispensing and prescribing. These should be limited to those in Box 3.5.

Box 3.5

Common abbreviations used in veterinary medicine prescription writing and labelling

a.c.	before meals	o.m.	in the morning
ad. lib.	at pleasure (ad libitum)	o.n.	at night
amp.	ampoule	p.c.	after meals (post cibum)
b.i.d.	twice a day (bis in die)	p.r.n.	as required (pro re nata)
cap.	capsule	q.	every (e.g. q12h means every
e.o.d.	every other day		12 hours)
g	gram	q.i.d./q.d.s.	four times a day (quater in die)
h or hr	hour	q.s.	a sufficient quantity
i.m.	intramuscular	s.i.d.	once a day (semel in die)
i.p.	intraperitoneal	Sig:	directions/label
i.t.	intratracheal	stat	immediately (statim)
i.v.	intravenous	susp.	suspension
l or L	litre	tab	tablet
m^2	square meter	t.i.d./t.d.s.	three times a day (ter in die)
mg	milligram	µl	microlitre
ml	millilitre		

Questions for Chapter 3

Convert the following:

1. 2.4 kg into grams

2. 1.02 g into milligrams

3. 0.6 mg into micrograms

4. 7.1 µg into nanograms

5. 250 ml into litres

6. 1 decilitre into ml

7. 900 µg into mg

8. 2 g into kg

9. 0.003 g into µg

10. 2400 µg into grams

How many mg/ml are the following solutions? (work out the % solution first)

11. 20 g dissolved in 100 ml

12. 25 g dissolved in 400 ml

13. 30 g dissolved in 1000 ml

14. A 7.5 kg dog needs two daily injections. If each injection is 15 ml, calculate the dose rate in mg/kg/d. What weight of drug in grams will be administered over a 5-day period if the solution used is of 2.5% concentration?

15. Convert the following:
    % into mg/ml
    – 2.5
    – 0.1
    – 1.25
    – 18
    – 33.3

    mg/ml into % solution
    – 1
    – 0.1
    – 10
    – 100
    – 3

16. Which of these three solutions is the most concentrated?
    - Solution A has 25 g of solute in 750 ml of solution
    - Solution B has 253 g of solute in 1750 ml of solution
    - Solution C has 2.56 g of solute in 78 ml of solution

    To work this out you need to first determine what % each solution is, i.e. divide the weight in grams by the volume in ml and multiply by 100.

17. A dog weighing 8 kg needs injections t.i.d. of a 4% solution. Calculate the weight in mg of the drug and the volume in ml that it receives per injection. Assume a dose rate of 6 mg/kg/8 h.

18. What do the following abbreviations stand for?

    u.i.d.
    u.d.s.
    o.d.
    p.r.n.
    a.c.
    p.c.
    o.m.
    o.n.
    q.s.
    c.i.
    d.i.

19. What volume of 2.5% thio would you give to a 10 kg dog if the dose rate is 10 mg/kg?
    a. 4 ml
    b. 14 ml
    c. 10 ml
    d. 7 ml

20. What volume of amoxicillin would you give a 5 kg cat if the dose rate is 5 mg/kg and the solution contains 5 mg/ml?
    a. 2 ml
    b. 3 ml
    c. 4 ml
    d. 5 ml

21. How many tablets would you dispense for a 5-day course to a 2.5 kg cat if the dose rate is 10 mg/kg q 12 h and tablets come in 50 mg and 250 mg?
    a. 10 × 50 mg
    b. 5 × 50 mg
    c. 2 × 250 mg
    d. 5 × 250 mg

22. How many mg/ml are there in 1.25% thio?
    a. 12.5
    b. 1.25
    c. 22.5
    d. 125

For answers go to page 238

CHAPTER 4

General Pharmacology

Four

Learning aims and objectives

After studying this chapter you should be able to:

1. **Describe the processes of absorption, distribution, metabolism and excretion**
2. **List the ways drugs act on their receptors**
3. **State the equation to calculate a drug's therapeutic index**
4. **List the drugs that should not be mixed with other agents**
5. **Describe how to safely store and handle hazardous drugs.**

Pharmacokinetics

This is the investigation of the fate of the drug. Basically, it concerns the effect of the body on the drug and takes into account the processes of:
- absorption
- distribution
- metabolism
- excretion.

Absorption

Firstly, the drug must be given in a suitable form at an appropriate site of administration. If local action is required, absorption from the site is a disadvantage, but when systemic effects are needed, absorption is essential. Unless given by the intravenous route, drugs need to penetrate the cell membranes that form a barrier between the drug and the circulation. Rate of absorption is governed by several factors:
- Dosage form – this is the form that the active pharmacological agent is introduced into the body. Drugs in aqueous solutions are more rapidly absorbed than those in oily solutions, suspension or solid form. For example, procaine benzylpenicillin has a duration of 24 hours in plasma; benzathine benzylpenicillin has a very low solubility and a duration of several days in plasma.
- Route of administration – there are two classes:
  1. *Enteral*. Oral, sublingual and rectal are all included in this category. Drugs are absorbed

all along the gastrointestinal tract and must cross the intestinal epithelium to enter the capillaries or lymphatics via the vessel wall. This passage is largely due to simple diffusion through the lipid membrane, but other mechanisms such as filtration and active transport do occur. The intestinal epithelium can even engulf large drug molecules by pinocytosis. There are several important features associated with oral administration:

- it is crucial that the drug is released from its dosage form, i.e. disintegration of capsules or dissolution of powders
- the presence of food may reduce absorption
- gastric acid secretion may affect the drug
- possible irritation of gastric mucosa
- microorganisms and gut enzymes may render the drug ineffective
- there will be some loss of drug due to the drug-metabolising enzymes in the liver that will inactivate some drug before its entry into the circulation; this is known as the first-pass effect.

2. *Parenteral.* This method includes intramuscular (i.m.), intravenous (i.v.) and subcutaneous (s.c.) injections. All of these methods bypass the gut and the desired plasma concentration of the drug is reached more quickly.

- The physical and chemical characteristics of the drug.
- Blood flow at the site of administration/absorption.

Distribution

Once a drug is in the bloodstream it distributes throughout the various body fluid compartments. Factors affecting this include the regional blood flow, the lipid solubility of the drug, the extent to which the drug becomes protein-bound and the existence of a suitable active transport system. Many drugs are protein-bound as they are so insoluble in water that they would not be transported in blood if it were not for this association. The most common protein involved is albumin and disease states that alter the amount of protein, such as uraemia and hypoproteinaemia, can affect the binding process.

There are also some functional barriers in the body, the blood–brain barrier being an example. This is a barrier between the plasma and the extracellular space of the brain and although it allows the passage of nutrients and lipid-soluble agents, some drugs (e.g. penicillin) have great difficulty in crossing unless inflammation is present. Other barriers to penetration include the walls of abscesses, penetration into bone and access to mammary tissue.

The body water percentage of newborns is 75–80%, about 20% higher than in the adult. This results in a larger volume of distribution, meaning water-soluble drugs may require larger initial doses to achieve the desired effect. There is also less muscle mass and decreased fat deposits, resulting in higher distribution of cardiac output to the vessel-rich organs such as the brain and heart. Drugs such as muscle relaxants or thiopentone that redistribute to muscle or fat therefore have a longer duration of effect.

Metabolism

Some drugs are excreted by the body unchanged, but most undergo one or more metabolic conversions. The purpose of this may be to render the drug more soluble to increase the ease of excretion. Occasionally a drug needs to be metabolised to its active form before it can have its effect. An example of this is primidone (Mysoline), which is converted to phenobarbitone by the liver.

The enzymes that carry out drug metabolism are found throughout the body including the kidney, lung and plasma, but the major site of drug metabolism is the liver. The frequency of liver damage as a sign of toxicity indicates the active role this organ plays in removing the drugs from the blood. The liver enzymes are also responsible for drug tolerance, a situation where increasingly higher doses of a drug must be given to produce the same effect. This can be seen with the barbiturates and is called enzyme induction. Factors affecting drug metabolism include:

- Species differences – for example the cat has much slower hepatic drug metabolism than many other species. It is defective in its ability to form most glucuronide conjugates, which is the major method of drug metabolism in mammals and hence should not be given paracetamol, which remains at toxic doses within the body.
- Age – fetal and newborn animals have a limited capacity to metabolise drugs as hepatic enzyme systems are functionally immature at birth. As puppies grow and hepatic blood flow increases, enzymatic systems mature and reach full activity by 5–8 weeks of age, around the time of weaning. The clinical effects of anaesthetic agents that require hepatic degradation for termination of action may last longer and be more intense in animals less than 8 weeks old and reduced doses should be used. Serum concentrations of albumin and other proteins used for protein binding also do not reach mature levels until 8 weeks of age, resulting in more unbound active drug in the circulation. Combined with the reduced renal function in

animals less than 8 weeks of age (due to low perfusion pressure and immature glomerular and tubular function), this means that drugs often have an increased duration of action.

- Sex – in rats it has been shown that females metabolise drugs more slowly than males due to a depressive effect of oestrogens.
- Nutrition – dietary deficiency leads to a decrease in enzyme metabolising activity.
- Pregnancy – certain aspects of maternal drug metabolism are decreased.
- Disease – liver pathology can affect its metabolising ability.

Excretion

The lowering of plasma drug concentration is termed clearance. This occurs either by excretion of unaltered drug or by metabolism followed by excretion. The principal organ of excretion is the kidney, where water-soluble material is removed. Quantitatively the next most important is the liver, which eliminates metabolised drugs in bile. There are also contributions from the sweat glands, the mammary glands and the salivary glands. Volatile agents are excreted via the lungs.

A small number of drugs, such as fat-soluble drugs and toxins, remain in the tissues where they can accumulate and cause tissue damage. Some of the drugs excreted in the bile are reabsorbed from the intestine – this is termed enterohepatic recycling and is shown in Figure 4.1. Factors affecting excretion:

- protein binding prolongs drug persistence in the body
- tubular reabsorption in the kidney, of lipid-soluble drugs when the concentration in the tubule rises

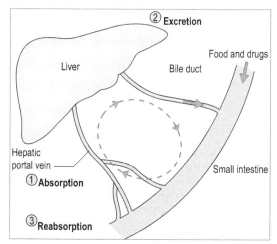

Fig. 4.1 Enterohepatic recycling

- tubular secretion of a drug increases its loss into urine, e.g. penicillin
- renal blood flow
- enterohepatic circulation.

Pharmacodynamics

This is the study of the action and effect of a drug on the body.

Drug–receptor complex

Most drugs work by associating with specific macro-molecules called receptors. Often the receptor is a histologically recognisable specialisation on the cell, e.g. the motor end plate on a skeletal muscle cell. The union of drug and receptor forms a complex that is responsible for the initiation of activity.

- If a response is elicited, then the drug is known as an *agonist*, having the right shape to fit in the receptor and the efficacy to start a biological action.
- *Antagonists* are drugs that have affinity for a receptor, i.e. they bind with it, but do not elicit a response as they lack efficacy. Atropine is an example of a drug that works in this way, blocking the receptors for acetylcholine (a neurotransmitter found in many synapses), and this is how the morphine antidote naloxone works.
- *Partial agonists* are drugs that have affinity for a receptor but only produce a weak response, i.e. have reduced efficacy. In the presence of an agonist these drugs will compete for receptors and actually antagonise the response to the pure agonist.

Once bound to a receptor, the drug works in one of four ways:

1. Lipid-soluble drugs cross the cell membrane and activate intracellular receptors, e.g. corticosteroids.
2. Some receptors cross the membrane and directly activate enzymes in the cell.
3. Receptors that are bound to transmembrane ion channels produce very quick responses to the binding of a drug to its receptor.
4. Some drug–receptor complexes activate internal proteins that in turn activate an enzyme or ion channel.

Side effects and toxicity

A side effect, or an adverse drug reaction, is defined by the World Health Organization as 'any response to a drug which is noxious, unintended and occurs

Box 4.1

Therapeutic and toxic levels

The margin of safety of a drug is termed its therapeutic index. This is worked out by the equation:

Therapeutic index (TI) =

$$\frac{\text{The dose that was lethal in 50\% of experimental animals}}{\text{The dose that was effective in 50\% of animals}}$$

The higher the TI the safer the drug.

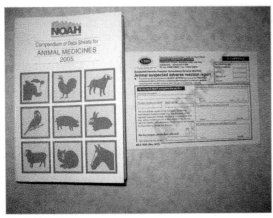

Fig. 4.2   The Noah Compendium

Box 4.2

Some of the common side effects of drugs

Gastrointestinal
- dry mouth
- metallic taste
- oesophageal reflux
- nausea and vomiting
- diarrhoea
- constipation

Nervous system
- depression
- mania
- confusion
- collapse

Dermatological
- pruritis (inflammation)
- pruritus (itchy)
- urticaria (hives)
- photosensitivity

Blood disorders
- anaemia
- thrombocytopaenia

at doses used for prophylaxis, diagnosis and therapy'. Box 4.1 shows the way the safe dose of a drug is calculated. Side effects are always listed in the data sheets and should always be reported to the drug company and the Veterinary Medicines Directorate for inclusion in future drug information leaflets. Yellow forms for reporting incidents can be found in the back of the NOAH compendiums (Fig. 4.2). Side effects can affect any body system and careful clinical monitoring of patients should be carried out during all drug therapy. Some of the more common side effects are listed in Box 4.2.

The skin is one of the most commonly affected organs and the most implicated drugs are sulphonamides and penicillins. The signs are often due to degranulating mast cells causing histamine release. It may be the intended pharmacological action of the drug that causes skin complications, e.g. immunosuppressive drugs causing poor wound healing, alopecia and increased susceptibility to secondary pyoderma. Hypersensitivity reactions are unpredictable and unrelated to the pharmacological action of the drug. These are more serious as they will persist and cross-reactions can occur with related compounds.

Most side effects that result from large doses or long-term therapy gradually subside once the drug is discontinued. Haematology and biochemistry should be performed where indicated. Side effects and toxicities should be managed according to the clinical signs shown. For example, a dog showing uncontrolled running movements after sulphonamide therapy may need sedating or a dog vomiting after digitalis glycoside (digoxin) therapy might require intravenous fluids.

Some side effects may not be as noticeable and require careful observation of the patient. Digoxin can cause visual disturbances and depression which is made worse by any poor health such as hypercalcaemia (high blood calcium) or hypokalaemia (low blood potassium). Managing a digoxin toxicity requires specific treatments including giving drugs like phenylbutazone or a barbiturate anaesthetic which increase the rate of detoxification. Some drugs, such as the antibiotic neomycin, act to decrease the absorption rate of digoxin by acting on the gut to destroy the bacteria responsible for absorption of the drug.

Adverse drug reactions are either a direct toxicity, resulting from the interaction between the drug and its metabolites or tissues, or a hypersensitivity reaction, which is immune-mediated. Drug-induced fevers are thought to be immune-mediated due to release of endogenous pyrogens. Drugs that are low molecular weight must combine with serum proteins in order to be immunogenic; a type III or IV hypersensitivity reaction is responsible and a genetic predisposition to sensitisation may be the reason some animals show adverse reactions.

At the extreme end of the adverse drug reaction spectrum is poisoning. For a general management plan the following should be considered:
- maintain respiration
- maintain circulation
- maintain body temperature
- maintain fluid and electrolyte levels
- remove the drug (gastric lavage/emesis/active elimination)
- inactivation of the drug (activated charcoal to adsorb it)
- correction of metabolic disturbances caused.

Direct drug–drug interactions

A drug interaction occurs when the effects of one drug are altered by the effects of another. Occasionally these interactions are beneficial, e.g. when using diuretics and angiotensin-converting enzyme (ACE) inhibitors in the treatment of hypertension, but most of the time we regard them as a problem. Box 4.3 shows the drugs that are likely to be involved in interactions.

When pharmaceutical preparations are mixed for administration by virtually any route, interactions may occur between the active ingredients or the adjuncts in the formulations. Incompatibilities may result in precipitation, chemical inactivation, and a change in colour, taste or the physical form of the preparations. A few examples of drugs with many incompatibilities are listed below; these drugs should not be mixed with any other drug preparations:
- semisynthetic penicillins
- benzylpenicillin
- aminoglycosides
- barbiturates
- diazepam
- vitamin B complex.

There are many pharmacokinetic interactions between drugs where one agent affects the absorption, distribution, biotransformation or excretion of another. The data sheets should be consulted before using more than one drug at a time to check compatibility. Competition for plasma-protein binding sites is quite common, e.g. non-steroidal anti-inflammatories (NSAIDs) displace sulphonamides

---

Box 4.3

Drugs likely to be involved in interactions

Highly protein-bound drugs

These are likely to displace other drugs from protein-binding sites:
- aspirin
- phenylbutazone
- sulphonamides

Drugs that stimulate or inhibit the metabolism of other drugs
- phenytoin
- phenobarbital
- griseofulvin
- chloramphenicol
- cimetidine
- erythromycin
- metronidazole
- ketoconazole

Drugs that affect renal function
- diuretics alter the renal clearance of other drugs

Drugs with a low therapeutic index
- aminoglycoside antibiotics
- anticoagulants
- anticonvulsants
- antihypertensive agents
- cardiac glycosides
- cytotoxic and immunosuppressive drugs

---

and phenylbutazone displaces warfarin. Some drugs, such as ketoconazole, do not absorb as well if the stomach is less acidic and therefore can not be given with antacids, H_2 blockers or omeprazole.

Some drugs interact even within the body and their concurrent use should be avoided. For example kaolin binds lincomycin in the GI tract and aminoglycosides inactivate certain penicillins at sites of infection – despite the synergistic action of the penicillins and aminoglycosides in some instances.

Pharmacodynamic interactions are sometimes desirable but may induce toxicity. For example, the toxicity of cardiac glycosides is enhanced by hypothyroidism and halothane sensitises the myocardium to the arrhythmogenic effects of catecholamines such as adrenaline. Fatal renal failure has been reported following the combined use of methoxyflurane and tetracyclines.

Drug–food interactions

Whether the drug can be given with food is an important dispensing point that owners must be made aware of – too often, a drug's efficacy is compromised by owners not complying with this instruction. The gastric pH of the dog and cat varies from 1 to 6 depending on the relationship to feeding stimuli and so those drugs that rely on an acid environment for dissolution may have drastically different effects in fasted animals compared to those dosed post-prandially. A few examples are listed below.

- Griseofulvin has a low water solubility and absorption is enhanced when given with a fatty meal.
- Fluoroquinolones given with food take longer to be absorbed but the overall result is the same and so they can be given with or without a meal.
- Drugs that require an acid environment for absorption, such as the antibiotic rifampin, should be given on an empty stomach.
- Other antibiotics that should not be given with food include lincomycin, erythromycin and oxytetracycline. Tetracyclines easily bind to calcium ions and so absorption is decreased with the co-administration of food and dairy products.
- Food can impair the oral absorption of some NSAIDs or contribute to drug interactions for others, e.g. phenylbutazone sticks to hay in the gut of horses and has reduced availability and delayed absorption.
- Sometimes the same drug can have different bioavailabilities depending on its presentation, e.g. the antifungal drug fluconazole (Diflucan) is best absorbed on a full stomach if in tablet form, but on an empty stomach in its liquid state.

Effects of disease states on therapy

Renal disease

The glomerular filtration rate falls with age and tubular function decreases, so even if clinically, elderly animals appear normal, special considerations apply. Many drugs are excreted in the urine or have active metabolites that are so excreted and require reduced doses in renally compromised patients, examples include digoxin, gentamicin and other aminoglycosides. Tetracyclines accumulate when renal function is poor, causing nausea and vomiting and their antianabolic action worsens the uraemia and promotes muscle wasting.

Hepatic disease

As the liver is often the main site for metabolism of a drug, reduced doses may be required when hepatic dysfunction is diagnosed.

Shock/dehydration

Patients with reduced circulating blood volume or decreased peripheral circulation will not absorb drugs injected subcutaneously or intramuscularly as quickly as expected.

Nephrotic syndrome/malnutrition

These disorders reduce the amounts of plasma proteins available for distribution of the drug.

Owner drug abuse

Box 4.4 lists the chemical agents most commonly subject to abuse. The adverse effects of drug abuse can be split into physical and psychological effects and again into the acute, chronic and withdrawal effects. If a benzodiazepine is taken for a few weeks or longer, dependence can occur. When the drug is withdrawn, signs of anxiety occur within 2–3 days and can be severe enough to produce shaking, nausea and headaches.

Anabolic steroids are most often taken by those who want to increase their strength and endurance in competitive sport, but there is a growing trend amongst young people to take them for their euphoriant effects and intravenous use is increasing. Alterations in sex drive and gonadal function, mood changes and aggression are observed and hypertension and abnormal liver function are seen in regular users.

Drugs used in diagnostic tests

- *Tetracosactide* (Synacthen) is a synthetic version of ACTH with the same pharmacological effects

Box 4.4

Commonly abused drugs

- opiates
- CNS stimulants
- benzodiazepines
- barbiturates
- anabolic steroids

but a shorter duration of action. It acts on the adrenal gland, stimulating the production of glucocorticoids, but has little effect on the production of aldosterone. It is used in the diagnosis of hyperadrenocorticism (Cushing's disease).

- *Desmopressin* (DDAVP) is a vasopressin (antidiuretic hormone) analogue with a longer duration of action than vasopressin and no vasoconstrictor activity. It is used in the diagnosis and treatment of central diabetes insipidus (CDI) and to help increase clotting factors in patients with haemophilia A or von Willebrand's disease. The drug is administered intravenously, intramuscularly or as drops into the eye or nose. The urine specific gravity (USG) is measured before and 2 hours after treatment. An increase in USG is consistent with CDI, whereas nephrogenic diabetes insipidus or medullary washout should be considered if it remains low.
- *Dexamethasone* is a corticosteroid with high glucocorticoid but low mineralocorticoid activity. It is used as an anti-inflammatory and in the diagnosis of hyperadrenocorticism. Box 4.5 shows the protocols for the two tests.

Box 4.5

Dexamethasone screening test

Low dose dexamethasone screening test

- Use: diagnosis of hyperadrenocorticism (HAC)
- Protocol: Assess blood cortisol levels at 0, 3 and 8 hours. Give the dexamethasone intravenously (0.01–0.015 mg/kg) after the 0 hour sample.
- Results:
  - Normal if the cortisol is suppressed to < 50% of the basal level after 3 hours and < 40 nmol/l after 8 hours
  - HAC if failure to suppress at 3 and 8 hours.

High dose dexamethasone suppression test:

- Use: to differentiate between pituitary-dependent (PDH) and adrenal-dependent HAC
- Protocol: as above using 1 mg/kg dexamethasone i.v.
- Results:
  - PDH will suppress to < 50% of the basal level after 3 hours and < 40 nmol/l after 8 hours
  - Adrenal tumours will fail to suppress at 3 hours.

Box 4.6

Xylazine stimulation test

Used to assess growth hormone production:

- take an EDTA blood sample at 0 minutes
- administer 100 μg/kg xylazine i.v. immediately
- take an EDTA blood sample at 20 minutes post-injection
- separate the plasma and store at −20°C

- *Thyroid stimulating hormone (TSH)* and *thyrotrophin releasing hormone (TRH)* (Protirelin) stimulate thyroid hormone production. The TSH stimulation test is the best test for hypothyroidism but no licensed preparation is available in the UK and recombinant human TSH is imported on an STA. The TRH stimulation test is of limited value.
- *Xylazine* is an α_2 adrenergic receptor agonist. It is a sedative and muscle relaxant that also stimulates growth hormone production and so is used to assess the pituitary's ability to produce this hormone. Box 4.6 outlines the procedure.

Factors affecting choice of therapy

When you assess a patient, you evaluate their need for medication based on the clinical signs shown and the history from the owner. It is important to know past medication history to ensure the animal is not currently taking any over-the-counter medications, prescription drugs or herbal remedies and to identify any problems relating to drug therapy. The decision is based on:

- a subjective analysis, which involves your opinion of the animal's condition, e.g. if it is dull or bright and alert
- an objective examination, where you can record specific data such as temperature and heart rate
- secondary sources of information, such as a report from the owner that the clinical signs only occur after eating
- tertiary sources of information, such as a literature search to help choose a suitable therapy.

When choosing a therapy, we must be aware that the patient has individual needs and that the plan of care must be adapted accordingly. For example the culture and sensitivity from a wound might indicate that a penicillin-based drug is suitable for treating the infection but if the owners are penicillin sensitive, an alternative therapy must be chosen to avoid any health and safety issues. It is also important to reassess the need for a particular therapy throughout the treatment period, monitoring vital signs, observing the therapeutic effects and checking for side effects or signs of toxicity.

How to handle a hazardous drug

There are some drugs, notably the chemotherapeutics, which potentially could cause harm to those who handle and administer them so great caution and good technique should always be observed. Accidental exposure via the skin, respiratory system or digestive system must be prevented by strict adherence to specific safety protocols as laid out in your practice's risk assessments. Box 4.7 shows some suggestions to avoid contacting hazardous agents.

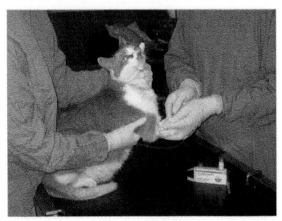

Fig. 4.3 Administration of vincristine

Box 4.7

Reducing the hazards of handling chemotherapeutics

1. Two pairs of latex gloves or one pair of heavy autopsy gloves should be worn during administration of any chemotherapeutic drug regardless of the route of administration (Fig. 4.3).

2. Intravenous administration should be performed through a well-placed indwelling catheter. Liberally flush the catheter before administration of the drug to ensure proper placement and patency of the catheter.

3. Perivascular injection (extravasation) of some agents will result in severe tissue necrosis. Flushing with saline after administration of the drug will remove residual drug from inside the catheter.

4. To reduce drug aerosolisation or to capture leakage from the needle after administration is completed, place an alcohol-moistened cotton ball under the needle before withdrawing the needle from the catheter.

5. Recapping, crushing, or clipping used needles and/or syringes should be avoided since this may aerosolise drugs or cause injury.

A chemotherapy/hazardous drug spill kit should be kept near the site where chemotherapy drugs are mixed or administered. Each spill kit should contain at least the following: 2 pairs of latex gloves; plastic-backed absorbent pad; zip-lock bag for disposal. The addition of a gown, mask and eye protection is also recommended. If a spill occurs:

- absorb the spilled liquid with absorbent pads or cat litter
- wearing gloves, use paper towels to clean up the remaining liquid
- place the contaminated materials in an appropriate sealed receptacle marked 'Chemotherapeutics'
- clean the contaminated area with water and detergent.

Chemotherapy safety should be discussed with clients prior to discharge of the patient. There is a fine line between protecting clients and alarming them unnecessarily. While it is important to point out potential hazards associated with human exposure to these drugs, it is equally important to avoid frightening people. Assure the client that the pet is safe to be around all of the family members. Being with family members is an important part of a pet's life and enjoying normal activities together, hugging, and even kissing the pet are all safe activities. Provide each client with an easy-to-understand information sheet about how to prevent exposure to chemotherapeutic agents. Then, review the information with the client to make sure there is a clear understanding of the hazards and precautions. Explain to each client that excretions from their pet receiving chemotherapy may be hazardous. Inform clients that potentially hazardous materials (faeces, urine, vomit) should be collected using appropriate protective equipment and disposed of in labelled bags for incineration.

Table 4.1 Drugs that can be used as adjuncts for control of pain

Drug	Indications for use to control pain/discomfort
Amitriptyline	Pain of neuropathic origin; an antidepressant that calms the patient
Dexamethasone	When inflammation is causing nerve compression or where there is raised intracranial pressure; also stimulates appetite which can help demeanour
Diazepam	Augments the sedation and relaxes the muscles
Metoclopramide	Relieves nausea and vomiting and stimulates GI motility

Getting the best results from your drug

- Administering the drug correctly and at the ideal time ensures the agent will be most efficacious. For example, there is evidence to suggest that once-a-day steroids should be given to dogs in the morning and cats at night. This is because cats are nocturnal and produce their normal body steroids at this time.
- Polypharmacy can be employed to reduce the amounts of an individual drug needed. As an example, Table 4.1 lists drugs that can be used as adjuncts for control of pain that reduce the dose of opioid required significantly and thereby reduce the side effects.
- Always consult the data sheets to check drug compatibility when using more than one agent. For example, bacteriostatic antibiotics (those that stop the replication of bacteria) should not be given with bacteriocidal antibiotics (those that kill actively replicating bacteria) as one will decrease the efficacy of the other.

Non-therapeutic methods of relieving pain

Good nursing skills can reduce or alleviate the need for drug therapy completely. The following list includes some of the ways you should consider:
- TLC – stroke, groom, talk to your patients; provide comfortable bedding
- warmth – postoperative analgesia is far more effective in a patient with good peripheral circulation
- massage and physiotherapy where appropriate
- support dressings
- transcutaneous electrical nerve stimulation (TENS)
- acupuncture
- good plane of nutrition
- well hydrated
- ensure the patient has an empty bladder
- quiet environment
- freedom from fear.

Questions for Chapter 4

1. Which intravenous anaesthetic used routinely in cats causes a fatal anaphylactic reaction in dogs due to histamine release?
   Halothane
   Ketamine
   Isoflurane

2. Which of the following drugs would be safe to give to a dog on long-term theophylline (Corvental-D) therapy?
   Phenobarbital
   Cimetidine (Tagamet)
   Erythromycin
   Fluoroquinolone antibiotic (e.g. Baytril)
   Beta blockers (e.g. propranolol)

3. Which of the following listed antibiotics is not suitable to give concurrently with amoxicillin/clavulanate (Synulox)? Oxytetracycline or enrofloxacin (Baytril)

4. Which of the following groups of drugs' effects are enhanced by the use of the antihistamine chlorphenamine (Piriton)? Antibiotics, sedatives or steroids

5. Which antibiotic can cause a potentially fatal clostridial enterotoxaemia in rabbits, guinea pigs and hamsters? Clindamycin (Antirobe), enrofloxacin (baytril), oxytetracycline

6. Which drugs antagonise the effects of insulin?

7. What is a potential side effect of diuretics such as furosemide that is made worse by the use of corticosteroids?

8. Which parasite treatment can cause irreversible paralysis in chelonians (tortoises, turtles and terrapins)? Ivermectin, fenbendazole (Panacur), praziquantel (Milbemax), piperazine (Endorid)

9. Which drugs are known to be human carcinogens?

10. Which drugs are teratogenic (cause fetal abnormalities)?

Multiple choice questions

1. What is pharmacokinetics the study of?
   a. the way drugs act on the body
   b. the way the body acts on the drug (i.e. absorption, metabolism, excretion)
   c. both of the above
   d. the level of toxicity of the drug

2. What is a contraindication?
   a. a situation in which a drug should not be used
   b. an off licence use of a drug which is known to be safe in another species
   c. use of a drug in the same species but for another condition
   d. a side effect

3. Which of the following describes a synthetic drug that can treat bacteria, fungi, viruses and protozoa?
   a. antibiotic
   b. fluconazole
   c. antimicrobial
   d. anticyclic

4. Which name is given to a drug in its chemical form (i.e. not the drug company's name)?
   a. generic
   b. proprietary
   c. brand
   d. trade

5. If a drug is capable of stopping bacterial multiplication but not killing the organism, e.g. oxytetracycline, it is called:
   a. bactericidal
   b. antidivisional
   c. bacteriostatic
   d. bacteriological

6. What term is applied when two antibiotics work together to produce more effects than when used alone?
   a. additive
   b. complementary
   c. successional
   d. potentiation

7. Which of these drugs would treat a *Toxoplasma gondii* infection?
   a. antifungal
   b. antiviral
   c. antiprotozoal
   d. all of the above

8. Which antibiotic has the broadest spectrum of activity?
   a. oxytetracycline
   b. metronidazole
   c. benzyl penicillin
   d. neomycin

9. What term is applied to a drug that binds to a receptor but does not stimulate it?
   a. agonist
   b. partial agonist
   c. antagonist
   d. mimic

10. Which of these drugs has anti-emetic properties?
    a. apomorphine
    b. liquid paraffin
    c. sulfasalazine
    d. acepromazine

11. Which of these drugs can produce deep sedation?
    a. antihypertensive
    b. tranquilliser
    c. narcotic
    d. sedative antagonist

For answers go to page 238

The Sciences

SECTION 2

CHAPTER 5

Biology

Learning aims and objectives

After studying this chapter you should be able to:

1. **Describe the structure and function of proteins, carbohydrates and lipids within the body**
2. **Describe how cells produce their energy.**

Major biological chemicals

Scale

In considering molecular structure it is important to have a sense of scale (Fig. 5.1). Nanometers (nm) are used as the measure of length at the atomic level, where 1 nm is equal to 10^{-9} meters:

- small biomolecules such as sugars and amino acids are typically less than 1 nm long
- biological macromolecules, such as proteins, are at least 10-fold larger, e.g. haemoglobin, the oxygen-carrying protein in red blood cells, has a diameter of 6.5 nm
- macromolecules, such as ribosomes (the protein synthesising machinery of the cells), have diameters of 30 nm
- most viruses range from 10 nm to 100 nm
- cells are a hundred times as large, in the range of micrometers (μm); a red blood cell measures 7 μm long.

It is important to note that the resolution of the light microscope is about 0.2μm, which corresponds to the size of many subcellular organelles. Mitochondria, the major generators of adenosine triphosphate (ATP – see below), can just be resolved with a light microscope. Most of our knowledge of biological structure has come from electron microscopy.

Protein structure and function

Proteins are made up of large numbers of amino acids (Fig. 5.2) linked into chains by peptide bonds

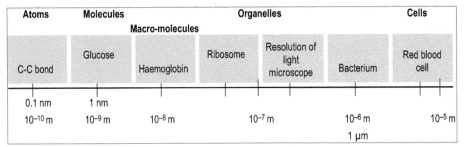

Atoms	Molecules	Organelles		Cells
	Macro-molecules			
	Glucose	Ribosome	Resolution of light microscope	Red blood cell
C-C bond	Haemoglobin		Bacterium	

0.1 nm 1 nm

10^{-10} m 10^{-9} m 10^{-8} m 10^{-7} m 10^{-6} m 10^{-5} m

1 µm

Fig. 5.1 Dimensions of some biomolecules and cells

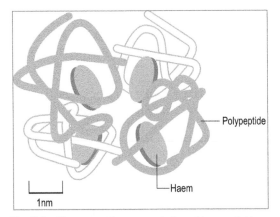

Fig. 5.2 Amino acid structure and formation of peptide bonds. The dotted lines show how the peptide bonds are formed with the production of H_2O. R is the remainder of the amino acid. For example, in glycine, R = H; in glutamate R = $-(CH_2)_2-COOH$ (bonds)

joining the amino group of one amino acid to the carboxyl group of another. In addition, some proteins contain carbohydrates (glycoproteins) and lipids (lipoproteins). Smaller chains of amino acids are called peptides or polypeptides.

The order of the amino acids in the chain is called the primary structure of the protein. The chains are twisted and folded in complex ways and the term secondary structure refers to this spatial arrangement. The tertiary structure of a protein is the arrangement of the twisted chains into layers, crystals or fibres. Many proteins are made of subunits, e.g. haemoglobin, and the term quaternary structure is used to refer to the arrangement of the subunits (Fig. 5.3).

Proteins play crucial roles in virtually all biological processes.

Enzymes

Nearly all chemical reactions in the body are catalysed by macromolecules called enzymes. They increase reaction rates by at least a million-fold and are highly specific for the reaction catalysed. Proteolytic enzymes, for example, catalyse the hydrolysis (breaking of a bond by the addition of water) of peptide bonds in proteins, examples including trypsin and thrombin (Fig. 5.4).

Some enzymes are synthesised in an inactive form, which is activated at an appropriate time and place. The digestive enzymes show this kind of control, e.g. trypsinogen is synthesised in the pancreas and is activated in the small intestine to form the active enzyme trypsin. Much of the catalytic power of enzymes comes from their ability to bring substrates together in a favourable way by creating enzyme–substrate complexes. The substrates are bound to a specific region of the enzyme called the active site (Fig. 5.5).

Enzymes can be inhibited by specific molecules resulting in a major control mechanism in biological systems. Also, many drugs and toxic agents act by inhibiting enzymes. For example, the action of nerve gas on acetylcholinesterase, an enzyme that plays an important role in the transmission of nerve impulses, demonstrates irreversible inhibition – as does penicillin. Penicillin was discovered by Alexander Fleming in 1928, when he observed by chance that bacterial growth was inhibited by a contaminating

Fig. 5.3 Diagrammatic representation of haemoglobin molecule showing the arrangement of the four subunits (quaternary structure)

Polypeptide

Haem

1nm

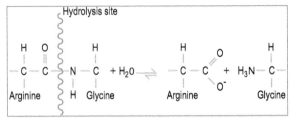

Hydrolysis site

Arginine   Glycine   Arginine   Glycine

Fig. 5.4 Thrombin catalyses the hydrolysis of this protein by breaking the bond as shown

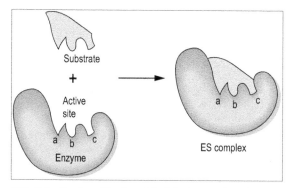

Fig. 5.5 'Lock and key' model of the interaction of substrates and enzymes. The active site of the enzyme is complementary in shape to that of the substrate

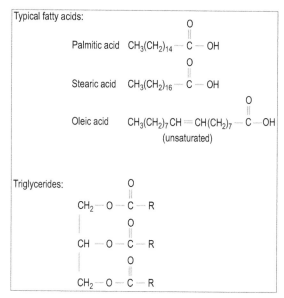

Fig. 5.6 Structure of a triglyceride where 'R' represents a fatty acid. Some typical fatty acids are shown

mould (*Penicillium*). Penicillin blocks the last step in bacterial cell wall synthesis by inhibiting the transpeptidase enzyme that catalyses the cross-linking between the protein strands. The enzyme catalysing the first step in a biological pathway is usually inhibited by the final product.

Transport and storage

Many small molecules and ions are transported by specific proteins. For example, haemoglobin transports oxygen in erythrocytes, whereas myoglobin, a related protein, transports oxygen in muscle. Iron is carried in the plasma of blood by transferrin and is stored in the liver as a complex with ferritin, a different protein.

Coordinated motion

Proteins are the major components of muscle. Muscle contraction is accomplished by the sliding motion of two kinds of protein filaments. Also, the movement of chromosomes in mitosis and the propulsion of sperm by their flagella are produced by contractile assemblies of proteins.

Mechanical support

The high tensile strength of skin and bone is due to the presence of collagen, a fibrous protein.

Immune protection

Antibodies are highly specific proteins that recognise non-self antigens (bacteria, viruses and cells from other organisms).

Generation and transmission of nerve impulses

Receptor proteins receive and interpret stimuli to produce a nerve cell response. For example, rhodopsin is the photoreceptor protein in retinal cells.

Control of growth and differentiation

The activities of different cells are coordinated by hormones. Many of them, such as insulin and thyroid stimulating hormone, are proteins.

Lipid structure and function

The biologically important lipids are the fatty acids and their derivatives, the neutral fats (triglycerides), the phospholipids and related compounds, and the sterols. The triglycerides are made up of three fatty acids bound to glycerol (Fig. 5.6). Naturally occurring fatty acids contain an even number of carbon atoms; they may be saturated (no double bonds) or unsaturated. The phospholipids are constituents of cell membranes and the sterols include various steroid hormones, bile acids, cholesterol and various vitamins. Fatty acids have three major roles:

Building blocks of phospholipids and glycolipids

These are important components of biological membranes.

Hormones and intracellular messengers

The phosphoinositide cascade converts extracellular signals, like the binding of a hormone to a cell surface receptor, into intracellular ones and evokes a wide variety of responses in many kinds of cells (Box 5.1). The eicosanoids include prostaglandins, thromboxanes and leukotrienes. Leukotrienes are

Effects mediated by the phosphoinositide cascade

- glycogenolysis in liver cells
- histamine secretion by mast cells
- serotonin release by mast cells
- aggregation of blood platelets
- insulin secretion by pancreatic islet cells
- epinephrine secretion by adrenal chromaffin cells
- smooth muscle contraction
- visual transduction in invertebrate photoreceptors

mediators of allergic responses and inflammation and their release is provoked when specific allergens combine with IgE antibodies on the surface of mast cells. Thromboxane is synthesised by platelets and promotes vasoconstriction and platelet aggregation.

Fuel molecules

Fatty acids are stored as triglycerides and are highly concentrated stores of metabolic energy because they are reduced and anhydrous. The yield from the complete oxidation of fatty acids is about 9 kcal/g, in contrast with about 4 kcal/g for carbohydrates and proteins. A gram of anhydrous fat stores more than six times as much energy as a gram of hydrated glycogen, which is the reason that triglycerides rather than glycogen were selected in evolution as the major energy reservoir. In mammals, the major site of accumulation of triglycerides is the cytoplasm of adipose cells (fat cells).

Structure and function of carbohydrates

Carbohydrates (CHO) are one of the four major classes of biomolecules, the other three being proteins, nucleic acids and lipids. CHO are aldehyde or ketone compounds with multiple hydroxyl groups. They make up most of the organic matter on earth because of their multiple roles:

- *Energy stores, fuels and metabolic intermediates.* Starch in plants and glycogen in animals are polysaccharides that can be rapidly mobilised to yield glucose, a prime fuel for the generation of energy. ATP, the universal currency of free energy, is a phosphorylated sugar derivative, as are many coenzymes.
- Ribose and deoxyribose form part of the *structural framework of DNA and RNA.* The

conformational flexibility of these sugar rings is important in the storage and expression of genetic material.

- Polysaccharides are *structural elements in the cell walls of bacteria and plants and in the exoskeleton of arthropods.* In fact, cellulose, the main constituent of plant cell walls, is the most abundant organic compound in the biosphere.
- CHO are *linked to many proteins and lipids.* For example, the sugar units of glycophorin give red blood cells a highly polar coat and CHO units on cell surfaces are key participants in cell–cell recognition during development.

Monosaccharides are the simplest carbohydrates. These are aldehydes or ketones that have two or more hydroxyl groups; their empirical formula is $(CH_2O)_n$. The smallest ones, for which $n = 3$, are glyceraldehyde and dihydroxyacetone; they are trioses. Glyceraldehyde is also an aldose because it contains an aldehyde group, whereas dihydroxyacetone is a ketose because it contains a keto group (Fig. 5.7). There are two stereoisomers of the glyceraldehyde molecule because it has a single asymmetric carbon – the prefixes L and D designate the absolute configuration.

Disaccharides consist of two sugars joined by a glycosidic bond. Common examples are sucrose, lactose and maltose (Fig. 5.8). Sugars with 4, 5, 6 and 7 carbon atoms are called tetroses, pentoses, hexoses and heptoses. Two common hexoses are glucose and fructose. The predominant forms of these sugars are not open chains, rather, they form into rings.

Animal cells store glucose in the form of glycogen, a very large branching polymer of glucose residues. These branches serve to increase the solubility of glycogen and make its sugar units more readily mobilised. Dextran, a storage polysaccharide in

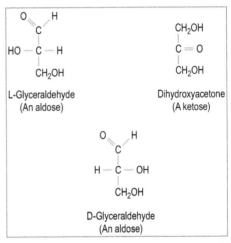

Fig. 5.7 Structure of two monosaccharides. The L & D isomer are glyceraldehyde are shown

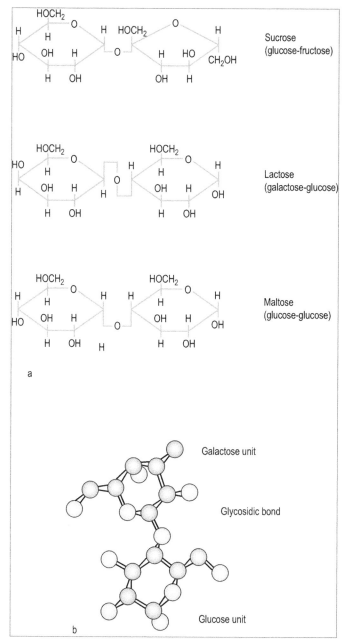

a

b

Fig. 5.8 (a) Formulae of three disaccharides. (b) A three-dimensional model of disaccharide lactose

yeasts and bacteria, also consists only of glucose residues but differs in its linkages.

Structure and function of nucleic acids

DNA is a very long thread-like macromolecule made up of a large number of deoxyribonucleotides, each composed of a base, a sugar and a phosphate group. The bases of DNA carry genetic information, whereas the sugar and phosphate groups perform a structural role (Fig. 5.9). The sugar is a deoxyribose and the base is a derivative of purine or pyrimidine. The purines are adenine (A) and guanine (G) and the pyrimidines are thymine (T) and cytosine (C) (Fig. 5.10).

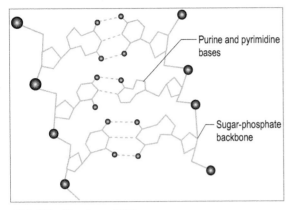

Fig. 5.9 Structure of DNA

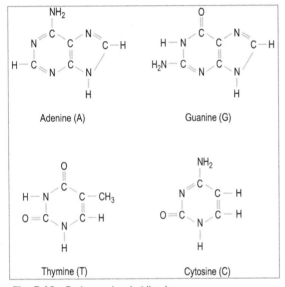

Fig. 5.10 Purine and pyrimidine bases

In 1953, James Watson and Francis Crick deduced the three-dimensional structure of DNA. The important features are that:

1. Two helical chains are coiled around a common axis. The chains run in opposite directions.
2. The purine and pyrimidine bases are on the inside of the helix whereas the phosphate and deoxyribose units are on the outside.
3. Adenine is always paired with thymine. Guanine is always paired with cytosine.
4. The sequence of bases carries the genetic information. DNA molecules must be very long to encode the large number of proteins present in even the simplest cells.

Genes in all prokaryotic and eukaryotic organisms are made of DNA. In viruses, genes are made of either DNA or RNA (ribonucleic acid). The sugar units in RNA are riboses and the other difference is that the base T is replaced with uracil (U). A number of RNA viruses produce malignant tumours after being injected into susceptible animal hosts; these are also called retroviruses.

Metabolism

How do cells extract energy from their environments and how do they synthesise the building blocks of their macromolecules? These processes are carried out by a highly integrated network of chemical reactions which are collectively known as metabolism. Living things require a continual input of free energy for three major purposes:

- the performance of mechanical work in muscular contractions and other cellular movements
- the active transport of molecules and ions
- the synthesis of macromolecules from simple precursors.

The free energy is obtained by the oxidation of foodstuffs and the carrier is adenosine triphosphate (ATP). It is the breaking of the bonds between the phosphates that releases the energy. The basic strategy of metabolism is to form ATP for consumption in energy-requiring processes:

- anabolism – biosynthetic processes
- catabolism – degradative processes

(derived from the Greek words *ana,* up; *cata,* down).

Aerobic/anaerobic glycolysis

Muscle contraction requires energy and muscle has been called 'a machine for converting chemical energy into mechanical work'. The immediate source of this energy is the energy-rich organic phosphate derived from muscle, the ultimate source is the intermediary metabolism of CHO and lipids. At rest and during light exercise, muscles utilise lipids in the form of free fatty acids as their energy source. As the intensity of exercise increases, the utilisation of CHO becomes the predominant component in the muscle fuel mixture. Thus during exercise, much of the energy for building up the muscle's energy stores comes from the breakdown of glucose to CO_2 and H_2O. This aerobic glycolysis can only occur in the presence of oxygen. If oxygen is absent anaerobic glycolysis takes over, resulting in the production of smaller quantities of energy-rich phosphate bonds and the production of lactate.

Structure and function of water

Water profoundly influences all molecular interactions in biological systems. Two properties are especially important in this regard:

- *Water is a polar molecule*. The shape of the molecule is triangular, so there is an asymmetrical distribution of charge.
- *Water molecules have a high affinity for each other*. A positively charged region in one water molecule tends to orient itself towards a negatively charged region in one of its neighbours. Ice has a highly regular crystalline structure in which all potential hydrogen bonds are made. Liquid water has a partly ordered structure in which hydrogen-bonded clusters of molecules are continually forming and breaking up.

The polarity and hydrogen-bonding capacity of water make it a highly interactive molecule. It is an excellent solvent for polar molecules. The existence of life on earth depends critically on the capacity of water to dissolve a remarkable array of polar molecules that serve as fuels, building blocks, catalysts and information carriers. High concentrations of these molecules can coexist in water, where they are free to diffuse and find each other. However, the excellence of water as a solvent poses a problem, for it also weakens interactions between polar molecules. Biological systems have solved this problem by creating water-free microenvironments where polar interactions have maximal strength. There are many examples of the critical importance of these specially constructed niches in protein molecules.

Water also functions as a lubricant and a temperature buffer.

Structure and function of cells

Arising from a single fertilised egg, each cell develops structural attributes to suit its function through the process of differentiation. Cells can be classified into groups based on their main function (Table 5.1).

- A *tissue* is an assembly of cells that are arranged in a regular formation. Some are simple tissues such as cartilage and some are termed compound tissues as they contain a mixture of cells, e.g. nervous tissue contains neurons and glial cells.
- An *organ* is an anatomically distinct group of tissues, usually of several types, which perform specific functions, e.g. heart, liver and kidney.
- The term *system* has two uses:
  - it describes cells with similar function but widely distributed in several anatomical sites, e.g. the specialised hormone-producing cells scattered throughout the gut and the lungs (diffuse endocrine system)
  - a group of organs which have similar or related roles, e.g. the tongue, oesophagus, stomach and intestines are all part of the alimentary system.

The relationships between cells, tissues and organs are shown in Figure 5.11. Cells have many common features (Fig. 5.12):

- an outer membrane
- they are composed of a solution of proteins, electrolytes and CHO (cytosol), divided into

Table 5.1 Modern functional cell classification

Cell group	Example	Function	Special features
Epithelial cells	Gut lining	Barrier, absorb, secrete	Tightly bound together by cell junctions
Support cells	Cartilage, bone	Maintain body structure	Produce and interact with extracellular matrix material
Contractile cells	Muscle	Movement	Filamentous proteins contract
Nerve cells	Brain	Cell communication	Release message onto surface of other cells
Germ cells	Sperm, ova	Reproduction	Half normal chromosome content
Blood cells	RBCs and WBCs	O_2 transport, defence	Proteins bind oxygen and destroy bacteria
Immune cells	Lymphoid tissues	Defence	Recognise and destroy foreign material
Hormone-secreting cells	Thyroid and adrenal	Cell communication	Secrete chemical messages

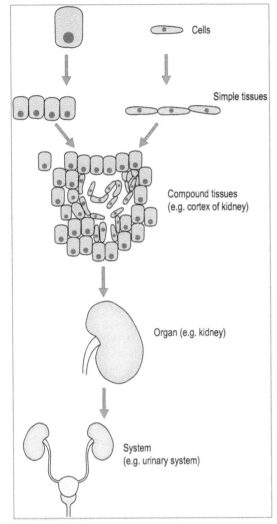

Fig. 5.11 Cells, tissues, organs and systems

specialised functional areas (organelles) by inner membrane systems
- their shape and fluidity are determined by the arrangement of internal filamentous proteins (intermediate filaments, actin and microtubules) which form the cytoskeleton.

Cell membranes

The outer membrane surrounding each cell and the membranes surrounding internal cellular organelles have a common basic structure of a lipid bilayer containing specialised proteins in association with surface CHO (Fig. 5.13):
- the membrane is a fluid, allowing lateral movement of membrane proteins and facilitating cell mobility

- the lipid composition leads to differential permeability to different substances, being highly permeable to water, oxygen and small hydrophobic molecules but impermeable to charged ions such as Na^+ and K^+
- membrane proteins are placed to perform functional roles in processes such as transport, enzymic activity, cell attachment and cell communication.

Transport in cells

- Protein diffusion through the membrane is slow.
- Areas of the cell have tight junctions that restrict protein diffusion to only certain areas of the cell membrane. Tight junctions are prominent in the epithelia lining the gut (Fig. 5.14).
- Gap junctions are integral membrane proteins that link cytoplasm of one cell to that of its neighbour, providing a water-filled pore that crosses both bilayer membranes (Fig. 5.14). These gap junctions allow metabolic support of neighbouring cells, electrical synchronisation and sharing of hormone messengers.
- Endocytosis and exocytosis: material from the extracellular space may be incorporated into the cell by invagination of the cell surface, termed endocytosis. The invaginated membrane fuses to form an endocytotic vesicle or endosome (Fig. 5.15). The term pinocytosis is used when cells take up fluids and form endosomes about 150 nm in diameter, while the term phagocytosis is used when cells ingest large particles. Exocytosis is the reverse and describes the fusion of a membrane-bound vesicle with the cell surface to release its contents into the extracellular space.
- Receptor-mediated endocytosis (Fig. 5.16): a coated pit has surface receptors that bind specific extracellular particles. Once internalised, the coat protein is shed and returns to the surface to form new coated pits. This form of transport is a feature of internalisation of iron, low-density lipoprotein and some growth factors.

Extracellular matrix

This is composed of two major materials – glycos-aminoglycans (GAGs) and fibrillar proteins:
- GAGs are large polysaccharides divided into four groups depending on their structure: hyaluronic acid, chondroitin sulphate, heparin and keratan sulphate
- the four proteins that form the extracellular matrix are collagen, fibrillin, elastin and fibronectin.

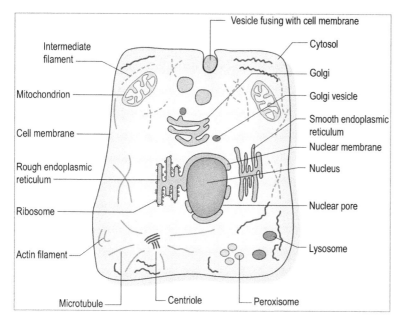

Fig. 5.12 Cell structure

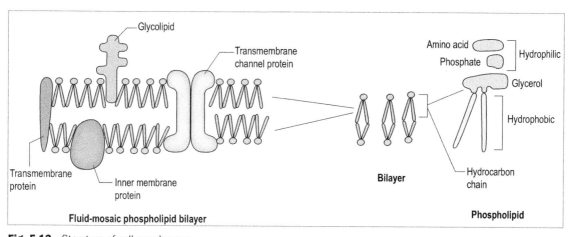

Fig. 5.13 Structure of cell membranes

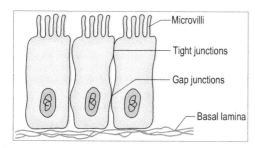

Fig. 5.14 Tight and gap junctions

Cell organelles

Ribosomes

These are complexes of protein and RNA molecules. They can be found lying free in the cytoplasm or attached to the endoplasmic reticulum. Their function is to synchronise the alignment of both messenger RNA and transport RNA during protein synthesis.

Nucleus

- This is the largest organelle and its function is to store the DNA.

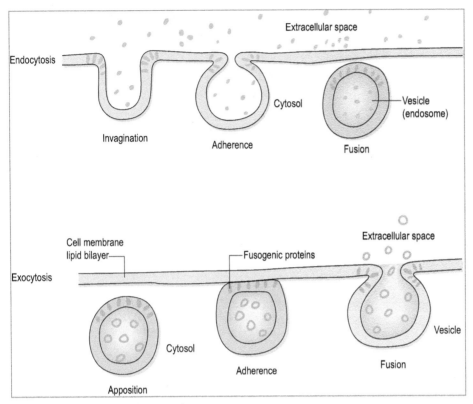

Fig. 5.15   Endocytosis and exocytosis

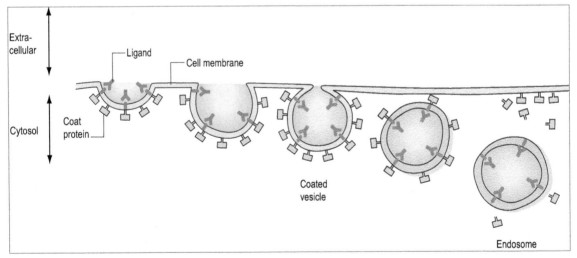

Fig. 5.16   Receptor-mediated endocytosis

- The nucleolus is a dark-staining region of the nucleus which synthesises ribosomal subunits.
- Nuclei have two membranes: an inner membrane to attach to filamentous proteins to give the nucleus its spherical shape and an outer membrane which creates a space that is continuous with the endoplasmic reticulum. The membrane contains pores that allow the diffusion of small molecules between the cytosol and the nucleus.
- DNA is wound around proteins called histones which form strings to make the structure of

chromatin. Further condensation is possible during cell replication to form distinct chromosomes.

Mitochondria

- These organelles are the site of energy production through oxidative phosphorylation (the use of oxygen to regenerate ATP).
- They have an outer and inner membrane which is folded into pleats or cristae, to increase the surface area (Fig. 5.17).
- The matrix is 50% protein gel containing enzymes to oxidise fatty acids and mitochondrial DNA.

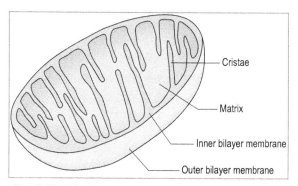

Fig. 5.17 Mitochondria

Endoplasmic reticulum (ER) and Golgi bodies

- This membrane-bound compartment is involved in the biosynthesis and transport of cellular proteins and lipids. The amount present depends on how active the cell is in secreting protein and lipids.
- Rough ER consists of flattened parallel sacs (cisternae) which form an interconnected branching network with ribosomes attached to the cytoplasmic side of the membrane.
- Protein synthesis begins in the cytosol where messenger RNA attaches to free ribosomes and translation produces the new peptide. Newly made proteins then enter the smooth ER for transport to the Golgi bodies.
- Smooth ER processes proteins and synthesises lipids.
- From the smooth ER, further processing of macromolecules takes place in the Golgi bodies (Fig. 5.18). To reach it, vesicles bud from the smooth ER and travel in the cytosol to fuse with its inner face. Here, sugars are added to form oligosaccharides and molecules are sorted into those destined for secretion or for use within the cell.

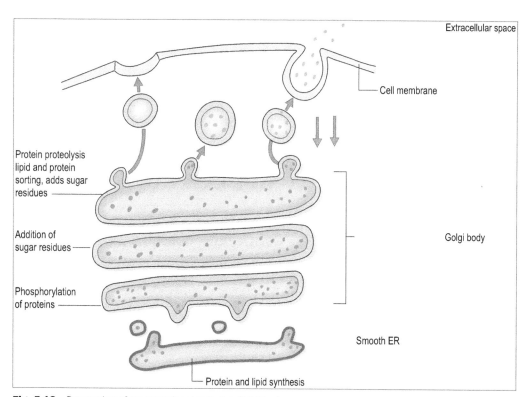

Fig. 5.18 Processing of macromolecules in the Golgi body

Cytoskeleton

Microfilaments, intermediate filaments and microtubules form a dynamic three-dimensional scaffolding in the cell. The cell spindle, along which chromosomes are organised in cell division, is constructed from microtubules and they form the basis for cilia.

Epithelial cells

These cover and line internal and external surfaces of the body such as body cavities, airways, gastrointestinal tract, blood vessels and skin. There are three main cell groups according to cell shape: squamous (flat), cuboidal (similar height and width), columnar (height greater than width). They can be then classified as simple (single layer of cells) and stratified (multiple layers of cells) (Fig. 5.19).

The urinary system contains a specialised type of stratified epithelia called transitional epithelium. Protection from hypertonic urine is provided by modified surface membranes and the balloon shape of the cells allows for great lateral stretching of the epithelium when the bladder fills.

Glands are cells whose main, if not only, function is the synthesis and secretion of material that has an extracellular function. They are classified according to the direction of secretion: exocrine secretion is towards the free epithelial surface and endocrine secretion is the secretion into blood vessels. Exocrine

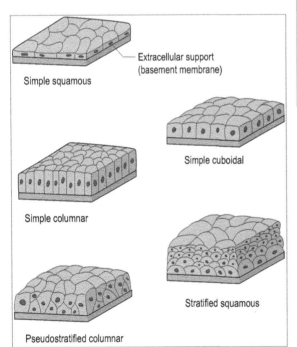

Fig. 5.19   Types of epithelial tissue

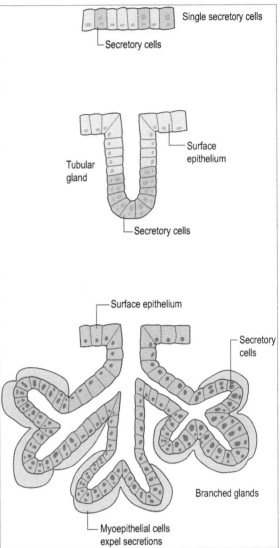

Fig. 5.20   Exocrine glands

glands can be simple alveolar, tubular or compound (Fig. 5.20).

Contractile cells

There are four types:
- muscle cells – striated or voluntary, cardiac and smooth or involuntary
- myoepithelial – form secretory glands
- myofibroblasts – secrete collagen
- pericytes – surround blood vessels.

Smooth muscle cells have a central nucleus and taper at each end; the cells interdigitate.

Skeletal muscle cells are long, thin cylindrical structures (myofibrils). In addition to contractile proteins,

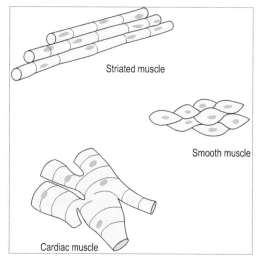

Fig. 5.21   Types of muscle tissue

the cytoplasm contains mitochondria and glycogen to provide energy.

Cardiac muscle is a type of striated muscle which is mononuclear and much shorter than skeletal muscle. Long fibres are produced by linking cells end to end. Unlike skeletal muscle, following damage, regeneration can not occur (Fig. 5.21).

Homeostasis

The actual environment of the cells of the body is the interstitial component of the extracellular fluid (ECF). Since normal cell function depends upon the consistency of this fluid, there are a number of regulatory mechanisms in place to maintain this. The buffering properties of the body fluids and the renal and respiratory adjustments to the presence of excess acid or alkali are examples of homeostatic mechanisms. Blood calcium regulation by parathormone and calcitonin and the blood glucose regulatory systems involving insulin and glucagons are other examples.

Many of these regulatory mechanisms operate on the principle of negative feedback; deviations from a given normal set point are detected by a sensor and signals from the sensor trigger compensatory changes that continue until the set point is again reached.

Structure and function of the circulatory systems

The main systems transporting oxygen, nutrients and waste materials from one part of the body to another are circulatory systems. The two main systems are:
- the blood circulatory system – transports oxygen, carbon dioxide, nutrients, metabolic breakdown products, cells of the immune system, hormones and blood clotting factors
- the lymphatic system – drains not only extracellular fluid from the tissues, returning it to the blood circulatory system after passage through lymph nodes, but also nutrients absorbed by the alimentary tract.

Cardiovascular system

There are three types of blood circulatory systems – systemic, pulmonary and portal. The first two depend on a central pump, the heart, to push the blood around (Fig. 5.22). Portal systems are specialised vascular channels that carry substances from one site to another, but do not depend on a central pump. The largest portal system (hepatic portal vein) runs between the intestines and the liver (Fig. 5.23).

The wall of the heart has three layers:
- an outer epicardium (visceral pericardium) covered with flat mesothelial cells to produce a smooth outer surface
- a middle myocardium composed of cardiac muscle, which is responsible for the pumping action of the heart
- an inner smooth lining, the endocardium, in direct contact with the circulating blood.

One homeostatic mechanism which helps to regulate blood pressure is the release of atrial natriuretic hormone. Atrial myocardial fibres contain small

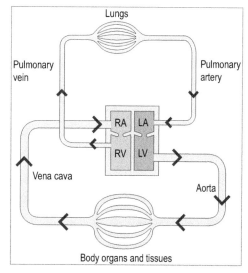

Fig. 5.22   Circulation

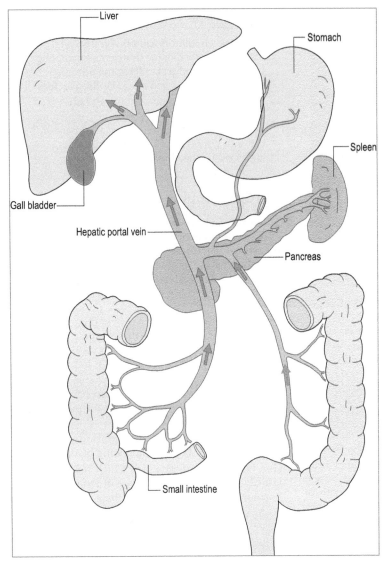

Fig. 5.23   Hepatic portal vein

neuroendocrine granules which secrete the hormone when the atrial fibres are excessively stretched. Atrial natriuretic hormones increase the excretion of water and sodium and potassium ions by the distal convoluted tubules of the kidney. They also decrease blood pressure by inhibiting rennin secretion by the kidney and aldosterone secretion by the adrenals.

The sinoatrial (SA) node of the heart is located where the anterior vena cava enters the right atrium. The impulse generated by the SA node passes quickly to the atrioventricular (AV) node, stimulating atrial contraction in the process. The AV node is located beneath the endocardium of the medial wall of the right atrium immediately above the AV valve. The bundle of His conducts the impulse to

the ventricles and then a network of specialised conduction fibres, the Purkinje fibres, carry the impulse through the ventricle walls. These are large fibres with vacuolated cytoplasm, due to a high glycogen content, and scanty myofibrils.

The left ventricle has a great oxygen demand and consequently a large arterial supply via the coronary arteries. Any interruption in the cardiac arterial supply particularly affects the structure and function of the left ventricle.

The systemic circulation is a high pressure system and the structural modifications to handle the high systolic pressure are most refined in the large elastic arteries, which receive the output from the left ventricle, i.e. the aorta and its large branches such as the carotid, subclavian and renal arteries. Distal to these, the arterial walls become more muscular. The walls of vessels have three layers:

- The intima is the thin inner layer of a blood vessel lined by endothelial cells which lie on a basement membrane.
- The media is the middle layer, which in muscular arteries is composed almost entirely of smooth muscle. These arteries are therefore highly contractile and controllable by the autonomic nervous system. A few elastic fibres are scattered throughout this layer.
- The adventitia is the outer layer and is composed of collagen. Small blood vessels are present in the thick-walled vessels called vasa vasorum to supply the media with blood.

Capillaries are the smallest vessels, being 5–10 μm in diameter. They form a complex interlinking network and are composed of endothelial cells, a basement membrane and occasional scattered contractile cells called pericytes. There are two types;

- those with continuous endothelium, which are the most common
- those with fenestrated endothelium, seen in the gastrointestinal mucosa, endocrine glands, and renal glomeruli.

Highly specialised vascular channels, called sinusoids, are seen in some organs such as the liver and spleen. They are endothelial-lined channels with a larger diameter than capillaries and absent basement membrane.

In addition to the microvasculature (i.e. arterioles emptying into a capillary network which drains into a venular system), there are additional vessels that bypass the capillary bed, so that arterioles can communicate directly with venules – these are arteriovenous anastomoses. Contraction of the smooth muscle coat in the arteriolar end closes off the lumen of the anastomosis at its origin and diverts blood into the capillary bed, whereas relaxation opens up the lumen allowing blood to flow directly into a venule, thus bypassing the capillary network. These anastomoses are widespread, but are most common in the peripheries and are thought to play an important role in the skin's thermoregulatory function.

Blood vessels have both an afferent and efferent innervation:

- Vessels that can significantly alter their lumen size by contraction and relaxation of their smooth muscle fibres have a major supply of adrenergic sympathetic fibres, stimulation of which causes muscle contraction and vasoconstriction. Some blood vessels in skeletal muscle also have a cholinergic sympathetic innervation capable of producing vasodilation.
- In certain areas blood vessels have an afferent innervation which supplies information about

the luminal pressure (baroreceptive information) and blood gas (i.e. carbon dioxide and oxygen) levels (chemoreceptive information). These are located in the carotid sinuses, and in the aortic arch, pulmonary artery and large veins entering the heart. Afferent fibres from the carotid sinus receptors travel in the glossopharyngeal nerve to the cardiorespiratory centres in the brain stem.

Lymphatic system

The intercellular spaces of almost all tissues contain small endothelial-lined tubes which are blind ending. These are lymphatic capillaries and are permeable to fluids and dissolved molecules in the interstitial fluid. In some areas the lymphatic capillaries have a fenestrated endothelium permitting entry of larger molecules such as large proteins, triglycerides and cells of the immune system.

The lymphatic capillary network acts as a drainage system, removing surplus fluid (lymph) from tissue spaces. Lymph is normally a colourless fluid but lymph draining the intestines is often milky because of its high lipid content and is called chyle. On its way to the larger vein-like lymphatics from the smaller ones, lymph passes through one or more lymph nodes, entering at the convex periphery and leaving it through one or two lymphatic vessels at the concave hilum (Fig. 5.24). During this passage, activated lymphocytes, important to immune defence, are added.

The larger lymphatic vessels have muscular walls and pump the lymph into the following main vessels:

- the thoracic duct, which empties lymph into the venous system at the junction of the left internal jugular and left subclavian vein

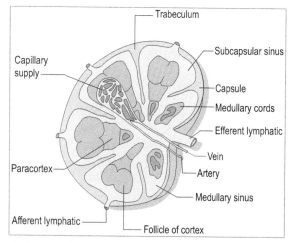

Fig. 5.24 Lymph node structure

- the right main lymphatic duct, which empties into the junction between the right internal jugular and right subclavian veins.

These two main lymphatic vessels run alongside the lumbar and thoracic vertebrae in the posterior abdominal and posterior thoracic wall, receiving lymph from lymphatics as they progress towards the jugular veins. All lymphatic capillaries from a particular area drain their lymph into lymph nodes serving that area (regional lymph nodes). Such drainage is particularly important to the spread of cancer, since cells can enter the lymph and be carried to other sites or be trapped in the lymph node.

Structure and function of the respiratory system

The main function of the respiratory system is to permit oxygenation of the blood and removal from it of carbon dioxide. In addition, it is also involved in the perception of smell and flavour and phonation. On its way to the lungs, where gaseous exchange takes place, the air is cleaned and moistened, and its temperature is approximately equated to that in the furthest reaches of the lung.

Air enters through the nares, the external aspect of which is covered by keratinising squamous epithelium. Most of the epithelium then changes to a pseudostratified columnar pattern, many of the cells being ciliated. Scattered throughout are glandular cells:

- mucus-secreting cells (goblet cells)
- serous cells which probably secrete small amounts of amylase
- serous cells which produce lysozyme.

The lamina propria also contains immune cells:
- lymphocytes
- plasma cells
- macrophages
- neutrophils
- eosinophils – numerous in animals with parasitic or allergic conditions.

Nasopharynx

This is a posterior continuation of the nasal cavities and becomes the oropharynx at the level of the soft palate. The Eustachian tubes from the middle ear open into its lateral walls. It is lined by columnar epithelium and stratified squamous epithelium. Beneath the epithelium is abundant mucosa-associated lymphoid tissue (MALT) which samples inhaled antigenic material and prepares defence mechanisms against them.

Larynx

Laryngeal architecture is maintained by a series of cartilaginous plates, the thyroid, cricoid, and arytenoid cartilages (Fig. 5.25). These are joined together by densely collagenous ligaments and are able to move by the action of small bands and sheets of striated muscle called the intrinsic muscles of the larynx. These cartilages maintain openness and shape of the airway and move to prevent food inhalation during swallowing, assisted by the epiglottis.

Trachea and bronchi

These consist of a series of incomplete circular rings of cartilage with a narrow strip of fibrocartilaginous

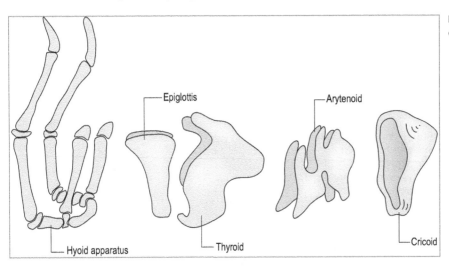

Fig. 5.25 Bones and cartilages of the larynx

Epiglottis

Arytenoid

Hyoid apparatus

Thyroid

Cricoid

ligament bridging the gap on the dorsal surface. The mucosa consists of pseudostratified ciliated columnar epithelia with scattered goblet cells. The bronchi which continue from the trachea have variable amounts of smooth muscle in their walls – hypertrophy of the smooth muscle is an important component of some lung diseases.

Lymphocytes and IgA-secreting plasma cells are closely associated with the bronchial glands and lymphoid aggregations are common, being most evident at the bifurcations.

The walls are innervated by the autonomic nervous system. There are abundant muscarinic receptors and cholinergic discharge causes bronchoconstriction. There is in addition a non-cholinergic, non-adrenergic innervation of the bronchioles that produces bronchodilation, with vasoactive intestinal peptide (VIP) being the mediator for the dilation. The leukotrienes are potent bronchoconstrictors.

Bronchioles

These distal airways are lined by ciliated columnar epithelium without pseudostratification. Occasional goblet and Clara cells can be found. The Clara cell is neither ciliated nor mucus producing – it contains numerous mitochondria and abundant smooth endoplasmic reticulum near the luminal surface. The function of these cells is not known but being rich in oxidative enzymes and lipoproteins, a role in surfactant production is suggested.

Alveoli

There are hundreds of millions of alveoli in a normal lung, providing an enormous surface area for gaseous exchange. Each alveolus is a polygonal air space with a thin wall containing pulmonary capillaries and forming an air–blood barrier. Macrophages lie on top of the lining cells phagocytosing inhaled dust (including carbon) and are therefore an important defence mechanism. There are also mast cells present that contain heparin, lipids, histamine and polypeptides that participate in allergic reactions.

Other functions of the respiratory tract

Pulmonary embolisation

One of the normal functions of the lungs is to filter out small blood clots and this occurs without any symptoms. When emboli block larger branches of the pulmonary arteries they provoke a rise in pulmonary arterial pressure and tachypnoea due to

activation of vagally innervated pulmonary receptors activated by serotonin release from the platelets at the site of embolisation.

Lung defence mechanisms

Bronchial secretions contain secretory immunoglobulins (IgA) and other substances that help resist infection. The pulmonary alveolar macrophages (PAM) help process inhaled antigens for immunologic attack and they secrete substances that stimulate granulocyte and monocyte formation in the bone marrow. The ciliary escalator moves debris away from the lungs at a rate of 16 mm/min. When motility is defective mucus transport is virtually absent, leading to sinusitis, recurrent lung infections and bronchiectasis.

Metabolic and endocrine functions

* Surfactant manufacture by the fibrinolytic system causes lysis of clots in the pulmonary vessels.
* Angiotensin I is converted to angiotensin II by the angiotensin converting enzyme in the pulmonary endothelium.
* Serotonin and norepinephrine are removed by the pulmonary circulation.

Genetics

Genetics is the science of heredity – the transmission of characteristics from one generation to the next. These characteristics could be eye colour, fur length or what sort of protein a cell produces. The basic unit of inheritance for any characteristic is the gene. They are lengths of DNA that contain a specific code for any particular protein and each gene is located at a particular position on the chromosome.

The DNA does not exist alone in a chromosome. It is tightly bound to a group of small basic proteins called histones which make up half the mass of a chromosome – this combination is called chromatin. Chromatin is made up of repeating units (each consisting of 200 base pairs of DNA) known as nucleosomes. Most of the DNA is wound around histones, the remainder joins adjacent nucleosomes and contributes to the flexibility of the chromosome fibre. Thus a chromatin fibre is a flexibly jointed chain of nucleosomes, rather like beads on a string. A seven-fold reduction in the length of DNA is achieved by organisation into nucleosomes, which are the first stage in the condensation of DNA (Fig. 5.26).

Our understanding of the architecture of chromosomes is at an early stage. Only a small proportion,

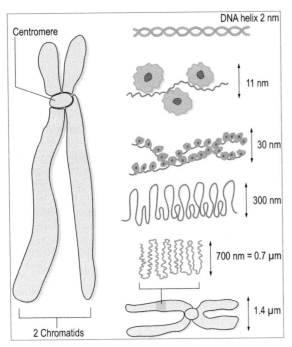

Fig. 5.26 Chromosomes and coiling of DNA

perhaps 2%, of the genome codes for proteins, the function of the remaining DNA remains an enigma.

Cell division

Nuclear divisions are of two types depending on the number of chromosomes in the daughter cell. Mitosis results in identical daughter cells with the same number of chromosomes as the parent cell. Mitosis takes place when growth occurs, e.g. red blood cell production. Meiosis results in four daughter cells, each containing half the number of chromosomes the parent cell had. For this reason it is also called reductive division. This process occurs in the production of gametes.

The cell cycle starts and ends with cell division and consists of the processes of mitosis and interphase. Interphase is when the cell carries out its normal functions and the genes are being read to produce active proteins. Energy stores are replenished and the DNA replicates.

Stages of mitosis (Fig. 5.27)

- Prophase – the chromosomes have replicated and the two chromatids are identical. The normal cell activity stops and the nuclear membrane breaks down. The centrioles move to opposite sides of the nucleus, where they form the spindle.

- Metaphase – the chromatid pairs attach themselves to individual spindle fibres and align themselves on the centre of the spindle. The chromosomes become attached at the centromeres and the chromosomes separate slightly from each other. The chromosomes arrange themselves on the spindle completely independently, with no influence on each other.
- Anaphase – the chromatids are pulled apart by the spindle fibres. The energy for this comes from the mitochondria which gather around the spindle. The newly separated chromatids are now called chromosomes.
- Telophase – the chromosomes reach the poles and become indistinct again. New nuclear membranes form and the cell divides into two. The daughter cells are now in interphase and ready for the next division.

Stages of meiosis (Fig. 5.28)

- Interphase – DNA replicates so there are four copies of each chromosome
- Prophase I – homologous pairs come together; crossing over occurs to give genetic make-up
- Metaphase I – the homologous pairs arrange themselves on the centre of the spindle
- Anaphase I – the chromatids are pulled apart and move to opposite poles of the cell
- Telophase I – the division of cytoplasm begins
- Interphase
- Prophase II – a new spindle forms
- Metaphase II – the chromosomes line up on the spindle
- Anaphase II – chromatids are pulled apart to opposite poles of the cell
- Telophase II – cytoplasm begins to divide; there are now four cells each with only a single chromosome, i.e. haploid.

Principles of Mendelian inheritance

Gregor Mendel was an Austrian monk alive in the nineteenth century. His study of the variation in the position of flowers on the plants in the monastery garden led him to the conclusion that the matings were not random, but could be predicted. By proving this he created his first law which states – the characteristics of an animal are determined by genes which occur in pairs and that only one of a pair of genes can be represented in a single gamete (i.e. ova or sperm). This law in its simplest form states that alleles separate to different gametes.

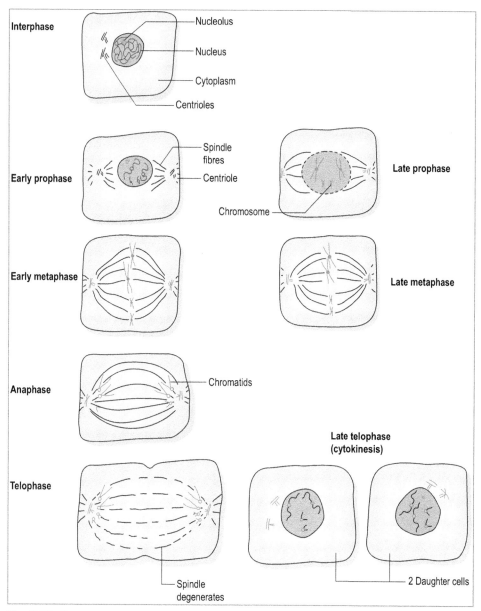

Fig. 5.27 The stages of mitosis

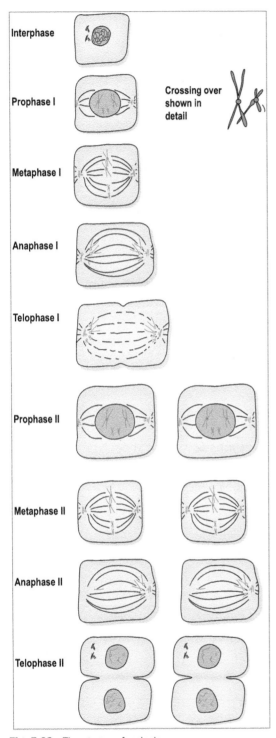

Interphase

Prophase I

Crossing over
shown in
detail

Metaphase I

Anaphase I

Telophase I

Prophase II

Metaphase II

Anaphase II

Telophase II

Fig. 5.28 The stages of meiosis

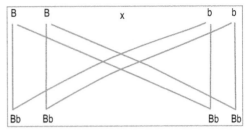

Fig. 5.29 Homozygous dominant crossed with homozygous recessive

Mendel's second law is the law of independent assortment. This states that members of different pairs of alleles assort independently during gamete formation.

The experiment Mendel carried out to investigate this inheritance involved using only a single pair of characteristics. Figure 5.29 shows an example of a cross of a homozygous dominant with a homozygous recessive. Note that the results of this cross would all be heterozygous, expressing the dominant phenotype.

Questions for Chapter 5

Short answers

1. What is a protease and what does it catalyse?

2. Which two of the following would hydrolyse the peptide bond on the carboxyl side of either an aromatic or an arginine residue? Lipase, trypsin, amylase, chymotrypsin, tropomyosin, lysozyme, galactosidase.

3. Explain the differences between plasma, interstitial fluid and intracellular fluid.

4. Why do red blood cells swell and burst when they are placed in a solution of 0.3% sodium chloride?

5. What are the functions of the proteins found in cell membranes?

6. What is receptor-mediated endocytosis?

Multiple choice questions

Select the single best answer:

1. Cell membranes
   a. consist almost entirely of protein molecules
   b. are impermeable to fat-soluble substances
   c. in some tissues permit the transport of glucose at a greater rate in the presence of insulin
   d. are freely permeable to electrolytes but not to proteins
   e. have a stable composition throughout the life of the cell

2. The primary force moving water molecules from the blood plasma to the interstitial fluid is
   a. active transport
   b. co-transport with H^+
   c. facilitated diffusion
   d. co-transport with Na^+
   e. filtration

3. Proteins that are secreted by cells are generally
   a. not synthesised on membrane-bound ribosomes
   b. found in vesicles and secretory granules
   c. moved across the cell membrane by endocytosis
   d. secreted in a form that is larger than the form present in the endoplasmic reticulum

4. Osmosis is
   a. movement of solvent across a semipermeable membrane from an area where the hydrostatic pressure is high to an area where the hydrostatic pressure is low
   b. movement of solute across a semipermeable membrane from an area in which it is in low concentration to an area in which it is in high concentration
   c. movement of solute across a semipermeable membrane from an area in which it is in a high concentration to an area in which it is in a low concentration
   d. movement of solvent across a semipermeable membrane from an area in which it is in a low concentration to an area in which it is in high concentration
   e. movement of solvent across a semipermeable membrane from an area in which it is in a high concentration to an area in which it is in a low concentration

In the following questions indicate whether the first item is greater than (G), the same as (S), or less than (L) the second item.

5. Hydrogen ion concentration in lysosomes
   G S L
   Hydrogen ion concentration in cytoplasm of cells

6. ECF volume 30 minutes after i.v. infusion of 1000 ml of isotonic (5%) glucose
   G S L
   ECF volume 30 minutes after i.v. infusion of 1000 ml of isotonic (0.9%) sodium chloride

7. Total body water 30 minutes after i.v. infusion of 1000 ml isotonic (5%) glucose
   G S L
   Total body water 30 minutes after i.v. infusion of 1000 ml isotonic (0.9%) sodium chloride

8. Calculated plasma volume when some of the dye used to measure it is unknowingly injected subcutaneously instead of i.v.
   G S L
   Calculated plasma volume when all of the dye is injected i.v.

9. Concentration of K^+ in intracellular fluid
   G S L
   Concentration of K^+ in interstitial fluid

10. Concentration of Ca^{2+} in intracellular fluid
    G S L
    Concentration of Ca^{2+} in interstitial fluid

True or false questions

1. 1 nm is equivalent to 10^{-10} meters

2. Examples of small biomolecules (less than 1 nm) are sugars and amino acids

3. Ribosomes synthesise proteins and fats

4. Amino acid chains contain peptide bonds

5. ATP is an energy source

6. Haemoglobin consists of four subunits

7. The breaking of a bond by the addition of water is called hydrazyme

8. Trypsinogen is an active enzyme in the small intestine

9. Myoglobin transports oxygen in blood

10. Ferritin and transferrin are the same protein, but found in different places – the blood and liver respectively

11. Collagen has high tensile strength

12. An antigen is a cell surface marker, usually a protein, which identifies a cell as self

13. The receptor protein in retinal cells is called rhodopsin

14. Sterols are made of three fatty acids bound to glycerol

15. Leukotrienes are fatty acids

16. Platelets are produced from thromboxane

17. Glycogen is the major energy reservoir

18. Glucose is derived from polysaccharides

19. Trioses are carbohydrates

20. Stereoisomers are different configurations of the same molecular structure

21. Hexoses have seven carbon atoms and are sugars

22. Each deoxyribonucleotide contains a base, a sugar and a phosphate group

23. Guanine is paired with adenine

24. Not all the genes in a dog are made of DNA

25. ATP stands for alpha-triose-protein

26. The basic strategy of metabolism is to produce ATP

27. Anabolism is a degradative process

28. All cells have an outer membrane and inner membranes round special functional areas

29. Actin is a filamentous protein found outside cells

30. The cell membrane is a fluid-mosaic structure consisting of proteins and lipids arranged in a bilayer

31. The epithelia lining the gut allow free protein diffusion between all the cells

32. Pinocytosis is the term used to describe the uptake of large particles by the cell

33. Iron is taken up by a cell by receptor-mediated endocytosis

34. Cytoplasm consists of GAGs and fibrillar proteins

35. GAGs are large proteins including hyaluronic acid and chondroitin sulphate

36. Fibronectin is found in the extracellular matrix

37. Histones are released by mast cells in the tissues

38. Oxidative phosphorylation is the process whereby energy is released from ATP

39. New peptides are translated in ribosomes

40. Lipids are synthesised in smooth endoplasmic reticulum

41. Endocrine secretion is towards the free epithelial surface and is how hormones are released

42. There are three types of contractile cells: muscle cells, myoepithelial cells and myofibroblasts

43. Following tissue damage skeletal muscle can regenerate

44. Homozygous is the maintenance of a steady state within a cell

45. The SA node is located where the caudal vena cava enters the right atrium

46. Purkinje fibres have no glycogen stores as they do not contract

47. Capillaries are 5–10 nm in diameter

48. Pericytes are scattered contractile cells around capillaries

49. Lymphatic capillaries are always blind ended

50. Goblet cells secrete lipid and some protein but no carbohydrate

51. Lysozyme is part of the body's non-specific immune system

52. Mucosa-associated lymphoid tissues are permanent aggregates of lymphocytes

53. The cricoid consists mainly of collagen

54. The trachea consists of incomplete C-shaped cartilages with a ventral collagenous ligament

55. Leukotrienes are potent bronchodilators

56. Clara cells are phagocytic cells found in the bronchioles

57. Bronchial secretions contain secretory immunoglobulins

58. Angiotensin I is converted to angiotensin II in the lungs

59. DNA only accounts for half the mass of a chromosome

60. Condensation of DNA involves uncoiling and spreading it out ready to be copied

61. Histones are carbohydrates that DNA is wound around

62. Alleles are alternative forms of the same gene

63. A homozygous individual carries two copies of the same gene

64. A gamete contains one of a pair of genes

65. The result of a cross between two heterozygous individuals would result in half the offspring being heterozygous

For answers go to page 239

CHAPTER 6

Chemical Sciences

Learning aims and objectives

After studying this chapter you should be able to:

1. **List the parts of an atom**
2. **Describe the make-up of the periodic table**
3. **State whether an agent is an acid or a base**
4. **Describe the common functional groups.**

Atomic structure

An atom is the smallest component part of an element. It consists of a small positive nucleus surrounded by negative electrons. For an idea of scale, think of Wembley stadium. If the centre spot on the pitch is the nucleus of an atom the electrons would orbit as far out as the back row of seats. Figure 6.1 shows the arrangement of these electrons as they orbit the nucleus. Most atoms have a radius of about 10^{-10} m or 0.1 nm and so are too small to see with light microscopes; they can, however, be seen with electron microscopy. Although they are too small to be weighed, it is possible to compare the relative atomic masses.

The sub-atomic particles

There are three sub-atomic particles:

Proton	RM = 1	RC = +1
Neutron	RM = 1	RC = 0
Electron	RM = 1/1836	RC = −1

where RM = relative mass, RC = relative charge.

The nucleus

The nucleus is at the centre of the atom and contains the protons and neutrons, which are collectively known as nucleons. Virtually all the mass of the

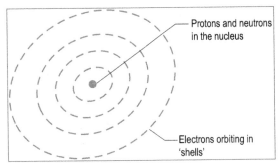

Fig. 6.1 Structure of an atom

atom is concentrated in the nucleus because the electrons weigh so little:

- number of protons = atomic number
- number of protons and neutrons = mass number (also called the nucleon number).

This information can be given in the following form:

$$_9^{19}F$$

The atomic number counts the number of protons (9), the mass number counts protons and neutrons (19) so there must be 10 neutrons. The atomic number is tied to the position of the element in the periodic table and therefore the number of protons defines what sort of element you are talking about. So if an atom has 8 protons it must be oxygen; likewise, if an atom has the atomic number 12, it must be magnesium.

Isotopes

The number of neutrons in an atom can vary within small limits. For example, there are three kinds of carbon atom: ^{12}C, ^{13}C and ^{14}C. They all have the same number of protons and are called isotopes. The fact that they have varying numbers of neutrons makes no difference to their chemical reactions.

Electrons

Atoms are electrically neutral and the positive charge of the protons is balanced by the negative charge of the electrons, so the number of electrons and number of protons are the same in a neutral atom. The electrons are found in a series of levels called energy levels or shells. The first level nearest the nucleus holds two electrons, the second and third hold eight, and the fourth (M shell) holds 18 electrons. An electron will always go into the lowest possible energy level (nearest the nucleus) provided there is space.

Electronic configurations

You can work out the electronic arrangement of an atom by looking up the atomic number in the periodic table – this tells you the number of protons and hence electrons. Arrange the electrons in levels, always filling up an inner level before going on to an outer one. To find the electronic arrangement of chlorine, for example, the periodic table gives you the atomic number of 17. Therefore there are 17 protons and 17 electrons – the arrangement of the electrons will be 2, 8, 7 (i.e. 2 in the first level, 8 in the second and 7 in the third).

Periodic table

In modern periodic tables the elements are in strict order of atomic number. The properties of the elements are related to their position in the table. Besides a division into vertical groups of similar elements, it is also useful to split the periodic table into five blocks of elements with similar properties:

- the reactive metals (elements in groups I and II)
- the transition metals
- the poor metals (metals in groups III, IV, V and VI)
- the non-metals in groups III, IV, V, VI and VII
- the noble gases.

In spite of its limitations, the classification of elements as metals, metalloids and non-metals is very useful. The commonest classification is based on electrical conductivity:

- metals are good conductors of electricity
- metalloids are poor conductors of electricity
- non-metals are non-conductors.

Other chemical properties that are shared are:

- metals, metalloids and diamond form giant structures; they have high melting points, high boiling points and high densities
- non-metals (except diamond) form simple molecular structures, have low melting points, low boiling points, low densities and are non-conductors.

The periodic table (Fig. 6.2) was arranged in 1869 by a Russian chemist called Mendeleev. At the time, although some elements had not yet been discovered, he was able to predict both their existence and properties. From left to right across the periodic table, elements change from being reactive metals through less reactive metals, metalloids, less reactive non-metals to reactive metals (on the extreme right are the noble gases). Another example of how properties change across the table is that the elements change

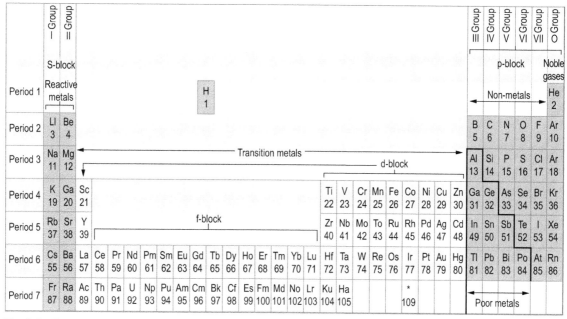

Fig. 6.2 The periodic table

from strong reducing agents (e.g. Na, Mg) through elements that are weak reducing agents, then weak oxidising agents to strong oxidising agents (e.g. Cl).

Elements in any column or group are similar. For example, the first column on the left (starting with hydrogen) contains the alkali metals; they are all soft metals that react violently with water to make hydrogen gas. The number of electrons in the outer shell is the same in each of the elements in the column and this contributes to their shared properties. In the alkali metals, there is one electron in the outer shell, meaning the energy needed to set that lone electron off into dizzying freedom is very small. That is why the alkali metals all react so violently.

Not all elements lose an electron in a chemical reaction. Sometimes the opposite happens. The second column from the right contains the halogens – they all have 7 or 17 electrons in their outer shell. The halogens are all highly reactive elements as the outer shell can take 8 or 18 electrons and so they attract any spare electrons. This means the halogens and the alkali metals form compounds together, e.g. NaCl.

The far right group are called the noble gases and they have a full outer level of electrons. As a consequence they never form compounds with other elements. In general, the arrangement of the outermost electrons, called the valence electrons, tells you about an element's chemical behaviour.

The elements in the middle of the table are called the transition metals – all of them have similar properties.

Ionic (electrovalent) bonding – the transfer of electrons

NaCl is formed because sodium has one electron in its outer shell and if it gave that away it would be a more stable structure. Chlorine has one electron short of a stable structure and so attracts the spare electron to make it more stable. However, now the sodium has lost an electron, it no longer has equal numbers of electrons and protons and therefore has a charge of plus 1. This positive ion is called a cation. The chlorine has gained an electron, has a negative charge of 1 and is called an anion. The sodium and chloride ions are held together by the strong electrostatic forces between the positive and negative charges.

Hydrogen bonding

These are particularly strong intermolecular forces that require:
- a hydrogen atom attached to a highly electronegative atom
- an unshared pair of electrons on the electronegative atom.

In the NH_3 molecule there are three N–H bonds and one non-bonded electron pair. This means there can be one H bond per molecule. In water however, there are two O–H bonds and two unshared electron pairs per molecule. This means that each H_2O

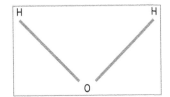

Fig. 6.3   The structure of water (H_2O)

molecule can form two hydrogen bonds (Fig. 6.3) and this helps to explain the three-dimensional lattice structure seen in ice. Water has unexpectedly high values for its melting point and boiling point and these are explained by the extra attractions between water molecules due to the formation of H bonds. It also explains the high surface tension of water, which forms a sort of 'skin' over the surface so small beetles can float on an undisturbed water surface.

Proportions by which chemicals react

Relative atomic mass

Chemists use a relative atomic mass scale to compare the masses of different atoms. Originally hydrogen was chosen as the standard against which the others could be measured as it had the smallest atoms. But when scientists discovered that one element could contain atoms of different masses (isotopes) it became necessary to choose a single isotope as the reference standard and carbon-12 was chosen. This is the isotope of carbon with a relative atomic mass of 12 and was chosen as carbon is a common element, is a solid and can be easily stored and transported.

The mole

Since the atomic mass in grams of all elements contains 6×10^{23} atoms, chemists refer to this number of atoms of an element as 1 mole. They also use the term mole to mean the relative atomic mass in grams. The mole is the amount of substance which contains the same number of particles (atoms, ions or molecules) as there are in exactly 12 grams of ^{12}C. The symbol of an element can be used to represent one mole of the element as well as one particle of the element – O represents one mole of oxygen atoms (16 g of oxygen) but O_2 represents one mole of oxygen molecules (32 g of oxygen). So it is important to specify which particles you mean

when discussing the number of moles of different substances.

To summarise, the relative atomic mass in grams of any element contains 6×10^{23} atoms and the relative molecular mass in grams of any compound contains 6×10^{23} molecules. The relative molecular mass is used to calculate molar quantities of compounds.

The mass spectrometer is used to weigh atoms and atomic masses are quoted to four decimal places. Mass spectrometers can distinguish between carbon monoxide and nitrogen, whose atomic masses are identical, on the strength of those decimal places. This has two practical uses: we can assemble the correct number of particles to react with each other to give a known compound; alternatively, we can count the number of particles reacting in an unknown reaction and deduce what has happened.

To get out of the language of grams and into the language of moles we use the following formulae:

Mass in grams = number of moles × relative atomic mass

$$\text{Number of moles} = \frac{\text{mass in grams}}{\text{relative molecular mass}}$$

therefore to work out how many moles of substance are in 60 g of silicon dioxide (SiO_2):

$$\text{moles} = \frac{60}{[28 + (2 \times 16)]} = \frac{60}{60}$$

60 g of silicon dioxide therefore contains 1 mole.

Proportions in chemical reactions

To convert word to symbol equations you need to know the chemical formulae: magnesium + oxygen = magnesium oxide is written as:

Mg + O$_2$ = MgO

However, counting the number of atoms on each side of the equation shows three atoms on the left and only two on the right, so the equation is not balanced. To correct this, the equation is written as:

2Mg + O$_2$ = 2MgO

Chemical reactions occur according to the number of particles reacting in proportion, not according to the masses of the different substances taking part.

Acids and bases

In 1661 Robert Boyle summarised the properties of acids as follows.
- acids have a sour taste
- acids are corrosive

- acids change the colour of certain vegetable dyes, such as litmus, from blue to red
- acids lose their acidity when they are combined with alkalis.

The properties of alkalis are:
- they feel slippery
- they change the colour of litmus from red to blue
- they become less alkaline when they are combined with acids.

Acids and alkalis (bases) were first identified as specific types of compounds because of their specific behaviour in aqueous solutions. An *acid* is a substance that produces H_3O^+ (H^+) when it is dissolved in water. It is a proton donor and an electron pair acceptor or a species that donates protons, e.g. HCl, NH_4, $AlCl_3$. A *base* is a substance that produces an OH^- when it is dissolved in water. It acts as a proton acceptor, or an electron donor, e.g. NaOH, KOH, CH_3NH_2.

Acids and bases relate to each other in conjugate pairs, for every acid there is a conjugate base and vice versa, and they relate to each other by the donating and accepting of a single proton. Water can act as an acid or a base because it gives protons back and forth within itself. All acid–water interactions can be written in the general form:

$$\begin{array}{ccccc} \text{HA} & + & \text{H}_2\text{O} & \Leftrightarrow & \text{H}_3\text{O}^+ & + \text{A}^- \\ \text{acid 1} & & \text{base 2} & & \text{acid 2} & \text{base 1} \end{array}$$

where HA is a general formula for an acid which gives its hydrogen ion away as a proton to water and where the A^- left behind represents the conjugate base of the acid in question.

If the equilibrium is overwhelmingly to the right, as it is when A is chlorine, then the acid is described as strong and the conjugate base is weak. If the equilibrium is to the left of the equation, as it is with the organic acid ethanoic acid, then the acid is described as weak but the conjugate base is strong. In this situation the acid will not dissociate much. Amongst the hundreds of acids in existence, there is a wide spread of strengths and these are given a quantitative form called the acid dissociation con-

tant (Ka). The weaker the acid, the smaller the Ka and the less it will dissociate. Strong acids completely dissociate into their component ions in aqueous solutions:
- strong acids: HCl, H_2SO_4, HNO_3, $HClO_4$
- weak acids: NH^{4+}, NCN, HF, HNO_2

pH scale

The pH scale ranges from 0 to 14 (Fig. 6.4). It measures the acidity or basicity of a solution. A pH of 7 means it is a neutral solution – pure water has a pH of 7. A pH of more than 7 means the solution is basic. The less pH, the more acidic the solution is. The more pH, the more basic the solution is. pH stands for the power of H, or the amount of H^+ ions acids or bases take, or contribute, in solution. pH equals the negative log of the concentration of H^+, i.e. when the concentration of H^+ ions in a solution is 10^{-14}, the pH is 14.

Acid–base reactions

Alkalis consume, or neutralise, acids. Acids lose their characteristic sour taste and ability to dissolve metals when they are mixed with alkalis. Alkalis are known as bases because they form the base for making certain salts. The characteristic properties of acids result from the presence of the hydrogen ion generated when the acid dissolves in water. It also explains why acids neutralise bases and vice versa. Acids provide the H^+ ion, bases provide the OH^- ion and these ions combine to form water:

$$H^+ + OH^- \rightarrow H_2O$$

In these reactions a hydrogen ion is transferred from an acid to a base. In the below examples, the first reactant is the acid and the second is the base:

$$H_2SO_4 + Ca(OH)_2 \rightarrow CaSO_4 + 2H_2O$$

$$HCl + NaOH \rightarrow NaCl + H_2O$$

$$H_2SO_4 + 2NH_3 \rightarrow (NH_4^+)_2SO_4^{2-}$$

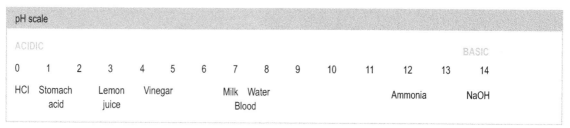

Fig. 6.4 The pH scale

Buffer solutions

Sometimes it is useful to have a system for preventing pH changes. This ensures the reagent in the system stays as we want it. Swimming pool water, for example, contains a 50:50 mixture of HOCl/ClO⁻. A reagent which opposes changes in the pH is called a buffer and it does this by either:

- taking the hydrogen ions out of circulation so that they cannot affect the pH, such as carbonate; or
- by having a reserve of hydrogen ions ready to be pulled off to neutralise the incoming OH⁻ ions.

Ethanoic acid is suitable for this. Every weak acid mixed with its conjugate base (in the form of the sodium salt) will operate as a buffer.

Experimental investigations

The fact that water dissociates to form H^+ and OH^- ions in a reversible reaction is the basis for an operational definition of acids and bases. An acid is any substance that increases the concentration of the H^+ ion when it dissolves in water. A base is any substance that increases the concentration of the OH^- ion when it dissolves in water. To decide whether a compound is an acid or a base we dissolve it in water and test the solution to see whether the H^+ or OH^- ion concentration has increased. The pH can be found by dissolving a small amount of the substance in deionised water and adding a few drops of Universal Indicator solution – the colour produced is compared with a pH chart.

Indicators

Acid–base indicators such as methyl orange, phenolphthalein and bromothymol blue are substances that change colour according to the hydrogen ion concentration of the solution to which they are added. Consequently they are used to test for acidity and alkalinity. It is not possible to say precisely when the two forms are at equal concentrations as the indicators effectively change colour over a range of about 2 pH units. Figure 6.5 shows the colour changes observed by some indicators.

Organic compounds

Hydrocarbons

Compounds that only contain carbon and hydrogen are called hydrocarbons. Carbon has four electrons in its outer shell and therefore can form four covalent bonds to other atoms. Methane (CH_4) is the main hydrocarbon in natural gas. Carbon can actually form single, double and even triple covalent bonds to other carbon atoms.

Alkanes

Hydrocarbons, in which all the carbon–carbon links are single covalent bonds, are known as alkanes (Table 6.1). The alkanes are a family of compounds

Table 6.1 Alkanes

Number of C atoms	Name	Formula	Boiling point (°C)
1	Methane	CH_4	−164
2	Ethane	C_2H_6	−89
3	Propane	C_3H_8	−42
4	Butane	C_4H_{10}	−1
5	Pentane	C_5H_{12}	+36

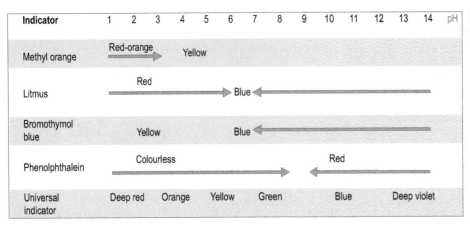

Fig. 6.5 Colour changes of some indicators

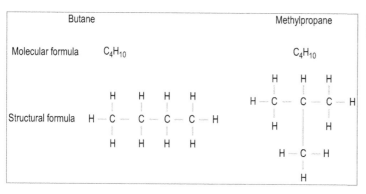

Fig. 6.6 The structures of butane and 2-methylpropane

with similar structures, similar properties and the same ending to their names -ane. There is a general formula for alkanes of:

$$C_nH_{(2n+2)}$$

where n = number of carbon atoms.

A family of compounds like this is known as a homologous series. Alkanes have the following chemical properties:

- burn very exothermically
- make good fuels
- when burnt they make CO_2 and H_2O.

Methane is a major part of natural gas; propane and butane are sold as liquefied petroleum gas (LPG). Propane is stored in tanks for those without a mains gas supply and butane is used for stoves and camping gas (e.g. Calor gas).

Alkenes

Alkenes (Table 6.2) have at least one double bond and are called unsaturated. Their formula is C_nH_{2n}. Alkenes are much more reactive than alkanes.

Table 6.2 Alkenes

Name	Molecular formula	Boiling point (°C)
Ethene	C_2H_4	−104
Propene	C_3H_6	−47
Butene	C_4H_8	−6
Pentene	C_5H_{10}	+30

Isomers

Molecules with the same molecular formula can have different structures. The same number of atoms can be connected in different ways – this is isomerism, e.g. C_4H_{10} can be butane or 2-methylpropane as shown in Figure 6.6.

Functional groups

The alcohols are a homologous series of compounds in the same way that the alkanes and alkenes are. All alcohols have an –OH group – this is known as the functional group. A functional group is a group of atoms in a structure that determines the characteristic reactions of that compound. The general formula is therefore:

$$C_nH_{2n+1}OH$$

Other examples of functional groups are shown in Figure 6.7.

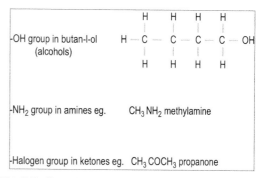

Fig. 6.7 Examples of functional groups

Questions for Chapter 6

Practical tasks

Identify the pH of the following substances and classify them as acids, bases or neutral substances.

- Soda water
- Milk of magnesia
- Salt
- Vinegar
- Lime
- Lemon juice
- Bicarbonate of soda

Apparatus and equipment required – test tubes, pH chart, beakers, spatula

Safety – wear gloves and eye protection where appropriate

Method – Place one spatula measure of solid or pour a few drops of liquid into a test tube. Half-fill the test tube with deionised water from a small beaker and shake to dissolve the solid or mix the liquid. Add a few drops of Universal Indicator to the test-tube. Make a note of the colour in a table. Compare it against the pH colour chart and record the pH of the nearest colour in the table.

Questions

1. Why might a scientist prefer to use Universal Indicator rather than a different indicator like litmus?

2. What would happen if equal amounts of vinegar and limewater were mixed?

3. Write out the symbol equations below the word equations (it is not necessary to balance the equations):

   Carbon + oxygen → carbon dioxide

   Calcium carbonate + sulphuric acid → calcium sulphate + water + carbon dioxide

   Potassium hydroxide + hydrochloric acid → potassium chloride + water

4. Balance the following equations:

   $CaCO_3 \rightarrow CaO + CO_2$

   $MgO + HCl \rightarrow MgCl_2 + H_2O$

   $SO_2 + O_2 \rightarrow SO_3$

   $Na_2CO_3 + HNO_3 \rightarrow NaNO_3 + H_2O + CO_2$

   $N_2 + H_2 \rightarrow NH_3$

5. If mass of substance = number of moles × Relative Formula Mass, what is the mass of 2 moles of carbon?

6. How many moles are there in 88 g of CO_2?

7. What is the difference between the molar mass, the relative formular mass and the mass of one mole?

8. What is a molecule?

9. Give another name for the joining together of two atoms.

10. What do atoms in covalent bonds share?

11. Why do atoms share electrons?

12. Which group of the periodic table do the atoms try to be like?

13. Write the formula for calculating moles.

14. What is an alkane?

15. What is an alkene?

16. Name three alkanes and their formulas.

17. Name three alkenes and their formulas

18. Name two chemical properties of alkanes.

19. What is a functional group?

20. Magnesium hydroxide is the active ingredient in some indigestion tablets, write an equation showing how this chemical reacts with acid in the stomach.

21. How do dock leaves relieve the sting from nettles?

22. What pH are wasp and bee stings and therefore what are suitable antidotes?

Practical pH investigation answers

- Exact colour and pH depends on concentrations
- Acids – soda water, vinegar, lemon juice
- Alkalis – milk of magnesia, lime, bicarbonate of soda
- Neutral – salt

For answers go to page 240

CHAPTER 7

Microbiology

Learning aims and objectives

After studying this chapter you should be able to:

1. **Understand the characteristics of micro-organisms by being able to explain the pathogenicity, life cycle and transmission of micro-organisms**
2. **Understand the growth of micro-organisms, be able to culture micro-organisms and perform cell counts**
3. **Understand the growth requirements of micro-organisms.**

Defences of the body

Bacteria, viruses, fungi, foreign proteins, cancer are all organisms or conditions which constantly pose a threat to the body. The body is equipped with an elaborate system of defence, known as the *immune system*, designed to protect it from these foreign invaders. There are two major components to immunity – recognition and discrimination.

Recognition

Recognition occurs when a foreign agent invades the body for the first time. The immune system recognises the agent as foreign due to its abnormal surface molecules, called antigens. Within a short time a series of reactions begin which eventually destroy the invader. Because it takes time for the immune system to launch its defence, first-time invaders usually will produce symptoms of illness, and severity will depend on the extent of exposure and invasiveness of the enemy agent. However, once the first-time invaders are destroyed, if that particular enemy agent attempts to invade at a later time, the immune response will occur much more rapidly and the body will experience few or no symptoms before the agent is destroyed. This is because of the memory response mediated by the lymphocytes.

Discrimination

The second component of the immune system is called discrimination. The immune system must be able to differentiate the normal tissues and fluids that make up the animal's body from the invading agent. To facilitate this, all cells have a unique set of molecules on their surface which allows the body's immune system to recognise them as its own cells. These molecules, known as antigens, are usually proteins but can be carbohydrates. The molecules on the surface of an invading agent will be different and will, therefore, allow the immune system to recognise the agent as foreign and initiate a defence.

Characteristics of micro-organisms and transmission

Micro-organisms can be defined as certain kinds of organisms, all of which are small and simple compared with higher forms of life. They comprise the following:
- bacteria
- unicellular algae
- fungi
- protozoa
- viruses.

Some of these, such as the protozoa, are classified as animals and some fall into the category of protista (bacteria and viruses). The more highly organised micro-organisms such as fungi have nuclei (Fig. 7.1), undergo mitotic division and have cytoplasmic organelles that are called eukaryotic cells.

Structure of bacteria

Figure 7.2 shows the range of shapes of bacteria while Box 7.1 lists the main points regarding their structure. Fungi and protozoa are eukaryotes and the main differences in their structure and function are listed in Box 7.2.

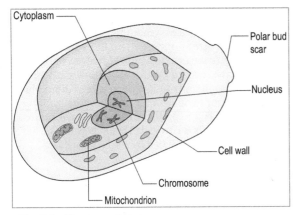

Fig. 7.1 Yeast morphology

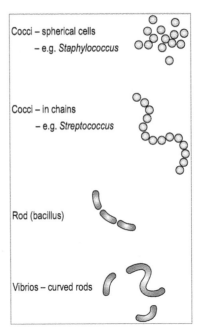

Fig. 7.2 Bacterial morphology

Box 7.1

Concepts of bacterial cell structure

- bacteria are small and simple in structure when compared to eukaryotes, yet they have characteristic shapes and sizes
- although they have an outer plasma membrane, which is required by all living cells, bacteria lack extensive internal membrane systems
- the cytoplasm of the cell contains ribosomes and the nucleoid with its genetic material
- most bacteria can be divided into Gram-positive and Gram-negative structures depending on their cell wall structure and the response to the Gram stain
- components like capsules and fimbriae are located outside the cell wall – one of these is the flagellum, which many bacteria use like a propeller
- some bacteria form resistant endospores to survive harsh environmental conditions in a dormant state

Fungi

Fungi have a true nucleus with several chromosomes. They are primitive plants but lack chlorophyll and therefore must gain nutrients by parasitism

Eukaryote cell structure and function

- have a variety of complex membranous organelles in their cytoplasm and the genetic material is within a membrane-enclosed nucleus
- a cytoskeleton composed of microtubules, microfilaments and intermediate filaments gives the cells their shape and is also involved in cell movements and intracellular transport
- genetic material is distributed by mitosis and meiosis

or by being saprophytes. They exist in a unicellular yeast form (e.g. *Candida, Cryptococcus*) or as a multi-cellular, filamentous mould colony (e.g. *Aspergillus, Microsporum*). Structural support is from a cell wall composed of polysaccharides, which is strongly antigenic and stimulates immune responses in patients very easily.

Microbial growth

Concepts

- Growth is defined as an increase in cellular constituents and may result in an increase in a micro-organism's size or number or both.
- When micro-organisms are grown in a closed system, growth remains exponential for only a short time, then enters a stationary phase due to factors such as nutrient limitation and waste accumulation.
- Water availability, pH, temperature, oxygen concentration, pressure and radiation all influence microbial growth – yet bacteria have managed to adapt and flourish under conditions that would destroy most higher organisms.
- Population growth is studied by analysing the growth curve of a microbial culture which has four distinct phases:
  - lag phase, where no growth takes place
  - exponential phase, where there is a maximum rate of growth
  - stationary phase, population growth stops
  - death phase, due to the build up of toxins.
- Dormancy occurs in some micro-organisms, e.g. anthrax, where the organism is inactive and not reproducing.

Oxygen concentration

- An organism able to grow in the presence of atmospheric oxygen is an aerobe.
- An organism that can grow in its absence is an anaerobe.
- If the organism is dependent on oxygen it is an obligate aerobe.
- Facultative anaerobes do not require oxygen for growth but do better in its presence.
- Organisms such as *Bacteroides, Fusobacterium* and *Clostridium* do not tolerate oxygen at all and die in its presence – these are obligate anaerobes.
- Campylobacter belongs to a group called microaerophiles, which require oxygen levels below the normal atmospheric range for growth.
- Fungi are usually aerobic.
- Yeasts are usually facultative anaerobes.

Osmotic effects on growth

- The cell wall that separates micro-organisms from their environment is a semi-permeable membrane, so micro-organisms are affected by changes in the osmotic concentration of their surroundings.
- If an organism is placed in a hypotonic solution, water will enter the cell and cause it to burst – unless something is done to prevent the influx.
- When an organism is placed in a hypertonic solution, water leaves the cell, it becomes dehydrated and the cell becomes metabolically inactive.

Temperature

- Environmental temperature profoundly affects micro-organisms as they are poikilothermic – their temperature varies with that of the external environment.
- Metabolism is more active at higher temperatures and the organism grows faster.
- High temperatures damage micro-organisms by damaging enzymes, transport carriers and other proteins.
- Some of the infectious organisms of animals, such as *Pseudomonas,* are psychrophiles (grow at 0–20°).
- Others, called mesophiles, grow best at 20–45°C; most pathogens fall into this category.

Sexual and asexual reproduction

- Yeasts reproduce either asexually by budding and transverse division or sexually through spore formation.

- Asexual spore formation occurs in individual fungi by mitosis and hyphae splitting to form cells that behave as spores. These cells are called arthrospores.
- Sexual reproduction in fungi involves the union of compatible nuclei. Some are self-fertilising.
- Most protozoa reproduce asexually. The most common method of asexual reproduction is binary fission. During this process the nucleus first undergoes mitosis, then the cytoplasm divides by cytokinesis to form two identical individuals.
- Sexual reproduction in protozoa is by conjugation. There is exchange of gametes between compatible types by them fusing together.

The viral replicative cycle can be divided into eight steps (Fig. 7.3):

1. attachment – virus attaches to host cell membrane, often to a specific protein receptor
2. penetration – penetrates host cell membrane
3. uncoating – viral protein coat is broken, releasing viral genetic material into host cell cytoplasm
4. transcription – an mRNA strand is made from the viral genetic material
5. translation – viral mRNA attaches to host ribosomes and nucleic acids are translated into viral proteins
6. replication – duplicate strands of genetic material are produced from the original viral template
7. assembly – viral proteins and newly formed viral genetic material combine to form mature viral particles
8. release – new virus particles either bud from the host cell membrane or are released as the host cell bursts, allowing infection of other cells.

Transmission of micro-organisms

- A carrier is an infected individual who is a potential source of infection for others.
- Zoonoses are diseases of vertebrate animals that can spread to humans.
- Vectors are organisms that spread disease from one host to another, such as mosquitoes, ticks, fleas or mites.
- Airborne transmission usually occurs from the respiratory system of one animal to another.
- Contact transmission can be direct (with the animal or its products), indirect (usually via an inanimate object such as a thermometer) or by droplet spread.
- Inanimate materials involved in pathogen transmission are called vehicles. In common vehicle transmission a single inanimate object spreads the disease to multiple hosts, e.g. a feeding bowl. These agents are called fomites.

Practical microbiology

Safety rules

1. Read instructions on all equipment – if you do not understand something ask your supervisor or contact the manufacturer.
2. Wear protective clothing including aprons, gloves and goggles where appropriate.
3. Wash hands and equipment with disinfectant and clear up any spillages immediately.
4. Label all cultures, plates and tubes correctly so that they can be identified. Details should include the type of plate used, your name and date, the organism's name (if a pure culture) or the source and dilution if unknown.
5. Ensure you follow your practice's SOP and risk assessments when using chemicals and Bunsen burners.

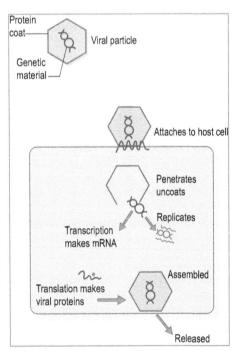

Fig. 7.3 Viral replication

Growing micro-organisms

If you wanted to do your own culture and sensitivity on swabs taken in your practice you must become familiar with the methods of growing bacteria and fungi in the laboratory. We can use either liquid or solid media as long as we provide the necessary nutrients for growth and ensure the following:

1. The medium contains no organisms except the ones we wish to grow, i.e. the agar plate is sterile.
2. The medium is inoculated so that only the organism we wish to grow is placed on the agar plate and that contaminants are excluded.
3. The organism must be incubated in or on its growth medium at a suitable temperature for it to grow.

Streaking a culture on an agar plate

The aim is to obtain single colonies of bacteria that are pure, since both cultures and colonies of bacteria growing on plates are made up of large numbers of cells and therefore may not be pure. As we streak out a drop of the culture, single cells will eventually be placed on the plate. The correct procedure is:

1. Sterilise your loop by holding the wire in the Bunsen flame until it is red hot.
2. If the broth culture is in a tube, remove the lid and flame the neck to ensure surface contaminants are killed off.
3. Introduce the loop into the tube, allow it to cool down first and remove a loop of solution.
4. Start the streaking at one end of the plate and continue as shown in Figure 7.4. Re-flame your loop before picking up culture from points 1, 2, 3 and 4.

Figure 7.5 shows some of the bacterial and fungal colony shapes you will see on agar.

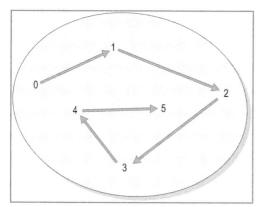

Fig. 7.4 Streaking an agar plate

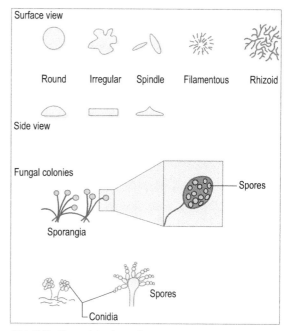

Fig. 7.5 Bacterial colony shapes on agar

Questions for Chapter 7

1. Which organisms are classified as protista?

2. Which exist as a unicellular fungi and which lives in mould colonies?
   a. *Candida*
   b. *Cryptococcus*
   c. *Aspergillus*
   d. *Microsporum*

3. Are fungal cell walls strongly or weakly antigenic?

4. What is an aerobe?

5. What happens to an organism in a hypertonic environment?

6. What range of temperatures do most pathogenic organisms grow at?

7. What happens to a virus during the uncoating stage of its replication?

8. What is a vector?

9. What is a fomite?

10. Is the capsule of bacteria found within or outside the cell wall?

For answers go to page 241

Applied Pharmacology

SECTION **3**

Disease categories

Diseases are described as one of the following:

- **Genetic – passed on through the DNA, may not be present at birth**
- **Immune mediated – the body attacks itself**
- **Traumatic**
- **Anomalous**
- **Degenerative – for example senility, where free radical damage affects nerve cells**
- **Toxic (poisoning)**
- **Overgrowth (hyperplasia) – epulis, benign oral growths are examples**
- **Infectious**
- **Inflammatory**
- **Congenital – an abnormality occurring during development**
- **Cancer**

CHAPTER 8

The Treatment of Infections

Learning aims and objectives

After studying this chapter you should be able to:

1. **Describe how antibacterials disrupt cell function**
2. **List commonly used antifungals and list sites of action of antifungal drugs**
3. **State how antiviral agents work**
4. **Explain the mechanism of action of antiparasitic drugs**

Antimicrobial drugs

Antibiotics

Antibiotics were discovered in the 1930s. They were produced initially by other micro-organisms and all have a detrimental effect on bacteria, viruses or fungi. Choosing an antibiotic is becoming increasingly difficult with the wide array available. Often broad-spectrum drugs like amoxicillin/clavulanate or enrofloxacin are chosen when the pathogen is unknown, but specific antibiosis based on culture and sensitivity is more appropriate. Broad-spectrum drugs are usually selected where the exact nature of the pathogen is unknown. Such choices take into account previous clinical experience and the likely flora known to cause specific infections (e.g. *Staph. intermedius* in canine pyoderma) as well as the specific indications of the chosen drug.

Antibiotic sensitivity of an organism can be tested by placing antibiotic-impregnated discs into cultures of the organism to see if growth is inhibited around the disc. This gives a good indication of sensitivity in vitro (in the laboratory) but does not necessarily mean the drug will kill organisms in vivo (in the body). This is because some drugs penetrate different areas of the body better than others. Neomycin is an example of an antibiotic that is poorly absorbed from the gut following oral administration and so is ideal for enteric infections but not appropriate for systemic infections. In-vitro results may suggest that penicillin is an appropriate drug for treating a streptococcal meningitis, but does not take into account the inability of penicillin to cross the blood–

brain barrier and enter the cerebrospinal fluid. It can not cross the physiological barrier unless it is damaged and so will not reach therapeutic levels in cerebrospinal fluid.

Antibiotics are either bactericidal or bacteriostatic, depending on whether they kill bacteria or stop their replication. The decision as to which antibiotic to use is also influenced by which of these groups it falls into. The list below shows a few examples of each:

- bactericidal
  - fluoroquinolones (e.g. enrofloxacin)
  - β-lactam antibiotics (e.g. penicillin)
  - aminoglycosides (e.g. gentamicin)
- bacteriostatic
  - sulphonamides (e.g. sulfasalazine)
  - tetracyclines (e.g. oxytetracycline)
  - chloramphenicol
  - erythromycin.

Antibiotic combinations are sometimes used in mixed infections, but the drugs must be chosen with care. Penicillin and streptomycin are two drugs that are often used together as they do not interfere with each other's mechanism of action. However, using a bacteriostatic drug with a bactericidal one may be antagonistic as bacteriostats inhibit multiplication whilst bacteriocides are active mainly against multiplying ones. Antibacterials can affect several processes within the cell:

- DNA synthesis, e.g. fluoroquinolones
- protein synthesis (most common), e.g. tetracyclines
- biochemical transformations, e.g. sulphonamides
- cell membrane function (most toxic, as damage may be caused to mammalian/vertebrate cell membranes, therefore rarely used systemically), e.g. polymyxins
- cell wall growth, e.g. penicillin; vertebrate cells do not have a cell wall therefore these are least toxic.

Fluoroquinolones

The fluoroquinolones have been shown to be effective in the treatment of a wide range of bacterial infections. These agents have a broad-spectrum bactericidal activity that includes Gram-negative and Gram-positive aerobic bacteria and mycoplasms. They are not active against anaerobes and are therefore not as broad spectrum as some might think. They should not be used as first-choice antibiotics in order to prevent the development of resistance. The fluoroquinolones in veterinary use include:

- enrofloxacin
- marbofloxacin
- orbifloxacin
- difloxacin
- ibafloxacin
- danfloxacin.

Ibofloxacin is a new fluoroquinolone that has been developed exclusively for veterinary use. These agents work by inhibiting the bacterial enzymes (DNA gyrases) that are required for DNA supercoiling to provide a suitable spatial arrangement of DNA within the bacterial cell.

The minimum inhibitory concentration (MIC) is a way of determining how sensitive a bacteria is to the antibiotic. *Pasteurella* species are very sensitive to the fluoroquinolones, as are Gram-negative bacilli (e.g. *E. coli*) and Gram-positive cocci (*Staphylococcus* spp.) as they have a low MIC. Enterococci, *B. bronchiseptica* and particularly streptococci have the highest MIC and are therefore usually classified as resistant. The minimum bactericidal concentration (MBC) is another interesting pharmacodynamic parameter. For bactericidal drugs it can be anticipated that MIC and MBC should be similar, while it is generally accepted that for bacteriostatic drugs MBC will be several times higher than MIC. Fluoroquinolones kill bacteria most rapidly when their concentrations are considerably above the MIC of the targeted micro-organism.

Enrofloxacin should not be given to growing animals as cartilage damage has been reported as a potential side effect.

Penicillins and related β-lactam antibiotics

- Penicillins and cephalosporins are the most commonly used agents in this group.
- The bactericidal effects are mediated by preventing bacterial cell wall synthesis and disrupting bacterial cell wall integrity. β-lactams bind to a series of enzymes involved in the final stages of cell wall synthesis. This leads to the formation of defective cell walls that are osmotically unstable and cell death usually results from lysis.
- The physical and chemical properties, especially solubility, of penicillins are related to the structure of the acyl side chain and the cations used to form salts.
- Hydrolysis is the main cause of penicillin degradation and can take place in the syringe when penicillin is mixed with another drug.
- Sodium or potassium penicillin salts suspended in an inert oil prolong absorption of penicillin from the site of injection for 18 hours.
- Incorporation of the poorly soluble procaine penicillin in oil prolongs absorption for 24 hours or more.

- Benzathine penicillin G is a repository salt of penicillin and absorption may be prolonged for 7 days or more.
- High concentrations of these drugs are achieved in kidneys, liver and lung.
- Penicillins do not penetrate the CNS unless there is inflammation present.
- Metabolites are inactive and are excreted in the urine.
- The cephalosporins are divided into four generations.
- Clavulanic acid augments the effects of β-lactam antibiotics by protecting them from breakdown by β-lactamases.

Aminoglycosides

- These are produced from strains of *Streptomyces* spp. and other bacteria.
- They have excellent water, but poor lipid, solubility and are thermodynamically stable over a wide range of pH values and temperatures.
- They are potentially nephrotoxic when given systemically and ototoxic due to binding to proximal tubules and inhibition of mitochondrial function.
- They function by irreversibly binding to bacterial ribosomes and interfering with mRNA translation.
- Gentamicin, streptomycin and neomycin are the most widely used agents in this group.

Sulphonamides

Susceptible organisms include:
- many bacteria (although resistance is growing)
- Coccidia
- Chlamydia
- protozoa, including *Toxoplasma* spp.

Sulphonamides are weak organic acids, relatively insoluble in water and vary in the degree of binding to plasma proteins. They tend to undergo crystallisation in the urine and to minimise crystalluria; they are often given in combination with each other.
- Mode of action – they are antimetabolites, interfering with normal production of RNA, protein synthesis and microbial replication mechanisms. They inhibit metabolism by interfering with the production of folic acid and are classed as bacteriostatic.
- Indications – urinary, CNS, joint, respiratory, prostatic infections. The drug is ineffective in the presence of necrotic tissue.
- Acetylation in the liver and lungs is the main route of metabolism and the metabolites are excreted by the kidneys.

- Sulfasalazine (Salazopyrin) – is a useful therapy for inflammatory bowel disease as one of its metabolites has a local anti-inflammatory effect in the colon. After oral administration, it is partly absorbed in the small intestine, where it undergoes enterohepatic circulation (unmetabolised by the liver) and is excreted in the urine. The majority of the drug (70%) remains in the intestine where it is active against the bacteria. The drug is composed of a sulphonamide (sulfapyridine) bonded to a 5-aminosalicylic acid; these are split apart by bacteria in the large intestine.
- Potentiated sulphonamides – the combination with other antimicrobial drugs (most commonly trimethoprim) reduces the minimum inhibitory concentration needed of both drugs and therefore reduces side effects. Trimethoprim is a lipid-soluble organic base that distributes to most tissues of the body and concentrates in tissues with a greater acidity than plasma, e.g. prostate.
- Adverse drug reactions should be suspected in any dog that develops new clinical signs or problems associated with the recent commencement of a new medication. They can affect single or multiple body systems simultaneously and therefore can mimic many different disease processes. Members of the sulphonamide group of antibiotics in particular have been implicated as a cause of adverse drug reactions in the dog with one survey reporting 82% of antibiotic reactions being due to sulphonamides. Other findings include a 4% incidence of lameness with their use and a predisposition for Dobermanns to be affected due to a difference in the metabolism of the drug compared with other breeds. Sulphonamide hypersensitivity is a type III hypersensitivity reaction causing signs such as sterile polyarthritis, blood disorders such as anaemia, neutropenia and thrombocytopaenia. Hepatopathy and glomerular disease have also been reported. One of the potential problems with therapy is that although the manufacturer's recommendations for maximum treatment is often 21 days, treatment of chronic bacterial skin conditions is often in excess of this. Usually there is rapid resolution of clinical signs following withdrawal of the drug.
- Sulphonamides are no longer used in human medicine for safety reasons; trimethoprim is still commonly used however.

Oxytetracycline (tetracyclines)

- This group includes tetracycline, chlortetracycline, oxytetracycline and the synthetic drug doxycycline.

- The antimicrobial activity of the tetracyclines is produced by binding to the ribosomes of susceptible organisms and interfering with bacterial protein synthesis in growing or multiplying organisms.
- The drug easily chelates (i.e. it binds to divalent ions such as calcium); this decreases its absorption, especially when given with dairy products, and therefore should not be given with food. It also means that it concentrates well in bone but will also be deposited in growing teeth, causing potential discolouration.
- It is not metabolised in the body and 60% is excreted in the urine with 40% excreted in the faeces.
- Tetracyclines inhibit the growth of a wide variety of bacteria, protozoa and many intracellular organisms such as *Mycoplasma*, *Chlamydia* and *Rickettsia*.
- The most common side effect is gastrointestinal signs due to irritation of the stomach and the upper small intestine where the bulk of the drug is absorbed after oral administration.

Chloramphenicol

- Manufactured synthetically and has a broad spectrum of activity.
- Inhibits protein synthesis by its action on the ribosome and affects mammalian protein synthesis similarly. This results in side effects such as bone marrow suppression.
- It is metabolised by the liver.
- Inhibits cytochrome P-450 and therefore inhibits the metabolism of other drugs, and prolongs pentobarbital anaesthesia.
- Its use is strictly controlled in food-producing animals. If chloramphenicol is used to treat infections in food animals, it is possible that low concentrations of chloramphenicol in milk, meat and other edible tissues will cause aplastic anaemia in susceptible individuals. Even though the amount consumed may be small, the reaction is not concentration dependent, thus there is a public health risk for individuals consuming these products.

Macrolide antibiotics

- Erythromycin is the main example; other agents that have found clinical applications include tylosin and tilmicosin.
- They are weak bases that are poorly absorbed.
- Inhibit protein synthesis by binding to the ribosome.
- They are mainly effective against Gram-positive organisms.

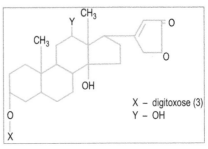

Fig. 8.1 Ribosomes moving along the mRNA-producing proteins. Lincosamides stop this process by binding to the ribosome.

- They are bacteriostatic at therapeutic concentrations, but can be slowly bactericidal, especially against streptococci.
- The antimicrobial action of erythromycin is enhanced by a high pH, with the optimum antibacterial effect at a pH of 8. Therefore, in an acidic environment, such as in an abscess, necrotic tissue or urine, the antibacterial activity is suppressed.

Lincosamides

- There are two agents in this group: lincomycin and clindamycin.
- Used primarily to treat Gram-positive infections where there is resistance or intolerance to penicillins.
- Inhibit protein synthesis by binding to the ribosome (Fig. 8.1).
- They penetrate bone well and are indicated in osteomyelitis and peridontitis.
- Toxic in small mammals, where they can trigger a clostridial overgrowth.

Antibiotic resistance and the prudent use of antibiotics

Therapeutic antibiotics are widely used and this has resulted in the selection of resistant forms of micro-organisms to antibiotics. The appearance of multi-drug-resistant strains of bacteria (e.g. MRSA) in human medicine has, in part, been attributed to the use of drugs in food animal production and has focused attention on the veterinary use of these valuable medicines. Recent research has demonstrated that the genes and biological mechanisms that make hospital pathogens resistant are abundant in ordinary soil bacteria which have never encountered some of the new semi-synthetic antibiotics. This implies that many genes that turn ordinary bacteria into antibiotic-resistant 'super bugs' may come from the soil beneath our feet and not from over-prescription of antibiotics. The prudent use of antibiotics involves:

- accurate diagnosis
- effective levels of the appropriate product – avoid sub-therapeutic doses which can lead to a lack of efficacy and increase the risk of resistance
- only using products with established specific effectiveness
- not treating uncomplicated viral infections
- not changing antibiotic therapy too rapidly, assuming therapeutic failure prior to correcting all contributing factors
- complying with label or written instructions – insufficient duration of treatment can lead to recrudescence of infection, increasing the likelihood of selecting organisms with reduced sensitivity. On the other hand, antibiotic use should be stopped as soon as the animal's own host defence system can control the infection itself – limiting the treatment will minimise the exposure of the bacterial population to the antibiotic and minimise the adverse effects on the surviving bacteria.
- responsible farming practices: limiting disease challenge, reducing stress, promoting the development of a healthy immune system – the use of antibiotics in farm animal medicine should not be used to mask poor husbandry practices.

Antifungals

Antifungal drugs can be used topically to treat skin, mucous membrane or corneal infections caused by fungal organisms. Examples of common fungal infections include: aspergillosis, *Candida* and microsporum. Superficial fungal infections should be treated by clipping the hair from affected areas and clipping the nails to fully expose lesions before application of the antifungal agent. The clinical response to local preparations is unpredictable. Resistance is common to many of the available drugs and spread of infection adds to the difficulty of controlling superficial infections. Perseverance is often an essential element of therapy. Some topical antifungal agents that have been used with success include:

- iodine preparations: tincture of iodine, potassium iodide
- copper preparations: copper sulphate
- sulphur preparations: monosulfiram
- phenols: thymol
- fatty acids and salts: propionates
- organic acids: benzoic acid, salicylic acid
- dyes: crystal (gentian) violet, carbol fuschin
- nitrofurans: nitrofuroxine
- imidazoles: miconazole, clotrimazole, econazole, thiabendazole
- polyene antibiotics: amphotericin B, nystatin, candicidin
- miscellaneous: tolnaftate, hexetidine, triacetin, chlorhexidine.

Figure 8.2 shows the sites of action of the antifungal drugs.

Griseofulvin

Griseofulvin is a systemic antifungal agent effective against the common dermatophytes. It works by distorting the hyphae of the fungus and hence

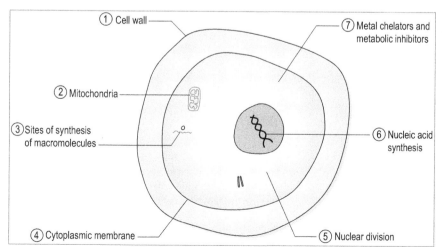

Fig. 8.2 Sites of action of antifungal drugs

① Cell wall
② Mitochondria
③ Sites of synthesis of macromolecules
④ Cytoplasmic membrane
⑤ Nuclear division
⑥ Nucleic acid synthesis
⑦ Metal chelators and metabolic inhibitors

is fungistatic rather than fungicidal. Its absorption from the gut is variable and is enhanced by high-fat meals, margarine and propylene glycol because of its low water solubility. The new growth of hair, nail and horn is free from fungal infection, but the infection persists in old hair until it is naturally shed. This means long courses of up to 6 weeks are recommended, combined with regular clipping of hair and disinfection of grooming equipment. Griseofulvin is contraindicated in pregnant animals because it is teratogenic; otherwise it has good selective toxicity as it is preferentially taken up by susceptible fungi rather than by mammalian cells.

Method of action – disrupts the mitotic spindle by interacting with the microtubules, stopping mitosis in metaphase.

Metabolism – mainly in the liver at a rate approximately $6\times$ faster in dogs than in humans, which is the reason why the dose rate is much higher.

Amphotericin B

This agent is a polyene fungicidal antibiotic used to treat serious systemic mycoses, fungal septicaemia or fungal urinary tract infections. It is also a useful treatment for leishmaniasis. Amphotericin is highly plasma protein bound and penetrates into body fluids and tissues relatively poorly. It acts by binding to sterols in cell membranes, thereby impairing cell membrane permeability – this allows the leakage of cell electrolytes, resulting in cell death.

The chemical structure of the drug is of a large macrolide lactose ring, one side of which is hydrophobic and the other side is hydrophilic, resulting in an amphipathic molecule. Once diluted in water, the drug is present in three forms: as soluble monomers (the active drug), soluble oligomers and insoluble aggregates (this last form is the most toxic). Amphotericin B is known for its nephrotoxicity, due to renal vasoconstriction, direct tubular damage and reduced glomerular filtration rate. One way to reduce its toxicity is to encapsulate the drug in liposomes or to dilute it in a solution of soya bean oil.

Azole antifungal drugs – imidazoles and triazoles

These are broad-spectrum antifungals including:
- clotrimazole
- miconazole
- ketoconazole
- fluconazole
- itraconazole
- enilconazole.

Mode of action – inhibit synthesis of primary steroid of the fungal cell membrane, ergosterol. They are fungistatic at therapeutic doses.

Ketoconazole is highly protein bound (> 98%) and therefore does not penetrate into the CSF, seminal or ocular fluid to a significant degree but does enter mother's milk. It is metabolised in the liver and excreted in the bile. It is only soluble in acid aqueous environments (pH < 3) and therefore antacids decrease oral absorption. The main adverse effects are nausea and vomiting. Drug interactions are common because ketoconazole inhibits metabolism of other drugs due to being an inhibitor of cytochrome P-450.

Fluconazole (Diflucan) – replacing the imidazole ring with a triazole ring increases activity of the compound by $4\times$. Due to different solubility characteristics, it is well absorbed regardless of the feeding circumstances. Unlike other members of this group, it is not highly protein bound, which allows it to be well distributed around the body. Due to its polarity, low molecular weight and metabolic stability, fluconazole is eliminated mainly by the kidney. A unique feature is that it is the only azole that is water soluble and excreted in the urine in an active form, making it suitable for treating fungal cystitis. It is a human preparation, commonly used for the treatment of thrush infections (candidiasis).

Enilconazole (Imaverol) has a residual effect after application.

Terbinafine (Lamisil)

This is a highly fungicidal drug which decreases synthesis of ergosterol and results in fungal death from disruption of the cell membrane. It is highly lipophilic and therefore accumulates in the stratum corneum, hair follicles and sebum-rich skin and nails. It is a human preparation.

Antivirals

Vaccination has always been the approach to controlling virus-induced diseases, but there are many where this is not possible. This may be due to either the vaccine inducing the disease, as in feline infectious peritonitis, or because the virus mutates too quickly for the vaccine to give protection. It is not easy, however, to find drugs that can impair the virus without damaging the host. This is because viruses are obligate intracellular parasites and use the host's genetic machinery to produce new virus. Damaging this process effectively without causing harm to the host is difficult – this is known as poor selective toxicity. Other complications include the infrequency with which definitive diagnosis is made attributing a disease to a virus. The antivirals are best grouped depending on which stage in viral replication they have their action.

Transcription

Idoxuridine and trifluridine incorporate themselves into viral and mammalian DNA strands, making them more susceptible to breakage. They are used topically in herpes keratitis. Toxic side effects include leucopaenia and hepatotoxicity.

Cytarabine and vidarabine are analogues of the nuclear bases cytosine and adenine respectively. Figure 8.3 shows the movement of a polymerase along a strand of DNA. These drugs competitively inhibit the DNA polymerase but have side effects including gastrointestinal, neurological and haematological toxicities.

Ribavirin is a purine analogue that inhibits a wide range of RNA and DNA viruses and its strongest activity is against RNA respiratory viruses (influenza A and B). It has several sites of action including inhibiting synthesis of guanine nucleotides. It can be given orally, i.v. and by aerosol – which produces the best results with the minimum side effects.

Acyclovir (Zovirax) and ganciclovir are only effective against herpes virus. Acyclovir has a good selective toxicity and a high therapeutic index and is available as a topical, oral and i.v. preparation. It is minimally metabolised with > 70% excreted in the urine. The mode of action is to selectively inhibit the viral DNA polymerase and to incorporate themselves into the viral DNA strands causing termination of elongation.

Zidovudine (AZT) is a thymidine analogue which has been extensively used to control HIV infection. It is phosphorylated by cellular enzymes which then inhibit viral reverse transcriptase (an enzyme important in the replication of DNA) 100× more than it inhibits the mammalian enzyme, therefore making the drug selective in its actions and ensuring a low mammalian toxicity. It has been used in cats to treat feline immunodeficiency virus (FIV), an incurable disease that is spread mainly through bites. The host remains asymptomatic for months to years before secondary infections cause illness. AZT produces at least temporary alleviation of clinical signs in some animals within 10–14 days of commencing treatment and should extend the life of FIV-infected cats. The drug has also shown promise in the treatment of FeLV.

Assembly

Amantadine and rimantidine are water-soluble cyclic amines with antiviral activity against a narrow range of RNA viruses, including influenza A. They inhibit late-stage assembly of the virus.

Host resistance through interferon production

Interferons are substances produced by the body to protect against viral infection. They inhibit the replication of a wide variety of viruses including togaviruses, reoviruses and paramyxoviruses. Interferons can establish an antiviral state in host cells and seem to modulate the immune system of the host as well as possessing anti-cancer properties. Three classes of interferons exist – alpha, beta and gamma, with the last being produced solely by T lymphocytes. Interferons affect RNA and DNA viral replication at various stages of the viral replication cycle. Being peptides, they are inactivated if given orally and must be administered parenterally. Penetration into CSF, brain and eye is poor. Therapy is useful in many viral diseases and has been licensed for the treatment of FeLV and parvovirus infection.

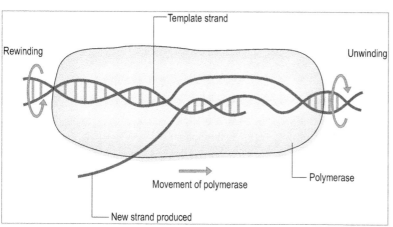

Fig. 8.3 Movement of polymerase along a strand of DNA

Template strand

Rewinding

Unwinding

Movement of polymerase

Polymerase

New strand produced

Anthelmintics/antiparasitics

The chemical control of ectoparasiticides can be grouped as follows:

1. Organochlorines, e.g. DDT, lindane. Long duration of action. Toxicity shows as CNS stimulation.
2. Organophosphates, e.g. diazinon, dichlofenthion, malathion. Persist in the coat for long periods. Some act systemically when given parenterally or orally but blood levels are only maintained for 24 hours. They are cholinesterase inhibitors and toxicity shows as salivation, dyspnoea, ataxia and muscle tremors.
3. Synthetic pyrethroids, e.g. deltamethrin, permethrin. They have a good repellent effect as they persist well on the coat or skin. They act as neurotoxins on the sensory and motor nerves of the neuroendocrine system and CNS of insects. They are all lipophilic and this means they act as contact insecticides. They have a high margin of safety.
4. Carbamates – mode of action similar to organophosphates.
5. Avermectins, e.g. ivermectin. They have a marked residual effect and a single treatment is still effective 3–4 weeks after application.

The move away from a reliance on organophosphate compounds for the control of ectoparasites has been prompted by an increase in the resistance to these products, as well as growing fears about the health risks to humans. A number of new products have made their appearance during the last 10–15 years. Fipronil (Frontline) is an effective adulticide against fleas, as is selamectin (Stronghold), which also kills adult sarcoptes, the mite responsible for 'fox mange'. Lufenuron (Program) and pyriproxyfen (Cyclio) are insect growth regulators and are widely used to control fleas in the environment. Both systemic and topical preparations are available but orally administered products have several advantages. For example, they reduce the exposure of the pet owners and the environment to the insecticides, their efficacy is not influenced by external factors such as rain, sunlight or animal behaviour and they make it easy to avoid over- or under-dosing, incomplete coverage or contamination of sensitive body parts like the eyes.

Fipronil

Fipronil is a synthetic molecule that has potent insecticidal and acaricidal properties. It belongs to the phenylpyrazole family and acts as an antagonist at the insect gamma-aminobutyric acid (GABA) receptor. In insects, GABA is a neurotransmitter that acts as the major inhibitor in the central nervous system and at the neuromuscular junction. Fipronil kills adult fleas by binding to a site within the chloride channel of their GABA receptors and inhibiting the GABA-regulated chloride influx into their nerve cells. Treatment with 10% fipronil solution has been shown to be effective not only in controlling fleas on animals, but also in significantly reducing the environmental burden. Three-monthly applications of fipronil results in a reduction in flea burden by 96.5% and the flea numbers in the environment were reduced by 98.6% without the use of an adulticide or insect growth regulator in the environment.

Avermectins and milbemycin

Avermectins and milbemycins are closely related macrocyclic lactones produced through fermentation by soil-dwelling actinomycetes. They are active against both internal and external parasites and are therefore called endectocides. Box 8.1 shows the parasites these drugs are effective against and those where the drugs have no activity.

Mode of action – they interact with chloride channels resulting in interference with synaptic transmission and paralysis and death in nematode and arthropod species. Ivermectin additionally stimulates the presynaptic release of GABA and increases its binding to postsynaptic receptors. These agents do not have activity against cestodes and trematodes because they do not use GABA as a neurotransmitter.

- Ivermectin – off label use of injectable ivermectin has been successful in cats and non-sensitive dogs for the control of sarcoptic and notoedric mange, *Cheyletiella* and *Otodectes* infestation. Doses necessary to kill parasites are toxic to certain genetic lines of collies.
- Mibemycin oxime – used once weekly for 3 weeks to control sarcoptic mange, even in sensitive dogs. One study showed better results

---

Box 8.1

Activity of the avermectins

- Susceptible parasites
  - Nematodes
  - Arthropods
- Resistant parasites
  - Cestodes
  - Trematodes
  - Protozoa

from oral alternative day therapy at 1 mg/kg for 10–14 days. Also effective against *Cheyletiella*, nasal mite infestation and generalised demodicosis. Side effects include transient vomiting and neurological signs.

- Moxidectin – oral doses of 0.4 mg/kg twice, every 15 days is effective against sarcoptic mange; daily administration is effective at this dose against generalised demodicosis.
- Doramectin – treats notoedric mange in cats.
- Selamectin – effective against *Cheyletiella* and notoedric mange.

In dogs, ivermectin has a half life of 1.8 days when administered i.v. When given orally it is rapidly absorbed, reaching peak plasma levels in 3–4 hours. In cats orally administered ivermectin is eliminated from plasma in 5 days with peak levels at 5.5 hours. When administered s.c. the non-aqueous bovine ivermectin formulation has a delayed peak action of 2 days and a prolonged half-life of 1 week, with persistence of therapeutic levels for up to 2 weeks.

Selamectin is licensed for topical use in dogs and cats and is absorbed percutaneously within a few hours, reaching peak plasma concentrations in 1–3 days. It has been shown to accumulate in the sebaceous glands. The plasma half-life is 8 days in the cat and 11 days in the dog, with efficacious plasma concentrations for 30 days. The main route of elimination is via the faeces (48–60% in cats and 18–20% in dogs), the rest being eliminated via the urine (1–3%) and cutaneous sebum.

Toxicity is low because mammals are less sensitive than parasites to these agents. This is because GABA-mediated nerve synapses are present only in the central nervous system and the drugs do not easily cross the blood–brain barrier, whereas in many invertebrates they regulate peripheral muscle activity. At high doses, toxicity shows as ataxia, tremors, mydriasis, depression, coma and death. Dog breeds sensitive to ivermectin include:

- Collies
- Australian Shepherd dog
- Old English Sheepdog
- Shetland Sheepdog.

This sensitivity does not occur in every animal, but in about half of them, due to a recessive autosomal gene that allows penetration of the drug across the blood–brain barrier.

Amitraz (Aludex)

This agent is used to treat generalised mite infestations including demodicosis, sarcoptic mange and cheyletiellosis (unlicensed use). It increases neuronal activity through its action on octopamine receptor sites in mites.

Endoparasiticides

Endoparasiticides are drugs used to treat helminth infestations, mainly nematode (roundworm) and cestode (tapeworm) infections. Each drug has its own indications and side effects. Some of the products currently available are listed in Table 8.1 together with an outline of their range of action.

Anthelmintics must be selectively toxic to the parasite. This is usually achieved by inherent pharmacokinetic properties of the compound, which cause the parasite to be exposed to higher concentrations of the drug than the host cells, or inhibiting metabolic processes vital to the parasite. Parasitic helminths must maintain an appropriate feeding site, and nematodes and trematodes must actively ingest and move food through their digestive tracts to maintain an appropriate energy state, which requires appropriate neuromuscular coordination. The pharmacological basis of the treatment for helminths generally involves interference with one or both of these energy processes, causing starvation of the parasite, or paralysis and subsequent expulsion of the parasite.

Table 8.1 Endoparasiticides and their range of action

Product name	Active ingredient	Worms treated
Droncit (Bayer)	Praziquantel	Tapeworms
Drontal plus (Bayer)	Praziquantel, Pyrantel embonate, Febantel	Tapeworms, roundworms
Lopatol (Ciba)	Nitroscanate	Tapeworms, roundworms
Panacur (Hoechst)	Fenbendazole	Tapeworms (not Dipylidium), roundworms
Canovel Endorid (Smithkline Beecham)	Piperazine	Roundworms

Fenbendazole (Panacur)

This popular wormer belongs to the benzimidazole family of safe, broad-spectrum anthelmintics which also includes albendazole and mebendazole.

- It comes as a white crystalline powder and is insoluble in water, which means it is poorly absorbed from the gut.
- Peak plasma levels take 6–30 hours after dosing and are never greater than 1% of the dose regardless of the type administered (paste, suspension, granules or bolus).
- It acts by binding to nematode tubulin which prevents the formation of many organelles and the processes of mitosis, protein assembly and energy metabolism.
- Adverse effects are rare. Attempts to cause poisoning in mice have been unsuccessful because they can tolerate the maximum quantities that can be physiologically given. Necrosis of the ear tips is an uncommon presentation that is usually associated with vasculopathies, particularly immune-mediated vasculitis, as the extremities are supplied by end-arterial systems with a limited capacity to develop a collateral supply. Causes of vascular damage include vasculitis associated with infections, neoplasia, vaccines and drug eruptions. Fenbendazole has been reported to cause ischaemic pinnal necrosis.

Febantel (Drontal Plus)

This agent belongs to the probenzimidazole family and is converted in the GI tract to fenbendazole. Its effects are seen in the larvae in eggs as well as in the different stages of the helminths.

Levamisole

This agent stimulates nicotinic acetylcholine receptors (nACh) and causes muscular paralysis by interfering with carbohydrate metabolism. It paralyses the worm and allows it to be expelled. Signs of toxicity include:

- salivation
- defecation
- respiratory distress.

Pyrantel (Drontal Cat)

This broad-spectrum anthelmintic belongs to the tetrahydropyrimidine family and is well absorbed after oral administration. It is a depolarising neuromuscular blocking agent which produces paralysis of the worms by producing contracture of the musculature similar to acetylcholine (ACh). The drug is free of adverse effects in all hosts at doses of up to 7× the therapeutic dose.

Piperazine

This agent belongs to the heterocyclic compound group which also includes phenothiazine. It is a diethylenediamine with a simple ring structure that is freely soluble in water and glycerol, less soluble in alcohol and insoluble in ether. It is a strong base and easily absorbs water and carbon dioxide, therefore containers should be closed tightly and protected from light. It is also very sensitive to moisture, but can be made more stable by the addition of salts such as hydrochloride and phosphate. It is readily absorbed from the proximal GI tract, some of the drug is metabolised in the tissues and the remainder is excreted in urine as early as 30 minutes after administration. Urinary excretion is complete within 24 hours.

The mode of action is blockage of transmission at the neuromuscular junction, producing flaccid paralysis of the parasite. Mature worms are more susceptible than lumen-dwelling larvae and so treatment in carnivores is advised to be repeated within 2 weeks.

Very young pups (from 2 weeks old) can be safely treated and there is a wide margin of safety. Large oral doses produce vomiting, diarrhoea, incoordination and head pressing in dogs and cats. It is effective against ascarids (*Toxocara canis*, *T. cati* and *Toxascaris leoninae*).

Organophosphate compounds

Examples are shown in Box 8.2. Their main effect on nematode parasites is inhibition of acetylcholinesterase (AChE) leading to interference with neuromuscular transmission and subsequent paralysis. Nematodes utilise ACh as a neurotransmitter and AChE stops transmission by breaking down ACh.

Box 8.2

Organophosphate compounds

- Dichlorvos
- Trichlofon
- Haloxon
- Coumaphos
- Naphthalophos
- Crufomate

Inhibition of this enzyme thus leads to persistence of the nervous impulses and coordinated feeding ceases. Animals should not be treated simultaneously (or within a few days) with other AChE-inhibiting drugs or certain sedatives, e.g. acepromazine. The margin of safety of the organophosphates is less than the broad-spectrum anthelmintics and strict attention to dosage is essential.

Other parasiticides

Leishmaniasis therapy

Amphotericin B is described above. Alternative treatments include the combination of the penta-valent antimony compound meglumine antimoniate (Glucantime; Merial) administered s.c. daily and the pyrazolopyrimidine allopurinol (Zyloric; Glaxo-Wellcome), which is given orally once or twice daily for the duration of the Glucantime treatment. Allo-purinol can then be given alone for up to 9 months afterwards to reduce the likelihood of relapse. Pain and local swelling may occur following injection of meglumine antimoniate. Zyloric inhibits growth of the parasites by blocking RNA synthesis and extends survival time to up to 4 years in 75% of cases.

Heartworm adulticides

Adult stages of *Dirofilaria immitis* cause the major damage associated with heartworm infection in dogs. Removal of adults is the key stage in therapy, but complete management involves elimination of microfilariae and prevention of new infections. Effective adulticides include:

- Thiacetarsamide sodium – a hepatotoxic and nephrotoxic arsenical agent, which must be administered i.v. because it is irritating to the tissues. Feeding the patient 1 hour prior to treatment is recommended and treatment should be stopped if the dog becomes anorexic or vomits. Arsenic toxicity is seen as persistent vomiting, icterus and orange-coloured urine. Severe toxic reactions can be treated with dimercaprol (8.8 mg/kg/d in 4 divided doses). Following four therapeutic injections of thiacetarsamide, adult worms die within 5–7 days and are swept out of the heart and lodge in pulmonary arteries where they are reabsorbed over the next 2–3 months. Dogs should be strictly rested to reduce the risks of pulmonary embolism for 6 weeks after treatment.

- Melarsomine – this agent is also an arsenical with activity against adult and 4-month-old heartworms in dogs. It is injected i.m. and a single, two-dose course kills all male worms and 96% of females. If clinical signs persist, the dose may be repeated after 90–120 days when 98% of dogs will be cleared of the infection. Melarsomine and its metabolites are free in the plasma, unlike thiacetarsamide, which binds to red blood cells. Over-dosage is seen as distress, salivation, tachycardia, abdominal pain, coma and death in severe cases.

- Selamectin – used to prevent heartworm. The drug should be administered within one month of first exposure to mosquitoes and the last dose must be given within one month of the last exposure.

Resistance to nematocides

- Resistance appears when drugs are used intensively against parasites, which have a good ability to survive in the host and where the host develops little acquired immunity.

- Nematodes develop cross-resistance to a mode of activity rather than a specific compound and so the entire family of drugs is at risk.

- Once use of the anthelmintic class stops, reversion back to sensitivity is slow.

- Drugs should be rotated and the frequency of treatment considered. Optimal impact from minimum number of treatments is the aim, timing them to disrupt key events in the annual cycle of the parasite.

Questions for Chapter 8

1. Which of these agents are suitable preventions or treatments for Leishmaniasis?
Sodium stibogluconate (Pentostam), amphotericin B, meglumine antimoniate and allopurinol, deltamethrin-impregnated collars (Scalibor; Intervet)

2. Explain why the spectrum of activity of the avermectins does not include the tapeworms.

3. Compare the modes of action of the different antiparasiticides.

4. Why is amphotericin B nephrotoxic?

For answers go to page 241

CHAPTER 9

Immunological Products

After studying this chapter you should be able to:

1. **State the reasons for vaccination**
2. **List the vaccines in common use**
3. **Explain the reasons for use of immunoglobulins**
4. **Describe the uses of immunostimulants.**

Introduction

Vaccination has long been used as a tool to control and fight infectious diseases in human and veterinary medicine. Smallpox was the first human disease to be eradicated by a mass vaccination programme. Polio is currently being targeted in the hope that it can be similarly eradicated. In the UK, distemper, leptospirosis and parvovirus are no longer the commonplace killers of dogs they were up until the early 1980s, thanks to the widespread use of vaccination. This chapter will present the case for continued vaccination of domesticated animals, the types of vaccine available, the factors affecting vaccine efficacy and the risks of vaccination.

Vaccination is often viewed with fear and distrust. The Animal Health Trust conducted a study to determine if there was any link between vaccination and ill health in dogs and they found no increase in the frequency of illness in recently vaccinated dogs.

The case for vaccination

Vaccination of animals seeks to make susceptible animals immune and thereby resistant to infectious disease. The aims of vaccination include:

- protection from clinical disease in individual animals
- transmission of temporary protection from the mother to offspring
- reduction of the amount of infectious agent produced following infection

- elimination of the infectious agent from a group of animals or a country.

Successful vaccination programs result in the disappearance of certain infectious diseases and the appearance of a certain amount of complacency amongst those who have never witnessed the devastation such diseases can cause. A drop in the uptake of vaccination will create a vulnerable unprotected population – introduction of an infectious disease into such a population results in the rapid multiplication and transmission of that disease, resulting in an epidemic.

Types of vaccine

Vaccines are of two general types (Box 9.1): modified live or non-living vaccines. It is generally considered that live vaccines produce a superior quality of immune response than non-living vaccines because they replicate in the animal. This can be explained by the following three features of live vaccines:

- live organisms express all of their proteins when replicating within the host – exposure of the host to the full range of viral antigens is thought to induce a better immune response
- by replicating within host cells, antigens are presented to the host's immune system and stimulate cell-mediated immunity through cytotoxic T cells, which subsequently recognise and kill infected cells – this allows infected cells to be targeted
- generation of mucosal immunity following intranasal or oral administration of a vaccine.

Live vaccines also possess a number of potential disadvantages:

- the extent of attenuation is inversely proportional to the quality of the immune response that the vaccine can be expected to induce
- reversion of the attenuated organism is possible, though fortunately very rare in small animal vaccines
- inactivation of the organism is possible and even common place – storage of such vaccines in a strictly monitored appropriate environment is required, both during storage and transportation to avoid death of the attenuated virus
- neutralisation of the virus is possible if it comes into contact with maternally derived antibody.

Non-living vaccines are derived from living and potentially virulent organisms that are then treated chemically to render them non-infectious, whilst not affecting their ability to stimulate an immune response. Subunit vaccines are derived by disrupting

Box 9.1

Types of vaccine

Live vaccines

- Live attenuated organisms
  - + rapid protection
  - + stimulate cell-mediated immunity
  - − can potentially revert to virulence
  - − can potentially cause disease without reverting to virulence
- Recombinant viruses
  - + produce good immunity, often with cell-mediated immunity
  - − expensive to produce
  - − need effective adjuvants

Non-living vaccines

- Inactivated organisms
  - + no reversion to virulence possible
  - + stable
  - − inappropriate responses
  - − lower antibody titres produced
  - − need adjuvants
- Subunit vaccines
  - + no reversion to virulence
  - + concentrated antigens in vaccine
  - − contamination possible with live virulent virus
  - − poor immunogens
- Recombinant proteins
  - + purity assured
  - − expensive to produce
  - − need effective adjuvants

the whole organism (e.g. with detergents) to release subunits that can stimulate an immune response. This has been used to generate some feline calicivirus and herpes virus vaccines. Genetic engineering has been used to generate an FeLV vaccine. The resulting vaccine contains the gene encoding a viral surface glycoprotein, inserted into bacterial cells – when expressed in the cat, this recombinant protein elicits an effective immune response.

All non-living vaccines require an adjuvant to provide an adequate immune response. The role of the adjuvant is two-fold – it slows the release of antigen by forming a depot of vaccine at the site of inoculation and attracts antigen-presenting cells such as macrophages to the inoculation site. These cells then process and present the antigen to lymphocytes.

The most significant advantage of non-living vaccines is that they are safer because they are unable to replicate. The most significant disadvantage is that higher doses of the organism have to be given and they do not present such a wide range of immunogens to the vaccinated animal. In addition, the adjuvant may provoke adverse reactions in the host.

Once an animal is immune to a particular disease it means the risks of becoming ill are reduced or negligible.

Factors affecting vaccine efficacy

A number of important factors can affect vaccine efficacy and should always be considered when considering the vaccination of an individual animal. Box 9.2 summarises the factors causing vaccine breakdown.

Vaccine factors

- Antigenic drift in wild strains of disease may render a vaccine ineffective against new emerging strains.
- Annual revaccination is generally recommended for most vaccines, especially where there is no evidence to suggest the likely duration of protective immunity. From observations on the persistence of antibody levels following vaccination with live canine viruses, it has been suggested that dogs do not require annual vaccinations but can be vaccinated every three years.

Host factors

- Maternal antibodies are passed on to newborn animals in utero and via colostrum. The starting levels of maternal antibody in the newborn will determine the length of protection conferred. This is therefore variable between individuals depending on factors such as the size of the litter, availability of colostrum and time spent suckling.
- Maternal antibodies are able to neutralise the small amount of live vaccine present in live virus vaccines.
- Vaccines given at the conventional times of 9 and 12 weeks may have some interference from maternal antibodies. This can be avoided by giving a third dose of vaccine after 12 weeks, by increasing the titre of virus in the vaccine or by establishing serum antibody levels. In practice this is rarely done.

Box 9.2

Causes of vaccine breakdown

- Disinfectant on syringe
  - can kill live vaccine
- Wrong route of administration
- Wrong timing of vaccination
  - e.g. delay between 1st and 2nd doses
- Exposing animal to infection at the time of vaccination
  - hence the need to clean all surfaces, including tables and weighing scales, when vaccinating young puppies and kittens
- Poor mixing
- Poor storage
  - temperatures above 4°C are likely to result in death of live vaccine
- Pre-existing infections
  - hence the need for a full clinical exam and health check prior to vaccination
- High titres of maternal antibodies
- Pyrexia, hyperthermia, hypothermia
- Immunosuppression
- Age
  - very young or very old
- Concurrent disease
- Pregnancy
- Malnutrition
- Stress
- Excessive attenuation of vaccine
- Wrong strain in vaccine
- Concomitant drug therapy

- Pre-existing infections can affect the host's immune system and impair its ability to respond to a vaccine. It is sensible to advise owners of a new puppy or kitten to isolate and monitor their new pet for one week prior to vaccination.
- A healthy and effective immune system is essential if an animal is to respond appropriately to a vaccine. Animals that are very old, very young, sick or receiving cytotoxic or immunosuppressive drugs may respond poorly to vaccination. It is suggested that low doses of glucocorticoids do not significantly reduce the response to vaccination. By contrast, a poor response to parvovirus vaccination has been demonstrated in hyperthermic puppies with temperatures greater than 103.6°F/39.8°C.

Human factors

- Vaccines must be stored at the recommended temperature during both transport and storage – usually 4°C. An approved pharmaceutical fridge is recommended and temperatures should be monitored and recorded daily. Aged fridges are to be avoided because of likely fluctuations in temperature.
- Expiry dates must be monitored closely and strictly adhered to. The amount of live vaccine decreases with time and it is therefore advisable that fresh vaccine be used where possible. Good stock management is therefore essential.
- The secondary anamnestic response requires that primary vaccination be given in the days preceding the second vaccination. If the interval is too short, then the primary response renders the second dose of vaccine ineffective. If the interval is too long, then the secondary response will not occur.

A course of two vaccines is given as maternal antibodies wane at different times, leaving young animals susceptible at different ages. The leptospirosis part of the canine vaccine regime requires the body to be primed with a first dose so that the second dose produces full levels of immunity due to the memory response of the lymphocytes.

Contraindications and adverse effects of administering vaccines

Effectiveness

The vaccine may not be effective in animals incubating the disease.

Hypersensitivity

Hypersensitivity reactions should be treated with an antihistamine, corticosteroid or epinephrine, without delay and by the most immediate route.

Antisera and immunosuppressive drugs

Animals that have received the corresponding antiserum or immunosuppressive drugs should not be vaccinated until 4 weeks has passed.

Adjuvants

In addition to the antigen, vaccines contain adjuvants, materials added to enhance their immunogenicity. Examples include other antigens, protein from tissue culture of egg yolk, preservatives such as antibiotics, and carrier substances such as aluminium. Animals may react to these substances.

Polyvalent vaccines

Polyvalent vaccines are those protecting against several infectious diseases, as such they are all-in-one vaccines. Concerns have been raised about whether this causes immunosuppression through antigen-overload, although this is yet to be substantiated. Immunosuppression may also occur as a result of one antigen component of the vaccine preventing the immune system from responding to another component – this is termed vaccine interference. Trials in dogs have demonstrated immunosuppression of 7–10-day duration post-vaccination with polyvalent vaccines but this would only be cause for concern if the dog was incubating an infectious disease at the time of vaccination. Alternatively, if a nutritional deficiency or hereditary immune disorder already compromises a dog's immune system, the added immunosuppression may result in clinical illness if the dog is exposed to a disease in the 7–10-day margin. The vaccine is not causing the disease directly, just making the underlying condition apparent. In light of this, animals suspected of harbouring infection or whose immune systems are already under stress (seasonal allergies, illness, taking certain medications) should not be vaccinated.

Immune complex disease

In some instances, when there is extensive formation of immune complexes, these large molecules may be deposited in certain organs of the body, resulting in inflammation of local tissue. An example of this occurred with the use of early Canine Adenovirus-1 (CAV-1) vaccines – shortly after being administered the vaccine, dogs developed a bluish cast to the cornea of the eyes. This abnormal condition was determined to be caused by fluid retention and inflammation of the corneal tissue resulting from the deposit of antibody–antigen complexes. The immune-complex disease was later found to be an effect not of the CAV-1 antigen, but of the high concentration of the carrier protein, bovine serum albumin (BSA), used in the early CAV-1 vaccines. Modern CAV-1 vaccines no longer cause 'blue eye'.

Vasculitis

Vaccine-induced vasculitis is an adverse reaction that occurs very rarely in dogs, but it has been most often associated with administration of the rabies vaccine. This condition may present as many as 3–6 months following immunisation. It has a distinct, consistent histological inflammatory pattern that may be helpful in differentiating this reaction from other underlying causes for vasculitis. In general, cutaneous forms of vaccine-induced vasculitis may be identified by areas of hair loss and large red or purple spots. The lesions may also appear as hives, a rash, or painful/tender lumps. In more severe cases, loss of blood flow to the skin may produce necrosis of the skin, which will appear as ulcers or small black spots at the tips of the ears or toes (i.e. the extremities – the blood supply to these areas is affected by immune complex deposition).

More specific symptoms of vasculitis will be dependent upon the organ or organ systems involved. These may include the brain and nervous system, GI tract, heart and lungs, and the eyes. It occurs in dogs that have abnormal T-cell function and more commonly in older dogs due to age-related compromise of the immune system. An aged immune system does not only increase risk for the older dog to contract and be more susceptible to infectious diseases, but also increases risk for adverse reactions to immunisation. The use of antihistamines in conjunction with vaccinations, however, may be indicated to reduce some components of the inflammatory response associated with immune-complex formation for which these older dogs may be at higher risk (since histamine has been found to play a role in platelet aggregation associated with allergic vasculitis).

Shedding of live virus

Live, attenuated viral components may be shed after immunisation. It is therefore recommended that any dog living with a sick or immunocompromised dog should only receive killed vaccines and not modified-live vaccines – to prevent possibility of infection in the immunocompromised dog.

Epilepsy and acute disseminated encephalomyelitis

Some forms of epileptic seizures may manifest as a direct effect of immunologic mechanisms and vaccination may trigger these mechanisms. An example is the modified-live canine distemper antigen. Similar to the actual disease process of canine distemper, where modified-live virus is introduced into the dog, if the immune system does not respond rapidly enough, then attenuated virus can cross the blood–brain barrier or enter the cerebrospinal fluid and gain access to the central nervous system, causing an inflammatory immune response.

Vaccine-induced hypertrophic osteodystrophy

Hypertrophic osteodystrophy (HOD) involves a change in osteoclasts (increased number and size) as a result of increased levels of interleukin-6 (IL-6 is a multifunctional cytokine produced by immune cells such as macrophages, T-cells, B-cells and endothelial cells).

Autoimmune disease

The immune system will attack the animal's own normal cells when surface proteins on a vaccine are similar to a self-antigen. This condition is known as molecular mimicry and a small population of individuals may have a genetic predisposition for developing autoimmune symptoms after immunisation.

Mixing

Though many vaccines are distributed as two vials, a lyophilised component and a diluent component (which must be mixed together prior to injection), it is important to note that different vaccine brands or types should not be mixed together or administered with the same needle or syringe used to administer another vaccine. Doing so may cause an interaction of the vaccine components, which may inactivate particular antigens and prohibit proper immune response. Additionally, although killed vaccines are also susceptible to improper handling, careful handling of modified-live vaccines is critical because vaccine efficacy is dependent upon the ability of the modified viruses to replicate.

Route of administration

Adhering to the route of administration recommended by the manufacturer is essential. Most modified-live vaccines are approved for s.c. injection, but the modified-live rabies viruses of some vaccines require nerve tissue to replicate – these vaccines will only produce sufficient antigens to induce an immune response if injected i.m. In some cases, killed vaccines also require a special route of administration. Vaccines such as those for protection against kennel cough stimulate local mucosal immunity against the disease in the respiratory tract and require intranasal administration. Furthermore, administration of some killed vaccines by a route other than directed may lead to severe systemic reactions since many of these vaccines contain adjuvant, or helper, components such as aluminium hydroxide which enhance the immune response to the killed antigen.

Subcutaneous injections of such vaccines can lead to localised tissue damage or to severe systemic allergic reactions. Alternatively, aerosolisation of a live s.c. vaccine, by squirting an air bubble out of a syringe (e.g. before injecting a patient), can lead to the patient inhaling the vaccine and developing the disease. Also, live vaccine injection sites should be swabbed with spirit after injection to prevent other animals from orally ingesting the vaccine through grooming. Box 9.3 lists some of the other adverse reactions seen following vaccination.

How often should we vaccinate?

- Yearly vaccination against viral infections associated with canine distemper virus, canine

> ### Box 9.3
>
> **Possible adverse reactions following vaccination**
>
> - Post-vaccinal encephalitis
>   - has been described in dogs given a live CDV vaccine
> - Polyarthritis and lameness
>   - reported following the administration of a live FCV vaccine
> - Plasmacytic pododermatis
>   - has followed the administration of FCV/FHV vaccines
> - Fibrosarcomas
>   - seen to develop at injection sites in cats, particularly in North America
>   - cause unknown but could be due to the adjuvant used
>   - injection of FeLV vaccine at a separate site (e.g. left abdomen) has been suggested to allow monitoring of response to vaccination; it has also been suggested, however, that increasing the number of injection sites may increase the risk of tumour formation

parvovirus and canine adenovirus are generally unnecessary since active immunity induced by these vaccines provides at least several years of protection. The only evidence for this, however, is based on antibody titres, not field challenges.

- This should not be generalised to bacterin vaccines, which immunise against *Bordetella bronchiseptica* (kennel cough), *Leptospira* (leptospirosis), and *Borrelia burgdoferi* (Lyme disease). They probably do not provide protective immunity for 12 months and therefore more frequent vaccination for these diseases is required.
- Owners need to be made aware that, whilst vaccination against certain viral diseases can be repeated every 3 years, this does not apply to bacterial diseases. The importance of an annual health check and vaccination boosters remains unchanged.

Types of vaccine

Homeopathic vaccines

Homeopathic vaccines, called nosodes, are prepared using high, serially agitated dilutions of infectious agents (i.e. infectious body fluids, vomitus, faeces, or other tissue) which are administered to the animal orally for the purpose of protecting against later infection with the respective pathogen. Controlled clinical studies exploring the ability of nosodes to protect animals that are directly challenged with infectious disease indicate that nosodes are not effective for this purpose. They do provide some benefits over not vaccinating dogs at all – the highest efficacy shown by a clinical trial was 22%, meaning 4 out of 5 dogs challenged after vaccination developed clinical disease.

Distemper, hepatitis, parvovirus and parainfluenza vaccination

These vaccines are usually live, attenuated, freeze-dried virus vaccines that require reconstitution and should be injected by the subcutaneous route. The duration of immunity to parainfluenza virus infection induced by vaccination is unknown – annual revaccination is recommended. Datasheets should be consulted for individual vaccine requirements but contact with infected animals is not usually recommended for 7 days after the completion of the course.

Leptospirosis vaccination

This is an inactivated, bacterial vaccine containing a liquid suspension of *Leptospira interrogans*, serogroups canicola and icterohamorrhagiae. The duration of immunity has been established as at least one year. Local reactions have been noted of limited size occurring during the first few days after vaccination.

Kennel cough vaccination

This is a live freeze-dried vaccine with accompanying diluent. Some combine *Bordetella bronchiseptica* strain B-C2 with canine parainfluenza virus strain Cornell. Protection is conferred within 72 hours of vaccination.

Two vaccines are licensed in the UK (Nobivac KC, Intervet; Intrac, Schering Plough). Both products should be administered into one nostril with the head in a normal position. With Intrac, it is suggested that half the volume be squirted into either nostril in small breeds (Fig. 9.1). Continental products are administered via the subcutaneous route. Vaccines should be used within one hour of reconstitution.

Rabies vaccination

The rabies vaccine can be given in some cases to animals from 4 weeks of age, with a single dose only required after 12 weeks of age. Rabies boosters are required every 1–2 years. The prescribed interval between vaccinations must be observed for the pet passport to remain valid. Where vaccination is delayed, a repeat serological test will become necessary. Some countries require annual vaccination – it is therefore advisable to renew rabies vaccination on an annual basis for all dogs travelling abroad

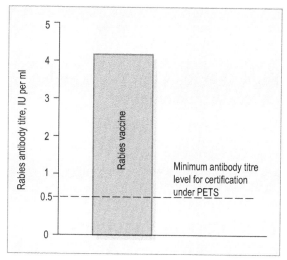

Fig. 9.2   Response to rabies vaccination

on the pet passport scheme. The vaccine is an aqueous suspension with aluminium phosphate as an adjuvant – it is usually an inactivated vaccine.

Recent DEFRA guidelines on rabies vaccination state that '…the manufacturer advises in its datasheet…the best time for a blood sample to be taken after the vaccination'. Rapid seroconversion to rabies vaccination has been demonstrated with the Quantum vaccine (Schering-Plough) with a group of 21 dogs all showing above the necessary antibody levels after just 14 days (Fig. 9.2).

Feline leukaemia vaccination

The antigen that stimulates the best immune response is known to be the envelope glycoprotein gr70, but early vaccines also included an envelope protein called p15E. This actually made cats more susceptible to infection and was subsequently withdrawn – this highlights the difficulties in producing an effective but safe vaccine. Some vaccine companies use the purified p45 FeLV envelope antigen (the specific fraction of the envelope glycoprotein gp70), obtained by genetic recombination of a strain of *E. coli*. The antigenic material is adjuvanted with aluminium hydroxide gel and 'Quil A' – a purified derivative of saponin. Prior to vaccination, it is advised that cats be checked for the presence of p27 circulating viral antigen, using the ELISA test. If the test is positive, vaccination will not be effective.

The vaccine's success is demonstrated by the following trial – 26 8-week-old cats were vaccinated s.c. with a commercially available FeLV vaccine; 26 others were given just the adjuvant. Each group was housed with five FeLV-positive cats – five of

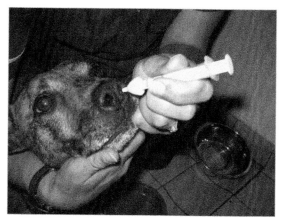

Fig. 9.1   Intranasal vaccination

the control group became infected (four of them only transiently), but none of the vaccinated group developed antigenaemia.

Feline herpes virus 1 and feline calicivirus vaccination

There are several types of vaccine available in the UK including:
- modified live systemic
- modified live intranasal
- inactivated adjuvanted systemic.

The future of vaccination

Many effective vaccines are being trialled that are live, genetically modified viruses. This makes their approval difficult and the only one to be licensed so far is the rabies vaccine. The vaccines are made by replacing the surface proteins on the virus that cause another disease, with proteins from the disease you want protection from. The altered viruses are not supposed to be able to cause disease but there are concerns that the viruses could mutate with unknown consequences.

Passive immunisation

Passive immunisation arises from:
- maternally derived humoral antibodies (colostrum)
- passive transfer of immune cells – by taking the lymphocytes from an infected animal and transferring them to an uninfected animal, the ability to respond to an infection is transferred
- passive transfer of hyperimmune serum – this is done by inoculating a species not usually susceptible to a disease, e.g. a horse with foot and mouth (which only affects cloven-hoof animals), and then harvesting the serum after the animal's immune system has produced antibodies to the organism. The serum will obviously contain antibodies to protect the recipient without them having to mount an immune response of their own.

Immunostimulants

This subject is covered in detail in Chapter 18. Levamisole is an antinematodal drug with an ability to enhance immune responsiveness. Its absorption and excretion are rapid following oral administration and 40% is excreted in urine within 12 hours.

Questions for Chapter 9

State whether the following statements are TRUE or FALSE:

1. The immune system responds much more quickly if it encounters an organism it has already encountered or been primed to meet.

2. Vaccination is a form of passive immunity.

3. Vaccination is the administration of an antibody complex.

4. Killed vaccines contain inactivated microorganisms.

5. Modified live vaccines have a higher frequency of adverse reactions than subunit vaccines.

6. Attenuated organisms are no longer capable of replicating and causing an immune response.

7. The FeLV vaccine is an example of a subunit bacterin vaccine.

8. Modern canine vaccines have an adverse reaction risk level of around 1 in 60 000.

9. It is not possible to vaccinate cats against Chlamydia or *Bordetella brochiseptica* respiratory infections.

10. Monovalent vaccines contain several different organisms or antigens.

11. There is no complete vaccine for kennel cough.

12. An example of attenuation of an organism would be to grow it for long periods of time in cells from a species other than its usual host.

13. Recombinant DNA technology provides the means to select attenuated strains of virus that are less likely to mutate back to

the original form and cause disease and are therefore safer to use.

14. Dogs receiving corticosteroid therapy should not be vaccinated.

15. Dogs suffering from hypoadrenocorticism (Addison's disease) should not be vaccinated.

16. Booster vaccines provide a more rapid immune response than the primary active immunisation.

17. A minimum of 1 week is required before a dog can be challenged with an infection after vaccination.

18. All maternal antibody has waned by 10 weeks of age in puppies and therefore will not interfere with vaccination after this age.

For answers go to page 241

Pharmaceutical Preparations used for the Respiratory System

Introduction

Disease processes affecting the respiratory system impede ventilation and alveolar gas exchange in many ways. Inflammation from infection, obstruction due to lungworms and constriction of the airways due to the release of inflammatory mediators such as histamine are all challenges that must be met therapeutically. The objectives in the management of respiratory disease are:

- support pulmonary defence systems (good circulation, cautious use of corticosteroids and immunosuppressants)
- promote tracheobronchial secretions to protect dry mucosa and use mucolytics and expectorants to aid their expulsion
- promote cilia beating to clear airways (cilia augmentors), thus ensuring the optimal functioning of the ciliary escalator that is responsible for mucociliary clearance
- suppress excessive and unproductive coughing (antitussives)
- enhance alveolar ventilation with bronchodilators and by reducing inflammatory exudate
- shrink swollen mucosa (decongestants)
- prevent and relieve pulmonary oedema
- minimise and counteract the destructive effects of inflammation
- treat infections.

The drugs to consider include:

- drugs acting on mucociliary clearance
- anti-inflammatory drugs

- bronchodilators
- mast cell stabilisers
- antibiotics.

Drugs acting on mucociliary clearance

The rate of removal of mucus from the airways is determined by a number of factors such as mucus viscosity, the amount of mucus produced, and ciliary activity. Mucociliary drugs can be divided into five groups according to their mechanisms of action:
- mucolytic drugs (sterile water, sterile saline, acetylcysteine, sodium bicarbonate, propylene glycol)
- surface-acting drugs (glycerol, ethyl alcohol)
- bronchomucotropic agents (expectorants such as bromexhine, potassium iodide, etc.)
- cilia augmentors (β sympathomimetics)
- bronchodilators (β sympathomimetics, xanthines).

Expectorants and mucolytics

These agents increase the volume and fluidity of secretions from the airway mucosa. Bromhexine is described as an expectorant by some authors, suggesting that the terms expectorant and mucolytic have a 'cross-over'. The mode of action is probably a combination of stimulation of:
- the gastro-pulmonary vagal reflex
- the vagal centre
- cholinergic fibres
- the bronchial glands.

Potassium iodide is capable of increasing secretions by 150%. There is direct stimulation of the submucosal bronchial glands because iodine accumulates in the gland. The drug should not be used in pregnant or hyperthyroid animals. Stimulant expectorants are used for coughing associated with chronic respiratory disease (however it should be noted that an irritant is likely to provoke further coughing). Guaifenesin is an example, as are carbon dioxide and certain sulphonamides. Guaifenesin is primarily a muscle relaxant used, in veterinary medicine, to provide balanced anaesthesia in conjunction with other anaesthetic drugs. It is added to cough mixtures in human medicine to help with the expectoration of airway secretions.

These substances thin airway mucus to increase airway clearance. Bromhexine and acetylcysteine as a 10% or 20% solution are the two most commonly

used mucolytics. Their method of action involves depolymerisation of glycoprotein molecules or hydrolysis of protein or nucleoprotein strands. By dissolving the chemical bonds in the mucus, it separates and liquefies, thereby reducing viscosity. Bromhexine also provokes an increase in immuno-globulins in respiratory secretions.

The viscosity of pulmonary mucus secretions depends on the concentrations of mucoproteins and deoxyribonucleic acid (DNA). While mucoprotein is the main determinant of viscosity in normal mucus, in purulent inflammation the mucoid concentration of DNA increases (due to increased cellular debris) and so does its contribution to mucoid viscosity.

Saline and acetylcysteine also have mucolytic properties – saline is a popular agent used for nebulisation, either on its own or as a carrier.

Cilia augmentors

These agents increase the beat frequency of airway cilia – salbutamol and clenbuterol are examples of adrenergic agents that work in this way. Other drugs include the expectorants and the cholinergic agents such as neostigmine that directly stimulate ciliary activity and bronchial secretions.

Antitussive agents

Antitussive agents:
- diminish the frequency of coughing
- should not be used to suppress productive coughs
- can be either locally acting (e.g. glycerin), or centrally acting (e.g. opiates)
- can be divided into opioid and non-opioid antitussives.

Butorphanol and codeine are potent opioid antitussives but may cause sedation, ataxia and excessive respiratory depression.

Dextromethorphan is a human licensed product and is the principal non-opioid antitussive available to veterinarians. It is almost as effective a cough suppressant as codeine but does not cause respiratory depression.

Diphenhydramine has anticholinergic, antihistamine and antitussive properties. Its antitussive mechanism of action remains unclear. It may cause mucus to dry out and the patient should therefore be encouraged to stay well hydrated. Recommended doses may provoke drowsiness and its value as an antitussive in veterinary medicine remains debatable.

Cough suppression may be indicated when clinical signs suggest that coughing is resolving and that further (chronic) coughing will only increase airway inflammation, increasing the risk of further mucosal irritation and further stimulation of cough receptors. Chronic coughing increases the risk of irreversible emphysema and there can therefore be a good reason for controlling coughing. Patients should be closely supervised and examined on a regular basis to ensure that secondary infections and other complications are detected early. These factors must be borne in mind when deciding on whether to issue a repeat prescription.

Anti-inflammatories

Both steroidal and non-steroidal anti-inflammatories play a valuable role in the management of respiratory symptoms and pathology. Rapid-acting steroid treatment is invaluable in the emergency treatment of acute respiratory distress and is indicated in severe pneumonia, anaphylaxis and inflammatory airway disease. Long-term treatment of chronic respiratory conditions will benefit from the judicious use of anti-inflammatories.

Bronchodilators

Bronchodilators are useful, as even a small reduction in airway diameter can have marked effects on expiratory effort. Bronchial tone is mediated by three physiological neuroendocrine systems:

1. The *parasympathetic* system. This is the dominant efferent (i.e. effector) pathway in mammals and is responsible for normal baseline bronchoconstrictive tone.
2. The *sympathetic* system. Bronchoconstrictive effects are mediated by $\alpha1$ adrenergic receptors and possibly by a $\beta2$-mediated reduction in parasympathetic bronchoconstriction. Bronchodilator effects are mediated by $\beta2$ adrenergic receptors.
3. The *non-adrenergic, non-cholinergic* system mediates bronchodilation via a number of neurotransmitters such as vasoactive intestinal peptide.

Bronchodilation can therefore be achieved via anticholinergic agents to counteract the effects of baseline parasympathetic tone. It may also be achieved using $\beta2$ adrenergic agonists. Methylxanthines and corticosteroids are also used for their bronchodilatory effects.

Anticholinergic drugs such as atropine decrease vagal tone in bronchiolar smooth muscle and so help some cases of bronchoconstriction. Their minimal efficacy is due to the fact that they only eliminate baseline vagal tone, which only accounts for a small amount of bronchoconstriction.

Terbutaline, albuterol and clenbuterol are $\beta2$ adrenergic agonists that act to produce smooth muscle relaxation and bronchodilation. They act on the sympathetic nervous system to cause relaxation of smooth muscle and bronchodilation but may cause nervousness, sweating and vomiting at high doses.

Caffeine, theophylline and theobromine are three naturally occurring methylxanthines. Aminophylline is the ethylenediamine complex of theophylline, which improves its solubility. Aminophylline and theophylline all possess the ability to relax smooth muscle. Side effects include vomiting and diarrhoea. Theophylline's method of action and effects are listed in Box 10.1.

The ability of corticosteroids to inhibit phospholipase enzymes in cell membranes prevents the formation of prostaglandins and leukotrienes, which are powerful bronchoconstrictives. The corticosteroids also counteract the effects of histamine.

Box 10.1

Methods of action and effects of theophylline

Methods of action
- increases intracellular cAMP levels (in bronchial smooth muscle)
- interferes with calcium mobilisation
- catecholamine release
- inhibits phosphodiesterase enzymes
- antagonises adenosine and prostaglandins

Effects
- produces bronchodilation through smooth muscle relaxation
- enhances mucociliary clearance
- stimulates the CNS (including the respiratory centre)
- increases sensitivity to $PaCO_2$
- increases diaphragmatic contractility
- stabilises mast cells and therefore reduces histamine release
- mild inotropic (stimulating) effect on the heart (it is a weak positive chronotrope and inotrope)
- mild diuretic

Mast cell stabilisers

Sodium cromoglycate is believed to inhibit the release of chemical mediators from mast cells in bronchial smooth muscle. In so doing, it can prevent the onset of bronchoconstriction. It has no direct effect on bronchial smooth muscle and does not directly antagonise inflammatory mediators. It is therefore predominantly used prophylactically.

Miscellaneous drugs acting on the respiratory system

- *Decongestants* produce vasoconstriction in mucous membranes, which reduces swelling and oedema. Phenylpropanolamine, a drug used to treat urinary sphincter incompetence, may also be useful in the management of nasal congestion due to its vasoconstrictive properties.
- *Antihistamines* such as chlorpheniramine and trimeprazine are used in the management of type 1 hypersensitivity reactions that are mediated by histamine. They also have a central action that can result in some relief of bronchospasm. The drowsiness seen in human patients is less commonly seen in dogs.
- *Respiratory analeptics* such as doxapram are occasionally used to stimulate the respiratory centres in the medulla. Their use is mostly limited to drug-induced respiratory depression and apnoea in the neonate. Over-dosage can excite the CNS and result in seizures. Naloxone is the antidote of choice in cases of opioid over-dosage and accidental etorphine injection.

Immunomodulators

Omalizumab has been developed for use in human patients suffering from asthma as it deals with the pathological processes triggered by airborne allergens. One of the causes of acute asthma is allergens entering the body, resulting in the production of IgE antibodies. A range of allergens can enter the body and bind to specific IgE immunoglobulins. They may gain access to the body via the digestive system (food items, e.g. peanuts), via the respiratory tree (airborne allergens) or across the skin and even ocular epithelium (e.g. pollen). The allergen–IgE complex binds to mast cells triggering the release of histamine – which can provoke severe broncho-constriction and inflammatory changes. Omalizumab is able to bind to the IgE and prevent it from interacting with mast cells, thus preventing the release of inflammatory mediators that lead to the symptoms of asthma.

Administering drugs by aerosolisation

Aerosol therapy or inhalation is a method of drug administration directly to the respiratory system. Because the drugs are deposited locally in the airways, aerosol therapy allows lower dosage, has a rapid action and minimises the incidence of side effects and systemic toxicity. The aerosol contains microdroplets of medication. It may be produced by nebuliser, metered-dose inhaler or dry powder inhaler relative to the physical aspect of the medica-tion (i.e. liquid, gas or solid, respectively).

Advantages

- Ensures the drug is delivered directly to the target organ, the respiratory mucosa and associated tissues.
- It helps to moisten the mucosa and encourages the mucus to move up the ciliary escalator.
- Systemic side effects are reduced.
- The problem of first-pass metabolism (when a drug is absorbed from the intestine and broken down in the liver before it reaches its target) is also eliminated.
- There is also the benefit to the compromised patient of minimal handling to administer the drugs. Figure 10.1 shows a cat receiving inhalation therapy via an Elizabethan collar covered with cling film.

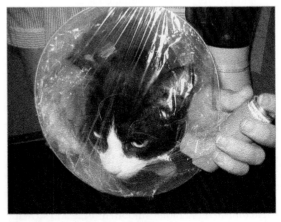

Fig. 10.1 Nebulisation of drugs

Disadvantages

- The irritant drug can cause reflex bronchoconstriction and therefore pre-treatment with a bronchodilator, 10 minutes prior to inhalational therapy, may be necessary. Products delivered by aerosolisation should be isotonic and should not contain certain irritant ingredients such as benzalkonium, EDTA, chlorbutol, edetic acid and metabisulphite.
- Much of the drug is deposited on the upper respiratory tract and oropharynx, nasal turbinates and oropharynx and little reaches the tracheobronchial tree.
- In chronic disease, respiration is shallow and rapid and most drug does not get further than the upper airways.

Indications

- Asthma
- Upper and lower respiratory tract infections
- Chronic bronchial diseases
- Diseases of the avian respiratory system (lungs and air sacs) – the poor vascularisation of air sac walls means that drug delivery to diseased air sacs is best achieved through nebulisation. Examples of drugs administered in this way include the disinfectant F10 and certain fluoroquinolone antibiotics.

Questions for Chapter 10

1. Prior to the administration of theophylline or aminophylline the patient's history should be checked for:
   a. use of antihistamines or nasal decongestants
   b. history of diabetes mellitus
   c. liver function tests
   d. history of glaucoma

2. An antitussive agent acts to:
   a. dissolve mucus
   b. suppress the cough reflex by acting on the medulla
   c. stimulate increased bronchial gland secretions
   d. reduce the release of leukotrienes

3. Guaifenesin is what type of drug?
   a. antitussive
   b. anti-inflammatory
   c. mucolytic
   d. β-adrenergic bronchodilator

4. Why does stabilisation of mast cells reduce signs of respiratory distress in allergic airway disease?
   a. prevents the release of histamine
   b. stimulates infiltration of basophils into the airways
   c. stimulates neutrophilic phagocytosis
   d. stimulates thrombocyte aggregation

5. Which of the following agents can be administered to avian patients by nebulisation?
   a. procaine penicillin
   b. lidocaine
   c. marbofloxacin
   d. neomycin

For answers go to page 242

Eleven

CHAPTER 11

Pharmaceutical Preparations used for the Cardiovascular System

Learning aims and objectives

After studying this chapter you should be able to:

1. **State the goals of therapy**
2. **Describe the treatment for arrhythmias**
3. **Describe how the different diuretics work**
4. **List the ACE inhibitors.**

Areas of cardiovascular medicine that benefit from medical therapy

Often the best treatment for cardiovascular (CV) disease is to remove the underlying cause, e.g. replacing a faulty valve. If this cannot be identified or surgically corrected then medical therapy is appropriate. The goals of therapy are shown in Box 11.1. Selection of an appropriate therapeutic agent depends on which aspects of the CV system are abnormal – the two main areas of therapy are cardiac arrhythmias and cardiac failure.

Medical management of arrhythmias

An arrhythmia is any variation from the normal heart beat. It may be caused by a faulty ignition system (diseased sinoatrial node) or damage to the specialised conducting system in the heart. A diagnosis should be made from an electrocardiogram before treatment is embarked on. A classification system of antidysrhythmic drugs was proposed by Vaughan Williams in 1970 – there are four classes:

1A. membrane stabilisers – quinidine, procainamide, disopyramide
1B. membrane stabilisers, increase ventricular fibrillation threshold and cause a shortened action potential – lidocaine, tocainide, mepivacaine, phenytoin

Box 11.1

Management of cardiovascular disorders

Control salt and water retention/relieve oedema

- low-sodium diets
- loop, thiazide, potassium-sparing diuretics
- venous and mixed vasodilators
- ACE inhibitors
- physical removal of fluid

Improve pump function

- improve diastolic filling
  - control heart rate
  - abolish arrhythmia
  - improve ventricular relaxation
- improve contractility
  - digitalis glycosides
  - calcium sensitisers
  - sympathomimetic drugs
- reverse or modify myocardial and vascular remodelling
  - ACE inhibitors
  - β-blocking agents

Reduce workload

- reduce workload
  - ACE inhibitors
  - arterial or mixed vasodilators
- reduce physical activity
- avoid environmental stressors
- weight reduction in the obese

2. adrenergic blockers – propranolol
3. prolong the cardiac action potential – rarely used in veterinary medicine
4. calcium channel blockers – verapamil, diltiazem.

Animals with symptomatic bradydysrhythmias typically present with syncope and exercise intolerance. Bradyarrhythmias are likely to require implantation of a cardiac pacemaker as animals with diseases of the cardiac pacemaking and/or conduction system are likely to be unresponsive to parasympatholytic agents. Where signs are mild, or if pacemaker implantation is not possible, medical therapy can be attempted. Suitable treatments include:

- atropine sulphate
- β sympathomimetics such as isoprenaline, dopamine and terbutaline.

Tachyarrhythmias may mean the heart beats too rapidly to permit filling in diastole or too irregularly to permit ejection of sufficient quantities of blood in systole. Drugs that slow atrioventricular (AV) nodal conduction are useful in converting to sinus rhythm. These include:

- the cardiac glycosides
- β-blocking agents
- calcium blocking agents
- lidocaine and quinidine (used to slow the impulse conduction velocity).

Medical management of cardiac failure

1. Rest and restricted dietary sodium intake
2. Preload reduction – dietary sodium restriction, diuresis, venodilation
3. Vasodilator drugs (venodilators and arteriodilators)
4. Angiotensin-converting enzyme (ACE) inhibitors
5. Positive inotropes
6. Negative inotropes.

Medications used to strengthen systolic force

Positive inotropes such as digitalis and dobutamine increase myocardial contractility. Digoxin is a cardiac glycoside derived from the purple foxglove plant (Latin name: *Digitalis*). The action of the therapeutic agent is to increase cytosolic sodium via inhibition of the sodium/potassium ATPase pump in the cell membrane. The build up of intracellular sodium inhibits a Na^+/Ca^{2+} pump due to the reduced sodium concentration across the sarcolemma, causing intracellular Ca^{2+} to build up. This causes an increase in the tension in cardiac muscle cells during contraction, without increasing the oxygen requirements of the heart.

Increased inotropy is also facilitated by the negative chronotropic property of the drug. Digoxin is therefore the drug of choice for dilated cardiomyopathy and atrial fibrillation, where both the positive inotropic effect and the negative chronotropic effect are beneficial. Digoxin has a narrow margin of safety/therapeutic index so thorough screening of patients is required prior to digoxin therapy. Monitoring serum drug levels helps to detect and prevent toxicity problems.

Pharmacokinetics of digoxin

In general, absorption across cell membranes and the extent of protein binding is directly proportional to the drug's lipid solubility and therefore inversely proportional to the drug's polarity. The number of hydroxyl groups on the steroid nucleus determines polarity – digoxin has only one steroidal hydroxyl group (Fig. 11.1) and is therefore relatively non-polar, meaning:

- it is well absorbed after oral administration
- it is highly bound to plasma proteins (about 25% is bound to albumin)
- it undergoes metabolic breakdown.

Digoxin is excreted by the kidneys, so any disease affecting the plasma protein levels or renal function will affect the dose required. Digitalis glycosides follow an enterohepatic recycling, in which compounds are excreted by the liver into the bile and some parent drug and its metabolites are reabsorbed, thereby potentiating the action of the drug.

The clinical signs of digitalis intoxication vary from mild GI signs to severe weight loss and life-threatening arrhythmias. Anorexia and loose stools are common side effects of digoxin therapy; vomiting occasionally occurs. Cardiac toxicity of digoxin is affected by the availability of electrolytes, especially calcium and potassium. As the drug competes with potassium, hypokalaemia will predispose to digoxin toxicity. Hypokalaemia can be induced by malnutrition, corticosteroid therapy and overuse of non-potassium-sparing diuretics. All these factors should be considered before deciding if toxicity is due to an actual digoxin overdose or a relative overdose caused by potassium disturbances. Clinical indications for digoxin therapy are:

- congestive heart failure
- atrial arrhythmias
- pre-treatment for heart surgery.

Dobutamine

Dobutamine is an agent that mimics the sympathetic nervous system, increasing the force of the heart's contraction and dilating the mesenteric and renal vessels. This means it is a better choice of drug in renally compromised patients. Dobutamine infusions are usually indicated for acute myocardial failure for positive inotropic support.

Diuresis

In cardiac failure, the ventricles fail to move blood from the venous circulation to the arterial circulation – consequently, 'backwards failure' occurs. The venous circulation becomes overloaded and its capillary beds become engorged with blood. Serum oozes out from the capillaries into the interstitial spaces. If the rate of oozing exceeds the rate at which the lymphatics can drain, tissue oedema occurs and the animal is in congestive heart failure.

Diuretics are drugs that act on the kidneys to increase the production of urine. The various classes of diuretics induce a diuresis and often a natriuresis. By preventing the reabsorption of sodium that is necessary to concentrate urine, an increased volume of urine is produced, reducing the circulating blood volume, ECF volume, preload and ultimately oedema and effusions. Blood pressure is also lowered. The diuretics available all work on a different part of the nephrons making up the kidney, as shown in Figure 11.2. The different diuretics vary in their ability to induce diuresis – some of the available drugs are discussed below.

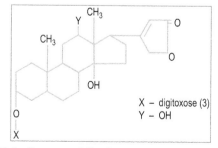

Fig. 11.1   Structure of digoxin

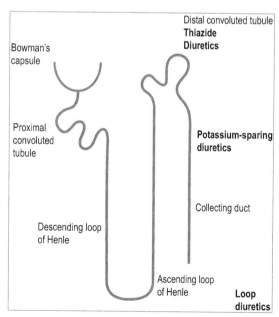

Fig. 11.2   Sites of action of diuretics on the kidney nephron

Thiazide diuretics

Thiazide diuretics, e.g. hydrochlorothiazide (Moduretic) and chlorothiazide (Saluric), act on the distal convoluted tubule, inhibiting resorption of sodium ions. They result in moderate diuresis and natriuresis and are associated with potassium loss, especially if combined with a loop diuretic. The thiazides are ineffective when the renal blood supply is low and so they are not very effective in severe congestive heart failure. They should be used carefully in animals with a prerenal azotaemia as they decrease glomerular filtration rate. They are also used to inhibit lactation in pseudopregnancy.

Loop diuretics

Loop diuretics, e.g. furosemide (Lasix), are very potent with rapid onset of action. They remain effective in the presence of reduced renal perfusion. Parenteral administration (i.v. or i.m. at 8 mg/kg) should be used in emergencies. It is often advisable to add a potassium-sparing diuretic to keep the dose of furosemide low. Loop diuretics act by inhibiting the resorption of electrolytes (Na^+, Cl^- and water) in the ascending loop of Henle. Furosemide also decreases reabsorption of sodium and chloride in the distal renal tubule. The diuresis results in enhanced excretion of sodium, chloride, potassium, hydrogen, calcium, magnesium and possibly phosphate.

Potassium-sparing diuretics

Potassium-sparing diuretics, e.g. spironolactone, are mild diuretics, used in combination with other diuretics to reduce potassium loss. The drug is well absorbed by the gastrointestinal tract and rapidly and extensively metabolised to the active product, canrenone, which is structurally similar to aldosterone. Its effects result from competitive binding to aldosterone binding sites in the distal tubule. It is thought that spironolactone can reduce myocardial fibrosis in patients with heart disease and may help to restore normal baroreceptor function in heart failure. However spironolactone interferes with the synthesis of testosterone and may result in endocrine abnormalities. Hyperkalaemia may result with concurrent use of NSAIDs, ACE inhibitors or potassium supplements.

Other examples of potassium-sparing diuretics include triamterene and amiloride, which have the additional effects of prolonging action potential duration and causing vasodilation. Potassium-sparing diuretics should generally be avoided if ACE inhibitors are also being used, as ACE inhibitors also act as aldosterone antagonists.

Vasodilators

These are drugs that relax vascular smooth muscle and reduce the afterload of the heart by decreasing the resistance of the systemic arterioles. Some agents act on the venous vessels, such as nitroglycerine 2% ointment (Percutol), some on the arterioles and some on both (termed balanced vasodilators). Table 11.1 shows the site and mechanism of action of the vasodilators. In veterinary medicine, these drugs are used to:

- reduce preload and afterload in patients with congestive heart failure
- reduce the regurgitant flow and left atrial pressure in patients with mitral valve disease
- manage systemic hypertension from a primary cause or secondary to disease such as hyperthyroidism.

Prazocin is an α adrenoceptor antagonist which is a short-acting but potent vasodilator. It causes a fall in arterial blood pressure and can be used to treat hypertension. Drugs that cause vasodilation should not be used in patients with hypotension (thready pulses, hypothermia, weakness) or those with outflow obstructions of the heart such as sub-aortic stenosis.

Table 11.1 Site and mechanism of action of the vasodilators

Site of action	Mechanism of action	Agent
Venodilators	Nitrates (direct acting)	Glyceryl trinitrate
Arteriolar dilators	Direct acting Calcium channel blockers	Hydralazine
Balanced vasodilators	Direct acting, alpha-adrenergic antagonists, angiotensin-converting enzyme (ACE) inhibitors	Nitroprusside Prazosin Enalapril Benazepril Captopril

Potential problems of treating congestive heart failure with vasodilators exist. It has been assumed that drug-induced vasodilation would automatically increase peripheral perfusion and thereby increase oxygen availability to all tissues. However, vaso-dilator agents of the nitroglycerin type exert a reduction in peripheral resistance and a pooling of blood in the venous beds. This does not necessarily mean the blood gets into all tissues. Furthermore, if arterial pressure is critically reduced, blood flow through coronary and renal vessels may be compro-mised further, causing injury to these organs. Reflex tachycardia and increased myocardial demand is another potential problem associated with a fall in blood pressure.

The ACE inhibitors are the most important balanced vasodilators.

Angiotensin-converting enzyme (ACE) inhibitors

In congestive heart failure both backwards and forwards failure are seen – these are intimately linked as a fall in cardiac output stimulates the juxta-glomerular apparatus in the kidneys and induces the renin–angiotensin–aldosterone system (RAAS). The net effect is sodium and water retention, which increases plasma volume, increases preload and ultimately results in pulmonary oedema and/or ascites.

ACE is a rather non-specific enzyme that cleaves dipeptide units off polypeptides. It is responsible for the conversion of angiotensin I to II and also for the breakdown of the potent vasodilator bradykinin. Inhibition of the ACE enzyme will therefore inhibit the production of angiotensin II and allow the build up of bradykinin. Angiotensin II is a potent vaso-constrictor. It is broken down further into angiotensin III, which stimulates aldosterone secretion and is involved with thirst.

When heart failure occurs the body attempts to compensate by activating the sympathetic nervous system to constrict the blood vessels and increase the heart rate to raise the blood pressure. The RAAS is also activated, further impairing the function of the heart. ACE inhibitors act by:

- preventing the conversion of angiotensin I to angiotensin II, stopping the release of aldosterone from the adrenal cortex and therefore lowering the blood pressure
- inducing vasodilation directly and improving haemodynamics by decreasing systemic vascular resistance by 25–30%
- protecting the kidneys – levels of bradykinin and renoprotective prostaglandins are allowed to accumulate

Box 11.2
ACE inhibitors

- Benazepril (Fortekor; Novartis)
- Enalapril (Enacard; Merial)
- Ramipril (Vasotop; Intervet)
- Captopril (Capoten; Squibb)

- preventing remodelling and fibrosis of the myocardium and vascular smooth muscle.

Box 11.2 lists the commonly used ACE inhibitors. It is difficult to determine the optimal dose for any ACE inhibitor or to compare the relative efficacy of the drugs available. It is suggested that once-daily dosing is sufficient, however giving an ACE inhibitor every 12 hours may be preferable to increasing the diuretic dose.

Calcium channel blockers

Calcium is necessary for the function of various excitable cells, therefore preventing its entry can be useful in a number of disorders. The drugs cause:
- arteriolar dilation in both coronary and peripheral arterial beds
- decreased force of contraction of the heart (negative inotrope)
- slowed AV nodal impulse conduction velocity (negative chronotrope)
- reduced oxygen demand by the myocardium
- reduced resistance to blood leaving the left ventricle.

The mechanism of action of the calcium channel blockers is to inhibit calcium influx and the asso-ciated calcium-dependent physiological responses of affected cells as shown in Figure 11.3. They do this in one of the following ways:
- interacting with specific calcium binding sites on cell membranes
- plugging the outer orifice of the calcium channel pores
- gaining access to the cytoplasmic side of the cell to interfere with channel operation.

Box 11.3 lists the clinical applications.

The two agents in this group of veterinary interest are diltiazem (Hypercard) and verapamil (Cordilox; Abbott). Diltiazem is a less potent negative inotropic than verapamil and may therefore be used more safely in animals with systolic dysfunction or con-gestive failure. Calcium channel blockers are pre-ferred to propranolol for the management of feline

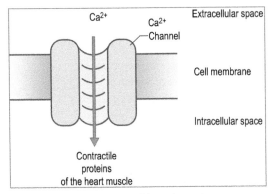

Fig. 11.3   Cell membrane calcium channels

Box 11.3

Clinical applications of the calcium channel blockers

- Supraventricular tachyarrhythmias – they do not convert the arrhythmia to normal sinus rhythm but effectively reduce the AV conduction and therefore reduce the ventricular rate
- Heart failure – myocardial contractile failure, valvular insufficiencies, obstructive cardiomyopathies
- Hypertrophic cardiomyopathy
- Circulatory shock and trauma

---

hypertrophic cardiomyopathy because they improve myocardial relaxation, optimise diastolic filling and dilate coronary vasculature. Verapamil is also effective in the management of hypertension, but to a lesser degree than amlodipine. In rabbits verapamil can be used perioperatively to minimise formation of surgical adhesions. The adverse effects include:

- hypotension (dizziness and fatigue are reported in humans)
- bradycardia (the most common side effect in dogs) or tachycardia
- nausea or vomiting (the most common side effect in cats) and constipation.

Use is contraindicated in patients with severe left ventricular dysfunction. It is also contraindicated in patients with severe hepatic disease as they may have a reduced capacity to metabolise the drug – the dose should be reduced by 70%. Cimetidine inhibits the metabolism of these agents, increasing their plasma concentrations. Verapamil and diltiazem

displace protein-bound drugs from plasma proteins, thereby enhancing their actions, and also increase cellular levels of vincristine by inhibiting its release from the cells.

Pimobendan (Vetmedin)

This inodilator agent has a dual method of action, acting:

1. directly on the heart as a calcium sensitiser to increase myocardial contractility (Fig. 11.4) and
2. on the peripheral circulation through selective phosphodiesterase III inhibition to produce both peripheral and coronary vasodilation.

It has shown promise in the treatment of dilated cardiomyopathy when used with other drugs such as furosemide, ACE inhibitors and digoxin.

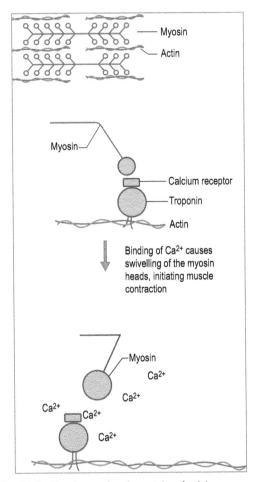

Fig. 11.4   How increasing the uptake of calcium increases myocardial contractility

Beta (β)-blocking agents

The β-blockers are in the class 2 anti-arrhythmic drug group and are negative inotropes and negative chronotropes. They may therefore be beneficial for cats with hypertrophic cardiomyopathy, restrictive cardiomyopathy and patients with pressure over-loaded ventricles (aortic stenosis, pulmonic stenosis, tetralogy of Fallot). They are the drug of choice in cats with hyperthyroidism as many of the cardio-vascular effects of this condition are mediated by catecholamines.

The aim of therapy is to reduce the heart rate and improve ventricular filling. In dogs with left ventricular hypertrophy secondary to severe aortic stenosis or right ventricular hypertrophy secondary to severe pulmonic stenosis, β-blockers remain the drug of choice. They improve filling by slowing the heart rate and they protect against malignant ventricular arrhythmias, a common cause of sudden death in animals with severe aortic stenosis.

Propranolol and the related β-blockers are similar in structure with an isopropyl-substituted second-ary amine on the carbon side chain, as shown in Figure 11.5. This is important for effective interaction with the β receptor. They cause minimal depression of heart rate, myocardial contractile force and cardiac output during normal conditions because at rest the heart is not under sympathetic tone. However, if the heart is stressed, a relative bradycardia, de-creased myocardial contractility and a reduction in cardiac output is produced. Propranolol prevents the positive inotropic and chronotropic effects of catecholamines in the heart and reduces their arrhythmogenic effects. Figure 11.6 shows the basic pathways involved in the medullary control of blood pressure and the mechanism by which propranolol stops the cycle. β-blockers affect blood pressure primarily through their effects on cardiac output rather than peripheral vascular effects and cause bronchiolar constriction by inhibiting sympathetic bronchodilator activity.

Clinical uses are in:
- hypertension
- cardiac dysrhythmias
- hypertrophic obstructive cardiomyopathies
- hyperthyroidism
- glaucoma
- lowering myocardial oxygen demand in chronic heart failure.

Adverse effects are most frequently seen in geriatric patients with chronic heart disease or in patients with rapidly decompensating heart failure because patients in congestive heart failure tend to be very dependent on their sympathetic drive. They include:
- bradycardia
- impaired AV conduction
- myocardial depression
- heart failure
- syncope
- bronchospasm
- diarrhoea
- peripheral vasoconstriction

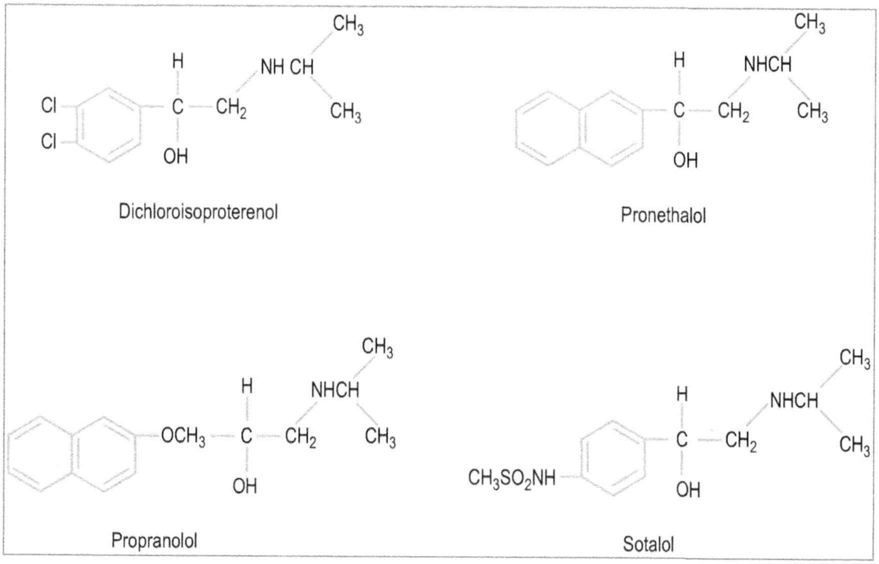

Fig. 11.5 Chemical structures of some β-adrenergic blocking drugs

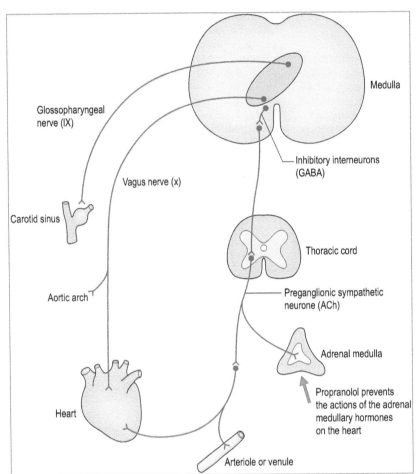

Fig. 11.6 The control of blood pressure by the medulla and the mechanism by which propranolol stops an increase from occurring

- enhancement of the hypoglycaemic effects of insulin
- depression and lethargy as a result of the high lipid solubility and penetration into the CNS.

Drug interactions occur with:
- anaesthetic agents – enhances the hypotensive effects of propranolol
- phenothiazines, antihypertensives, diazepam, diuretics, anti-arrhythmics
- calcium-channel blockers – increases the risk of hypotension
- digoxin – potentiates the bradycardia
- thyroid hormones – increases metabolism of atenolol, therefore reduces the dose of atenolol when initiating carbimazole therapy
- muscle relaxants – effects are enhanced
- phenobarbital – increases the rate of metabolism of atenolol
- theophylline – bronchodilatory effects are blocked by atenolol.

Strengthening muscles of ventilation

These may be weakened due to poor oxygenation and may be required to work harder to ventilate oedematous lungs. Aminophylline and digitalis both increase the strength of contraction of the diaphragm and aminophylline also causes dilation of the small airways.

Restoring blood volume

Haemorrhage and dehydration reduce the preload (the amount of blood returning to the heart). Because of the Frank–Starling relationship between the stretch of the heart chambers and the subsequent force of contraction of the heart, the cardiac output is reduced. Agents that can be used to ensure adequate preload include whole blood, plasma, crystalloid and colloid solutions.

Questions for Chapter 11

1. What is meant by inotropic stimulation of the heart?

2. What affects the heart's demand for oxygen?

3. What does the glycoside part of digitalis glycoside mean?

4. What are the therapeutic responses of the heart to digitalis therapy?

5. Would enalapril reduce or increase the following parameters?
   a. heart rate
   b. mean blood pressure
   c. pulmonary arterial pressure

6. What effect do the calcium channel-blocking drugs have on the heart?

7. Why is diuretic therapy alone not good for failing hearts?

For answers go to page 242

Twelve

CHAPTER 12

Pharmaceutical Preparations used for the Gastrointestinal Tract

Learning aims and objectives

After studying this chapter you should be able to:

1. **Relate the relevant physiology to the science of pharmacology**
2. **Describe how laxatives and cathartics work**
3. **Explain the mechanism of action of the anti-emetics**
4. **List the anti-ulcer treatments**
5. **List the antidiarrhoeal treatments.**

Digestive system

Major processes involved in digestion include motility of the gastrointestinal (GI) tract, glandular and epithelial secretions, absorption of end products and elimination of materials not absorbed from the gut. Several factors influence this including metabolic and electrophysiological responses in the glands and smooth muscle and haemodynamic events that occur in the GI circulation. In addition, the autonomic nervous system and circulating and locally acting hormones play a role. Agents are used therapeutically because of their influence on one or more of these physiological functions.

The stomach has many protective mechanisms against ulceration which can be exploited by drug therapy (Fig. 12.1). They include:

- bicarbonate secretion to neutralise gastric acid
- alkaline mucus to protect against hydrochloride and bile acids
- the rapid turnover of mucosal cells to repair any damage
- mucosal blood flow removing any H^+ ions that have penetrated the protective barriers
- mechanisms to control gastric hydrochloric acid secretion
- scavenging of mediators capable of cell damage.

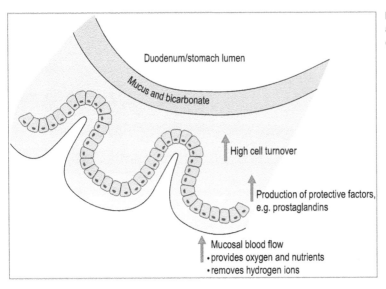

Fig. 12.1 Protective mechanisms against gastric ulceration which can be exploited by drug therapy

Laxatives and cathartics

These promote defaecation by increasing frequency or by altering faecal consistency. Laxatives promote elimination of a soft-formed stool whereas cathartics (purgatives) tend to produce a more fluid evacuation. Box 12.1 lists some drug interactions. Increasing the fluid content of the stool often helps to increase the volume and can be useful for cleansing of the bowel prior to radiography or endoscopy, to help eliminate a toxin from the gut or to decrease tenesmus after anal surgery.

Laxatives may be simple lubricants, such as paraffin and glycerine, or stimulant laxatives that work via an irritant effect on the mucosa, such as emodin and castor oil. These drugs have potent effects and over-dosage can result in excessive fluid and electrolyte loss. Lactulose works by increasing the osmotic pressure in the bowel, thereby drawing water into the gut. This causes a laxative effect and acidifies the colonic contents. It can be used orally or rectally but excessive doses cause flatulence and

cramping. Certain foods have laxative properties, including honey and prunes.

Emetics

Emesis is a protective reflex that is not well developed in all species; horses and rabbits, for example, are unable to vomit. Dogs and cats, by contrast, have developed a protective vomiting reflex and vomit readily in response to particular stimuli. Motion, acting via the vestibular apparatus, can trigger vomiting. Triggers act on the chemoreceptor trigger zone (CRTZ) to provoke the vomiting reflex. Common triggers include:

- inflammatory mediators/toxins such as those produced in uraemia and pyometra
- drugs such as apomorphine, digitalis and xylazine
- stimulation of the oropharynx and irritation of various visceral organs.

All these result in the emptying of the anterior portion of the digestive tract. Indications include induction of general anaesthesia if there is food in the stomach or after ingestion of non-corrosive poisons. Emetics can be split into:
- *Reflex emetics* – distension of the stomach with saline or hydrogen peroxide (3%) results in emesis. Ipecac syrup has been used for many years in children and cats but has been known to induce toxic effects including death. Box 12.2 illustrates the dangers of such preparations.
- *Centrally acting emetics* – opiates such as apomorphine are commonly used as they

Box 12.2

Important safety point

- Fatal aspiration of hydrogen peroxide foam after emesis is possible and this method of inducing emesis is not therefore recommended where safer options are available

produce little sedation and predictable vomiting after only a few minutes. Xylazine (Rompun) is an α2 agonist sedative drug that at low doses (0.05 mg/kg) produces emesis in dogs but is less reliable in cats. Apomorphine is difficult to obtain in the UK and xylazine is readily available in large animal practice but less so in small animal practices.

Anti-emetics

These drugs have a role to play both in gastrointestinal disease and as adjuncts to therapies that cause vomiting, such as some cancer treatments. Antiemetics are strongly indicated where:
- the patient is vomiting so severely that there is a risk of dehydration
- the vomiting is making the patient very distressed
- the client requests that the vomiting be stopped.

The most common veterinary example is metoclopramide. It is important when using these agents to determine the cause of the vomiting prior to administration as the signs of an intestinal obstruction may be masked by the treatment, or worse – stimulation of gastrointestinal motility at the site of blockage can result in damage to the wall of the GI tract and even cause perforation. The route of administration is important when using anti-emetics as GI disease may make oral absorption unreliable and may make the vomiting worse. Therefore where possible, these agents should be administered parenterally.

Vomiting is a reflex act that is coordinated through the vomiting centre in the medulla. Figure 12.2 illustrates the various ways in which vomiting can be triggered. Certain stimuli act directly on the CRTZ, others act via different parts of the central nervous system (CNS), such as the vestibular apparatus and cerebral cortex. Anti-emetics block one of the pathways involved and the choice of drug depends on the underlying cause.

Metoclopramide, a procainamide derivative, works both centrally, within the central nervous system, and locally, on the GI tract. In the CNS it acts on the CRTZ, blocking dopamine receptors. It increases oesophageal sphincter pressure and

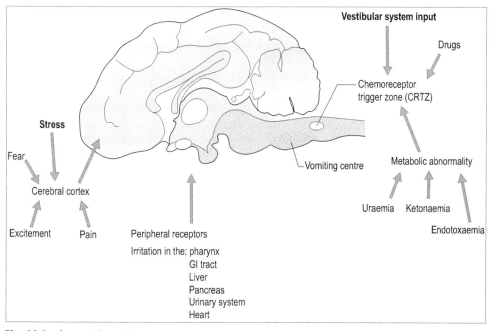

Fig. 12.2 Control of vomiting

increases peristaltic activity within the duodenum, thereby hastening gastric emptying. Adverse effects are rare, but restlessness and excitement have been reported and it should not be used in epileptics or in suspected cases of gastric obstruction. Due to its short half-life, a continuous i.v. infusion is recommended in acute, severe vomiting.

Antihistamines are effective anti-emetics in dogs and cats, when nausea is caused by motion sickness or dysfunction of the vestibular apparatus. They block vomiting at the CRTZ but may cause sedation. Diphenhydramine is an example of a drug in this category. Trimethobenzamide hydrochloride, another centrally acting anti-emetic, has actions similar to those of the antihistamines.

Anticholinergics are not very effective in controlling vomiting although they are occasionally used for this purpose. They are peripherally acting anti-emetics, effective in reducing gastrointestinal spasms and secretions. Atropine is one of the few agents that can penetrate the blood–brain barrier to act centrally. The side effects include:

- xerostomia
- mydriasis
- tachycardia
- urinary retention
- gastric retention (which can lead to vomiting itself).

Domperidone (Motilium) is a powerful anti-emetic with antidopaminergic actions, but does not easily cross the blood–brain barrier and so has few adverse CNS effects. It accelerates gastric emptying and increases gastric contractions.

Anti-ulcer drugs

Damage to the mucosal lining of the stomach, or gastric ulceration, can arise for various reasons but is most commonly associated with the administration of ulcerogenic drugs. Clinical signs include vomiting, anorexia and pain. Bleeding from the site of ulceration may be seen in the vomitus, either as fresh blood or as digested blood (coffee grounds). Digested blood may also be seen in the faeces, which can appear tarry black (melaenic). The aims behind treatment are to:

- remove the cause
- maintain mucosal perfusion to promote healing
- decrease gastric acidity because although pepsin and bile acids contribute to mucosal damage, ulcers do not usually occur if the pH is greater than 7
- protect the ulcer.

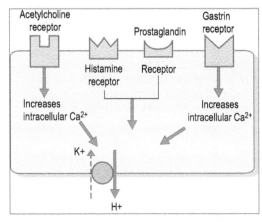

Fig. 12.3 Regulation of gastric acid secretion by the parietal cell

Figure 12.3 illustrates the control of gastric acid secretion by the parietal cell. Gastric acidity can be reduced medically by the following groups of drugs:

- anticholinergics
- histamine (H_2) receptor antagonists
- proton pump inhibitors
- prostaglandin E_2 analogues.

Box 12.3 details the adverse effects.

H_2-receptor antagonists

These block histamine receptors in the gastric parietal cells, thus reducing HCl production. Cimetidine (Tagamet) and ranitidine (Zantac) are the most commonly used in both human and veterinary medicine. Ranitidine is less hepatotoxic and more potent than cimetidine. Cimetidine is rapidly absorbed from the GI tract and undergoes hepatic metabolism before being excreted in the urine in an unchanged form. Ranitidine is less bioavailable following oral administration and is also metabolised in the liver. Both drugs have the potential to be hepatotoxic. Box 12.4 lists some drug interactions.

Cimetidine causes a reduction in hepatic blood flow – which has implications for the metabolism of other drugs that rely on the liver for their metabolism and excretion. Drugs such as lidocaine, morphine and propranolol should not therefore be administered

Drug interactions

- Cimetidine should not be given with food as this can delay the absorption process
- Ranitidine is unaffected by the presence of food and therefore can be given with meals
- Neither drug should be given at the same time as sucralfate, digoxin, ketoconazole or metoclopramide

Dispensing tip

- Clients must not sprinkle the contents of the omeprazole capsule onto food as the drug will be destroyed in the stomach

concurrently with cimetidine. Cimetidine also inhibits the liver enzyme cytochrome P-450, slowing the metabolism of many other drugs that are biotransformed in the liver.

Proton pump inhibitors

Omeprazole is a proton pump inhibitor that is 30× as potent as cimetidine in its ability to increase gastric pH. It is unstable in an acid environment and is formulated as encapsulated enteric-coated granules. The drug is released in the alkaline environment of the intestines. It takes up to 5 days before maximum effect is seen and the effects last for some time after the drug is discontinued. The drug can therefore be administered once a day (Box 12.5).

Antacids

By neutralising gastric acid and inactivating pepsin, antacids promote healing of gastric ulcers. To prevent rebound over-secretion of gastric acid they must be given frequently (every 2–4 hours). The most commonly used agents contain:
- sodium, aluminium, magnesium, bismuth or calcium as the cation
- hydroxides, carbonate or bicarbonate as the anion.

Side effects depend on the drug chosen and include:
- hypernatraemia and systemic alkalosis from sodium bicarbonate
- hypercalcaemia and constipation from calcium salts

Dispensing tip

- Sucralfate decreases the availability of antacids and should be given 2 hours before these drugs

- phosphate depletion and constipation from aluminium hydroxide
- hypermagnesemia and diarrhoea in patients on magnesium salts with renal insufficiency.

Other anti-ulcer medications

Cytoprotective drugs include misoprostol (Cytotec) and sucralfate (Antepsin). Misoprostol works by mimicking the action of the natural prostaglandins and increases mucus and bicarbonate secretion whilst increasing mucosal blood flow and epithelialisation of the mucosa. The main indication for use is for treatment or prevention of damage by NSAIDs.

Sucralfate is an orally administered disaccharide that binds to and protects the ulcerated site from acid, bile and pepsin activity (Box 12.6). It also binds epidermal growth factor, causing it to accumulate in the ulcer site, and increases blood flow to the mucosa. The only reported side effect is constipation. It binds more effectively in an acid pH so it should not be given at the same time as any drugs that lower acid production (such as cimetidine). It will also bind locally to several drugs and should not be given with tetracycline and phenytoin. A 2-hour gap between medications should be allowed if therapies must be given concurrently.

Antidiarrhoeal medications

Diarrhoea is an increased frequency, volume or fluidity of the faeces. Intestinal hypermotility is often incorrectly associated with diarrhoea when, in fact, intestinal hypomotility is often present – allowing the free flow of intestinal contents without the benefit of segmental contractions to delay transit and allow for more thorough digestion and absorption. Drugs used to treat diarrhoea are listed below.

Narcotic analgesics

Opiates and opioids are used to slow gastrointestinal transit time. Morphine has been widely used in conjunction with kaolin as an oral treatment for diarrhoea, but is now difficult to come by. Loperamide is a synthetic opiate available over the counter. Their effects on the GI tract include:

- increase segmental contractions
- decrease intestinal secretions
- increase intestinal absorption of luminal fluids, electrolytes and glucose.

Protectants and adsorbents

Protectants and adsorbents coat the GI mucosa and bind bacteria and toxins. An additional therapeutic benefit of increased intestinal absorption of fluid is seen with products containing bismuth subsalicylate.

These compounds are not absorbed from the GI tract and either line the mucosal surface (protectants) or adsorb toxic compounds which are then excreted in the faeces (adsorbents). They are often incorporated into antidiarrheal mixtures and include kaolin (aluminium silicate), bismuth salts, pectin and activated charcoal. Charcoal preparations vary according to the source of the base material, which may be lignite, wood or peat. Activation forms more pores and enlarges the surface area and therefore capacity for drug binding. Herbal tree bark is marketed for use in acute cases of diarrhoea.

Antibiotics

These are often inappropriate as they destroy the normal protective microflora and allow colonisation of the mucosa by potential pathogens.

- Primary pathogens include *Salmonella*, *Campylobacter jejuni* and *Yersinia enterocolitica*. Drug therapy should theoretically be based on culture and sensitivity.
- Bacterial overgrowth can be treated with penicillins or oxytetracycline.
- Metronidazole is useful for giardiasis, trichomoniasis and small intestinal bacterial overgrowth.

Anti-inflammatories

Inflammatory bowel disease is a common cause of GI signs in dogs and cats. The inflammatory infiltrate is usually lymphoplasmacytic and the condition is of multifactorial origin. Stress and dietary intolerance are incriminated as causative factors and should be addressed as part of the management of this condition. Where possible, patients should be managed without steroids as they might affect the interpretation and diagnostic reliability of any biopsies taken to confirm the diagnosis at a later date. Steroids can, however, be highly effective in conjunction with dietary and other therapies – both prednisolone and methylprednisolone can be used.

Methylprednisolone has less mineralocorticoid activity than prednisolone; it is therefore particularly indicated in cases with concurrent cardiovascular disease or in dogs that become excessively polyuric.

In animals that are poorly responsive, or require long-term treatment, steroid therapy can be administered per rectum as an enema, allowing high concentrations to be achieved locally whilst minimising systemic toxicity.

Budesonide is a steroid that shows considerable first-pass metabolism and can be used orally to treat intestinal disease with fewer side effects. It is unlicensed and the dose rate of 3 mg/m^2/day orally has been based on clinical experience.

Immunosupressants

These include the following:

- Ciclosporin (cyclosporine) (Atopica) is a fungal metabolite and potent immunosuppressant that acts as a T lymphocyte inhibitor. It can cause anorexia and allow opportunistic infections to develop.
- Azathioprine can be toxic in cats but is commonly used to manage irritable bowel syndrome in dogs. Haematological monitoring is required as severe bone marrow disease can occur in some patients.
- Chlorambucil is the treatment of choice in cats and non-steroid-responsive cases in dogs. Immunosuppression is a major side effect.
- Cyclophosphamide (Endoxana) treatment has the same side effects discussed above. These side effects are more commonly seen than with the other treatments. It remains a popular therapy despite being a potent cytotoxic drug.

Appetite stimulants

Appetite is controlled primarily by the hypothalamus and several neurotransmitters have been identified as stimulants or suppressants. In veterinary medicine it is often necessary to increase appetite, e.g. in renal failure cats or in cachexic, anorexic dogs with cancer. Drugs that promote gastric emptying such as metoclopramide (Emequell) have had some success in increasing appetite. In human medicine, megestrol acetate (Ovarid) is used in patients with advanced cancer in preference to anabolic steroids in order to avoid the adverse side effects associated with the latter group of drugs.

The benzodiazepines, such as diazepam (Valium), have been commonly used to stimulate appetite in cats due to suppression of the part of the brain that controls satiety. After i.v. administration of

Box 12.7

Contraindication

- Repeated oral administration of diazepam to cats results in hepatic necrosis (liver failure) and so should not be used as a method of assisted feeding long-term

0.5 mg/kg cats start to eat within a few seconds. However, sedation can be seen in some cats at this dose, whereas others can show no signs of sedation at doses of 2 mg/kg (Box 12.7).

Modulators of gastric motility

- Prokinetics enhance the transport of intestinal contents but their use is limited by their tendency to cause systemic effects.

- Metoclopramide effects are limited to the upper intestinal tract, promoting peristalsis in the duodenum and jejunum.
- Cisapride (Prepulsid) has the broadest spectrum of the prokinetic agents. It causes dose-dependent increased activity at all sites, including the colon, and hence has been used in the management of feline idiopathic megacolon. This drug is no longer available as it was marketed for use in humans and was withdrawn due to reported cardiac irregularities.
- Anticholinergic agents (parasympathetic antagonists) diminish motor and secretory activity of the GI tract through their action on muscarinic receptors. This often results in relaxation of spasm of visceral smooth muscle. These effects make them popular in antidiarrhoeal mixtures but care must be taken not to cause intestinal paralysis (ileus). Butylscopolamine (Buscopan) is an antimuscarinic advocated as a long-acting GI antispasmodic in horses and dogs.

Questions for Chapter 12

1. State whether the following cause vomiting (emetic) or suppress it (anti-emetic):
   a. apomorphine
   b. metoclopramide
   c. morphine
   d. digoxin
   e. phenothiazines
   f. stimulation of the vestibular apparatus
   g. antihistamines
   h. azotaemia
   i. bacterial endotoxaemia
   j. anticholinergics
   k. butyrophenones

2. Classify the following agents used as ulcer therapies into three groups: H_2 receptor antagonists (HA), antacids (A) and disaccharide protectants (DP).
   a. cimetidine
   b. sucralfate
   c. aluminium magnesium hydroxide
   d. ranitidine

3. What agent is a synthetic prostaglandin E analogue that decreases gastric acidity and promotes ulcer healing?

4. How do narcotic analgesics such as morphine aid diarrhoea?

5. What are the indications for antibiotic therapy in diarrhoea?

For answers go to page 242

CHAPTER 13

Pharmaceutical Preparations used for the Genitourinary System

Learning aims and objectives

After studying this chapter you should be able to:

1. **Describe the treatments for acute and chronic renal failure**
2. **Explain how to alter urine pH**
3. **List the treatments for feline cystitis**
4. **State the drugs used in urinary incontinence**
5. **List the medicines used for the reproductive system.**

Acute renal failure

Acute renal failure (ARF) is a medical emergency with non-specific presenting signs of anuria, anorexia, lethargy, vomiting and dehydration. Renal failure can be pre-renal, renal or post-renal. Hyperkalaemia is the most life-threatening complication of ARF and can be treated by removing the cause (e.g. relief of blockage causing post-renal failure). Further treatment of hyperkalaemia may be indicated and can include:

- calcium gluconate to protect the myocardium against the toxic effects of potassium
- sodium bicarbonate to correct the metabolic acidosis
- glucose/insulin therapy to stimulate the uptake of potassium into the cells.

Diuretic therapy is used in the anuric, or persistently oliguric, patient in an attempt to increase urine output. A number of drugs can be used to promote diuresis, including furosemide, dopamine and mannitol.

Anti-emetics may be of value in the uraemic patient suffering from nausea. H_2 antagonists, ulcer healing drugs and metoclopramide may be indicated for similar reasons.

Chronic renal failure

Diet is one of the cornerstones of management of chronic renal failure (CRF). Phosphorous accumulation must be avoided – necessitating low phosphorous, low-protein diets. The use of phosphate binders, such as ipakitine (Vetoquinol), will aid in the management of phosphorous levels.

Calcitriol is a vitamin D compound that can be used to influence calcium and phosphorous metabolism. It enhances intestinal absorption of calcium and is indicated to control the hypocalcaemia associated with CRF. It may, however, provoke hypercalcaemia.

Many cats with CRF are anaemic due to lack of erythropoietin and GI bleeding – treatment is indicated if the haematocrit falls below 20%. Iron deficiencies should be corrected and recombinant human erythropoietin (rhEPO) may be effective in restoring erythropoiesis to normal levels. Therapy involves s.c. injection of Epoetin beta at a dose of 50–100 IU/kg three times a week. The PCV should elevate rapidly (1% a day for the first month) and injections should be reduced to once weekly when PCV is normal, to avoid erythrocytosis. Potential side effects are listed in Box 13.1. The cost of treatment is around £100 a month but increases life expectancy by 6 months. Antibody development in about 30% of cats results in no response to therapy.

H_2 antagonists decrease gastrin activity and lower both hydrochloric acid and pepsin levels. In so doing, they improve patient comfort by alleviating uraemic gastritis. Famotidine has a longer duration of action and is 9× more potent than ranitidine and 32× more potent than cimetidine. All three are human medicinal products. Famotidine is, however, only 37% bioavailable after oral administration due to poor oral absorption. It is formulated as Pepcid AC 10 mg tablets, which should be given to cats at 0.25 tablet every 2–3 days. Pepcid 2 should not be used as it contains calcium.

Cyproheptadine (Periactin), a serotonin antagonist antihistamine, is often used as an appetite stimulant for CRF patients but may cause haemolytic anaemia, which is reversible following cessation of treatment.

B_{12} vitamin supplements are indicated as, being water soluble, they are lost into the urine and are therefore often depleted in CRF patients. Deficiency can contribute to anorexia, leading to catabolism of the body tissues and acidosis. Dose should be 0.25 ml once weekly for 6 weeks, then monthly.

Proteinuria is often associated with a urinary tract infection (UTI). Where a UTI is present, a one-month course of antibiotics active against *E. coli* is recommended. Clavulanate amoxicillin is a suitable first-choice drug. Fluoroquinolone use is inadvisable, particularly over such long periods, as it is easy for resistance to develop. In one study, 30% of cats presenting with CRF were found to have a UTI(s) (increasing to 75% if female).

ACE inhibitors are indicated for the treatment of CRF in cats. They are the first-line treatment for CRF hypertension in humans and are suitable for reducing blood pressure in mildly hypertensive cats. They also help to decrease proteinuria. In cats with severe hypertension, the calcium channel blocker amlodipine can be added to ACE inhibitor therapy.

Nausea and gastric ulceration may require management in uraemic cats. Sucralfate can be used as a gastric bandage but can be difficult to administer to cats. Metoclopramide can be used as an anti-emetic and may be administered orally, s.c., i.v. or as an i.v. infusion. Diazepam is no longer recommended as an appetite stimulant in anorexic cats as fulminant hepatic necrosis has been associated with repeated oral administration, even at the first dose.

Nandrolone (Laurabolin) is a testosterone derivative with anabolic and anti-catabolic actions. It is indicated for CRF patients where excessive tissue breakdown is present. It has also been advocated in the management of anaemia associated with renal failure. Haematology should be monitored to determine the efficacy of treatment when anaemia is being treated. Liver enzymes should also be monitored to detect any hepatotoxicity. It has a place in treating debilitating and wasting conditions and in terminal disease as it can improve appetite and promote wellbeing.

Feline idiopathic cystitis

Feline idiopathic cystitis (FIC) is a multifactorial problem that requires a multimodal approach to treatment. Research is ongoing into this problem and new ideas on therapy are likely to evolve over time. In addition to environmental change (stress reduction) and behavioural therapy (pheromones), the following medications have been recommended:
- GAG supplements have been proposed to protect the bladder epithelium through their effect on the protective mucus layer lining the bladder. Cats may therefore benefit from such nutritional therapy, e.g. Cystease (Ceva) or Cystaid (Vetplus).

Box 13.1

Potential side effects of rhEPO

- polycythaemia
- systemic hypertension
- vomiting
- seizures
- injection site discomfort
- allergic mucocutaneous reactions
- acute anaphylactic reactions

Benefits of the anti-spasmodic drug prazosin

- it is the most selective α antagonist for the α-1 receptor
- it leaves the α-2 receptors operational, therefore reducing side effects
- it reduces blood pressure due to peripheral vasodilation

- Tricyclic antidepressants such as amitriptyline (an agent that blocks norepinephrine and serotonin uptake in the brain), may be indicated. It may be useful in chronic or severe disease. Liver function should, however, be assessed prior to therapy and every 6 months whilst on treatment.
- Analgesia and anti-inflammatory drugs are probably more useful than antibiotics as 98% of cases are sterile. Buprenorphine oral solution is effective and can be dispensed to the owner to give q8h. Non-steroidal anti-inflammatory drugs may help relieve some of the symptoms associated with FIC, as may anti-inflammatory doses of corticosteroids (although these have been shown to be ineffective in some cases).
- Urethral spasm should be relieved with a smooth muscle (bladder to membranous penis) antispasmodic, e.g. prazosin (Hypovase) (Box 13.2). This is preferred to phenoxybenzamine (Dibenyline) which takes several days to take effect. For skeletal muscle relaxation (tip of penis) dantrolene is useful. Cats should be weaned off these medications when the disease is under control.

Fluid therapy is particularly important in the management of cystitis as regular flushing of the bladder will evacuate inflammatory mediators and reduce sludging and irritation of the bladder mucosa. Tips to promote oral fluid therapy include eliminating competition over water and increasing its availability by making it available throughout the house/environment.

Weight loss and an exercise program are advisable in obese cats.

Urinary acidifiers/alkalinisers

Hyperventilation secondary to stress is the most common cause of alkaline urine, so before therapy ensure the correct diagnosis. The urine of carnivores is usually acidic, whilst in herbivores it tends to be alkaline. In cases of UTI, the pH often becomes more alkaline. Urinary acidification is indicated in the management of struvite urolithiasis and some bacterial cystitis cases.

Ethylenediamine and methionine are urinary acidifiers that may be helpful in the management of cystitis and struvite urolithiasis, and to increase the efficacy of some antibiotics in urine. Methionine readily donates its terminal methyl group for methylation of various compounds. In addition, it contains a chemical group that protects the liver against certain toxins.

Vitamin C is an excellent urinary acidifier. It can be supplied as tablets of pure vitamin C or, alternatively, in the form of tomato ketchup or concentrate. It is particularly indicated in guinea pigs suffering from cystitis due to their reliance on a dietary source of vitamin C.

Potassium citrate alkalinises urine. It is used in the management of calcium oxalate and urate urolithiasis and fungal urinary infections.

Urinary incontinence

The main aim when treating urethral sphincter mechanism incompetence is to restore continence by increasing urethral tone. Oestrogens (Box 13.3) and drugs that act on the sympathetic nervous system can achieve this aim. Ephedrine and phenylpropanolamine (Propalin) act on urethral smooth muscle to increase the urethral tone, but the onset of action takes several days and animals can become restless and irritable. Ephedrine has been used in Oriental medicine for centuries but is now synthetically made. It has sympathomimetic effects by direct activation of adrenergic receptors (Fig. 13.1) and release of endogenous norepinephrine.

Animals that do not respond to treatment with the agents separately may respond to combined oestrogen and phenylpropanolamine therapy. Specific side effects of oestrogens are bone marrow suppression and anaemia, thrombocytopenia and leucopaenia. Oestrogens should not be used in

Hormones used to increase urethral tone

- diethylstilboestrol
- ethinyloestradiol
- oestradiol benzoate
- testosterone proprionate

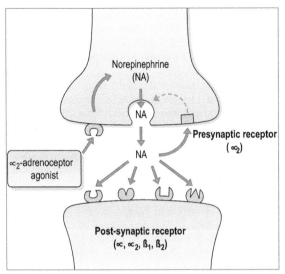

Fig. 13.1 Activation of the adrenoreceptor by adrenergic drugs

entire bitches before their first season as symptoms may improve without treatment, following the first season. Additionally, oestrogenic effects are seen in 5–9% of bitches receiving 2 mg/24 h. The possibility of ectopic ureters should not be overlooked in young dogs or dogs that fail to respond to therapy.

Benign prostatic hyperplasia

This condition occurs in 80% of dogs over 5 years of age and although castration is the treatment of choice, medical management is common:

- Delmadinone acetate (Tardak; Intervet) is a progestin with anti-androgen and anti-oestrogen effects. Adverse effects include polyuria and polydipsia, polyphagia and a coat colour change at the injection site.
- Megestrol acetate (Ovarid) decreases an enzyme in prostate tissue, thereby interfering with the conversion of testosterone to dihydrotestosterone – the agent causing the hypertrophy. The drug should not be given for more than 32 days and interferes with sperm production.
- Finasteride is another anti-androgen drug which will treat the condition but it is secreted into the semen. It is, however, teratogenic and should not therefore be used in breeding dogs.

Urinary retention

Bethanechol chloride (Myotonine) is a muscarinic agonist that increases urinary bladder detrusor muscle tone and contraction; it may be of value in urinary retention. It does not initiate a detrusor reflex and is ineffective if the bladder is areflexic. Also, it may increase urethral resistance and should not be used where urethral resistance is increased.

Preparations used in the reproductive system

Prevention of conception and treating infertility are the main aims of therapy. Drugs that alter the contractile state of the uterus are important in obstetrics. Some of the drugs used are described below.

Oxytocin

This hormone regulates myometrial activity by contracting the uterus and also contracts myoepithelial cells in the mammary gland, which causes milk let-down. It has a vasodilator action and a weak antidiuretic action, which may be of importance when considering therapy in patients with cardiac or renal disease. Oxytocin is used to induce or augment labour when the uterine muscle is not functioning adequately. It can also be used to treat post-partum haemorrhage. Oxytocin receptors are found not only in the uterus and mammary tissue, but also in the brain. Oxytocin has been shown to be important in mating and parenting behaviour.

Pessaries

Pessaries or other intrauterine products (e.g. Metricure; Intervet) are available.

Prostaglandins

Dinoprostone (Prepidil) is a topical gel which is used to relax the vagina and to induce uterine contractions in egg-bound birds. Application of the gel to the opening of the shell gland (uterus) within the cloaca may result in delivery of the egg within 30 minutes if it is a non-obstructive egg-binding. The treatment can be repeated if the egg is not delivered and the bird is not exhibiting signs of distress.

Progestogens (e.g. proligestone)

The endogenous hormone is progesterone. An example of a synthetic drug is medroxyprogesterone, a long-acting progestogen used to treat eosinophilic granuloma in cats and to prevent oestrus in bitches. Adverse effects can be of a serious nature and in some cases permanent (e.g. mammary neoplasia), therefore the risks versus benefits of therapy should be assessed.

Oestrogens

The endogenous oestrogen, oestradiol, is intended for the provision of short-term therapy. Indications include misalliance, hypogonadal obesity, hormonal urinary incontinence in bitches and the treatment of anal adenomas and prostatic hyperplasia in male

dogs. Oestrogens may be toxic to bone marrow and haematology should be performed when using high doses or in patients receiving chronic therapy. Other adverse effects include those listed in Box 13.4.

Anti-oestrogens

Tamoxifen citrate (Nolvadex) is used in humans to treat oestrogen-dependent breast cancer. It has found several indications in veterinary medicine, including the treatment of haemangiosarcomas.

Abortifacients

Abortifacients/treatments for misalliance:
- oestradiol benzoate (Mesalin; Intervet)
- aglepristone (Alizin; Virbac).

Pseudopregnancy and lactation

Treatment for pseudopregnancy and lactation involves anti-prolactin drugs. Cabergoline (Galastop) is a potent anti-prolactin drug which is also used in conjunction with a prostaglandin to terminate unwanted pregnancy. It should not be given with metoclopramide, which antagonises its effects.

Questions for Chapter 13

State whether the following are TRUE or FALSE.

1. The most common cause of alkaline urine is infection with *E. coli*

2. Phosphate should be supplemented in chronic renal failure

3. Anabolic steroids can be hepatotoxic and liver enzymes should be monitored in order to detect hepatotoxicity, if used

4. Whilst on rhEPO therapy, blood pressure and PCV must be monitored to avoid erythrocytosis

5. Famotidine is an H_2 antagonist that is a prescription-only human medicine

6. ACE inhibitors are the sole treatment for severe hypertension in CRF in cats

7. Amlodipine (Istin) has potential side effects including necrosis of digits and other extremities and collapse of the circulation in some animals

8. Buprenorphine is a useful analgesic to manage cystitis in cats but it can only be administered parenterally

9. Antibiotics should be given to all urinary catheterised cats

10. Certain ACE inhibitors and finasteride have all been proven to be teratogenic in animals and/or humans

For answers go to page 243

Fourteen

CHAPTER 14

Pharmaceutical Preparations for the CNS and Neuromuscular Drugs

Learning aims and objectives

After studying this chapter you should be able to:

1. **Describe how drugs affect the CNS**
2. **List agents useful in the management of seizures**
3. **List the useful neuromuscular blocking drugs.**

Blood–brain barrier in the CNS

The barrier between the blood and the CNS is less permeable to large molecules than that between the blood and other tissues of the body. It limits access of hydrophilic molecules and proteins into the brain and therefore stops many drugs from penetrating. The barrier exists in both the brain tissue capillaries and in the choroid plexus (i.e. the blood–cerebrospinal fluid barrier). Water, oxygen, carbon dioxide and most lipid-soluble agents can cross, including anaesthetic agents.

The neuromuscular junction

Physiology of the neuromuscular junction

An impulse travelling down the motor nerve causes depolarisation of the nerve terminal, triggering the release of acetylcholine (ACh), which crosses the junction to stimulate nicotinic receptors on the postsynaptic muscle membrane. Figure 14.1 shows an example of a neurotransmitter, in this case nor-epinephrine, crossing the synapse. If the stimulation of the muscle is of sufficient magnitude then a contraction is produced. The ACh is rapidly hydrolysed by the enzyme acetylcholinesterase so that the contraction is not maintained.

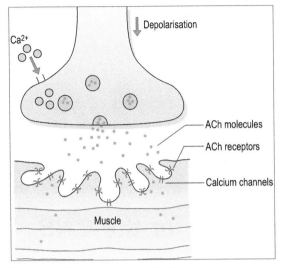

Fig. 14.1 The neuromuscular junction

In contrast to cholinergic receptors, an active re-uptake mechanism is present to stop the transmission of the impulse in noradrenergic neurons. Re-uptake is also prominent in neurones that secrete dopamine, serotonin and GABA. Figure 14.2 compares the biochemical events at cholinergic endings with those at noradrenergic endings.

There are several subtypes of receptor for each ligand. For example, norepinephrine acts on α-1 and α-2 receptors as well as β 1, 2 and 3 subtypes. This multiplies the response a ligand has and allows selectivity within different cell types. There are receptors on the pre- as well as the postsynaptic membrane. These presynaptic receptors or auto-receptors often inhibit further secretion of the ligand,

providing feedback control, stopping further release as shown in Figure 14.3.

The conversion of electric impulse into chemical signals is complex as it involves the manufacture of ACh, its parcellation into vesicles, the fusion of vesicles with the axolemma, hydrolysis of ACh and then recycling of both the membrane and neurotransmitter metabolites. The process of biosynthesis and catabolism of ACh is shown in Figure 14.4. ACh release is calcium dependent and the entire process involves many enzymes.

Diseases of the neuromuscular junction

Disease processes can be categorised according to whether they affect presynaptic function (causing a deficiency in ACh release) or postsynaptic function (causing a failure in the appropriate response to normally released ACh). Deficient release of ACh causes insufficient depolarisation of the postsynaptic membrane and therefore failure of muscle contraction. Botulism, for example, causes a presynaptic junctionopathy; the botulism toxins destroy proteins required for ACh vesicle exocytosis.

Myasthenia gravis is a postsynaptic disorder caused by a deficiency of ACh receptors as a result of immune-mediated destruction, congenital absence or congenital dysfunction. The immune-mediated destruction of ACh receptors can be associated with other disease processes, especially neoplasia and most notably thymoma.

Organophosphates are widely used as insecticides. As they interact with esterases, they impair the efficacy of acetylcholine esterase within the synaptic cleft. In toxic doses this allows intrasynaptic

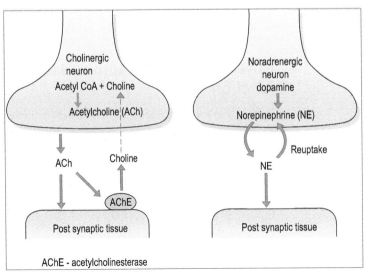

Fig. 14.2 Comparison of cholinergic and noradrenergic synapses

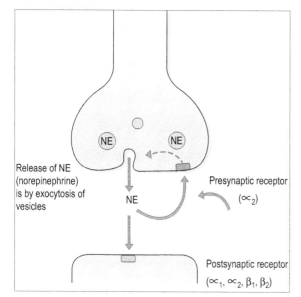

Fig. 14.3 Presynaptic and postsynaptic receptors at the ending of a noradrenergic neuron

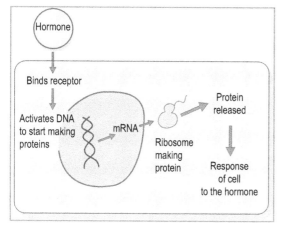

Fig. 14.4 Biosynthesis and catabolism of acetylcholine

accumulation of ACh, causing persistent post-synaptic depolarisation. This affects the cholinergic synapses in the autonomic, central and peripheral nervous systems and therefore causes a wide range of serious clinical problems.

Anticonvulsants

Anticonvulsant drugs are used to treat convulsions. The convulsions may be provoked by a number of possible causes, including toxicological, parasitic,

metabolic and idiopathic causes. Efforts should be directed at identifying the cause. This is essential if targeted therapy is to be provided.

Primary epilepsy is the most common neurological disorder in the dog, accounting for 2–3% of total hospital neuro-admissions. Anticonvulsants are indicated in the management of a fitting patient and in the long-term management of epilepsy. Management of fitting patients and those with status epilepticus is indicated to control acute seizure disorders:

- propofol infusions
- medetomidine
- diazepam
- phenobarbital
  - 5–30 mg/kg; maximum anti-seizure activity may take up to 30 minutes
  - dose may be increased and repeated at 30-min intervals.

Long-term (chronic) seizure therapy is generally indicated for seizures:

- seizures lasting for more than 5 minutes
- cluster seizures
- seizures that occur more frequently than once per month.

Control of canine epilepsy can be achieved in up to 80% of cases with one drug only and often this success rate can be improved further by combining agents.

Phenobarbital/phenobarbitone

This first-choice agent depresses the motor centres of the cerebral cortex, giving it excellent anticonvulsant properties. It increases the seizure threshold required to produce a seizure and decreases the spread of discharge to surrounding neurones. The primary means of action is to enhance the effects of GABA (an inhibitory neurotransmitter) as well as inhibition of the excitatory neurotransmitter glutamate.

Phenobarbital is a weak acid and is therefore absorbed well after oral administration, reaching peak plasma levels in 6 hours; it is 45% bound to serum proteins in dogs. It is metabolised in the liver, excreted in the urine and is a potent inducer of hepatic drug-metabolising enzymes. This means it increases the rate of clearance of other drugs metabolised in the liver, including itself, resulting in more drug being required to produce a given effect over time. If doses of > 4 mg/kg/day are used to initiate therapy, some dogs appear depressed or ataxic for a month but this resolves and doses can be increased without the sedation occurring again. Polyphagia and PUPD are also seen and likely to persist throughout therapy.

Phenobarbital is used adjunctively for the emergency treatment of acute seizure disorders due to other causes (e.g. strychnine toxicity and meningitis). It is used in the management/treatment of behavioural signs of limbic epilepsy and also in combination with propranolol in the management of fear and phobia-related behaviour problems.

It is a Schedule 3 controlled drug and is known to have hepatotoxic effects – serum biochemistry should be regularly performed along with serum drug levels.

Interactions – the effect of phenobarbital may be increased by other CNS depressants (antihistamines, narcotics and phenothiazines). Cimetidine, ketoconazole and chloramphenicol increase serum phenobarbital concentration through inhibition of the hepatic microsomal enzyme system. Phenobarbital may increase the metabolism of corticosteroids, β-blockers, metronidazole and theophylline.

Potassium bromide

Some 20–50% of epileptics will eventually be classified as 'refractory epileptics' and will be inadequately controlled on phenobarbital (PB) therapy. Another subpopulation will develop life-threatening hepatotoxicity, which means they must be weaned off phenobarbital. Potassium bromide (KBr) is an effective anti-epileptic drug when used in combination with PB and may be effective as monotherapy in some patients. There is a synergistic effect when using PB and KBr together and preparations containing both preparations are available on the continent.

Bromide ions suppress neuronal excitability, probably by replacing intracellular chloride and hyperpolarising nerve cell membranes. It is an anticonvulsant and sedative that has no hepatotoxicity and all the adverse effects can be reversed when the medication is stopped. The slow rise of plasma bromide levels after enteral administration limits its usefulness in status epilepticus.

It is slowly eliminated by the kidney in competition with chloride. KBr has a long half life in the body due to its reabsorption in the renal tubules. The rate of reabsorption is affected by the amount of chloride in the diet; restricted salt diets increase the reabsorption of KBr in the kidney and so result in reduced renal clearance and an increased half-life of the drug. KBr diffuses rapidly into tissues, including the brain, where it stays until plasma levels drop and it diffuses out again. Plasma drug levels should be monitored and therapy aimed at achieving values of approximately 1–1.5 mg/ml.

Adverse reactions are usually neurological and include ataxia and sedation. Escalating doses of KBr, however, may lead to therapeutic concentrations

that approach the toxic range. The characteristic clinical sign is tetraparesis that is more severe in the pelvic limbs. The pathophysiological basis for this is not well understood. Severe eosinophilic bronchitis, resulting in coughing, has been reported in cats and may be fatal.

Polyphagia is seen in most dogs and 25% of them will require low-calorie diets to maintain normal body weight. Polydipsia is also seen.

Primidone

Primidone is rapidly metabolised to the active metabolites phenobarbital and phenylethylmalonamide. In dogs, approximately 85% of anti-seizure activity is thought to be due to phenobarbital, with some potentiation by PEMA. The efficacy of primidone in patients refractory to phenobarbital may be the result of improved conversion following induction of hepatic microsomal enzymes – 3.8 mg of primidone is equivalent to 1 mg of phenobarbital. The hepatotoxicity seen is worse than with phenobarbital.

Phenytoin

Phenytoin depresses motor areas of the cortex without depressing sensory areas; it therefore decreases seizure threshold without causing sedation. Oral absorption is poor and the drug is 85% protein bound in the plasma. A short half life of 6–8 hours in dogs requires a high dosing frequency of 3–4 times a day. In cats, the drug is metabolised very slowly and toxicity easily develops. It is a potent inducer of hepatic enzymes and therefore has many drug interactions. Phenytoin is most effective if used in conjunction with phenobarbital or primidone.

Diazepam

Chronic dosing with diazepam leads to a shortened half-life due to activation of the hepatic microsomal enzyme system – tolerance to the anticonvulsant effects can therefore develop within a few weeks. Consequently, it is only useful in the short-term management of seizures in the dog. Benzodiazepines can provoke fulminant hepatic necrosis in cats and enhance the inhibitory effects of GABA in both the brain and spinal cord. They are well absorbed after oral administration (98% protein bound) but rapidly and extensively metabolised in the liver.

Chlorazepate

Chlorazepate is metabolised in the stomach to its active metabolite. It is less efficacious than diazepam but tolerance is slower to develop. Use with pheno-barbital will increase serum concentrations.

Gabapentin/valproic acid/carbamazepine

These agents have too short elimination half lives to permit maintenance of adequate drug concentrations in the plasma and CNS unless dosing is more frequent than four times a day.

CNS stimulants (analeptics)

Apomorphine stimulates the emetic centre in the medulla. Drugs that act directly on the respiratory centre counteract respiratory depression and can be used in barbiturate poisoning, drowning, neonatal asphyxia or respiratory collapse during anaesthesia. Doxapram is an example of such a drug; it works by directly stimulating chemoreceptors of the carotid and aortic regions. It may also stimulate the medullary respiratory centre – tidal volume increases as a result.

Antidepressants

Amitriptyline and clomipramine are tricyclic antidepressants that block serotonin and norepinephrine re-uptake in the brain, thereby increasing the effects of these neurotransmitters. Amitriptyline has been used in the management of feline retention cystitis and psychogenic skin complaints, seeming to calm anxious animals. Clomipramine (Clomicalm) is a similar drug used to control obsessive-compulsive disorders such as tail chasing and separation-anxiety disorders manifested by destructive behaviour. The drug is only effective when combined with behavioural therapy.

'Smart drugs' (nootropics)

Drugs that can boost brain power and memory are constantly improving what bodies and minds are capable of in the human field. A class of drugs called ampakines has been shown to improve memory by boosting the activity of glutamate, a key neurotransmitter that makes it easier to learn and encode memory. These drugs are finding their way into veterinary medicine to help with senile behavioural changes. They work by:
- increasing brain metabolism
- increasing cerebral circulation

- protecting the brain from physical and chemical damage.

Nicergoline (Fitergol)

Canine cognitive dysfunction is a medical condition and it is important to understand the changes that are occurring before embarking upon medication. During the normal ageing process behavioural changes can result from a compromising of the cerebral blood flow. Nicergoline is a neuroprotective agent that blocks serotonin and dopamine receptors and is an α-adrenergic antagonist, which results in cerebral vasodilation.

Propentofylline (Vivitonin)

Propentofylline is a potent potentiator of adenosine. It is a xanthine derivative that increases blood flow to the heart, muscle and CNS. This improvement in oxygenation improves demeanour in animals that are dull and lethargic. Other effects include:
- positive inotropic and chronotropic effects on the heart
- anti-arrhythmic action
- inhibits platelets
- reduces peripheral vascular resistance
- modifies glial cells.

Box 14.1 shows the licensed indications and the specific (non-licensed) indications where propentofylline can be used as an adjunct or solo therapy. The drug should be given on an empty stomach and it is best not to feed the animal for 1 hour after the dose.

Selegiline hydrochloride (Selgian)

In cases of canine cognitive dysfunction additional changes occur such as a depletion of brain dopamine levels and an increase in the presence of free radicals, leading to cell injury and brain pathology. Selegiline has three important actions in the management of canine dementia:
- enhances brain dopamine concentrations and metabolism through inhibition of monoamine oxidase B (IMAO B)
- decreases substances in the brain which are responsible for neural cell damage
- protects nerve cells, decreases cell death and promotes synthesis of nerve growth factors.

It can take up to 6 weeks for effects to be seen when treating emotional disorders but the effects on canine dementia are seen within 3 weeks. Side effects are minimal with mild GI signs occasionally reported. It may act on prolactin secretion and

Indications for use of propentofylline

Licensed indications

- increased eagerness to exercise
- increased exercise tolerance
- improved demeanour
- reduced dullness and lethargy

Non-licensed indications

- epilepsy
- incontinence
- arthritis (can halve the dose of NSAIDs)
- congestive heart failure
- wound healing (especially necrotic extremities)
- pyoderma
- senile dementias (especially in the cat)
- gonadectomy
- vestibular syndrome
- coughing (bronchodilator)
- improving working dog performance, e.g. greyhounds
- improving coat quality and alopecia
- 7 days pre-elective surgery to improve wound healing

should not be given to lactating or pregnant bitches. In long-standing cases combination therapy with propentofylline is preferred.

Treatment protocol for head injury

Oxygen and fluid therapy remain the priorities. Some authors advocate the use of glucocorticoids, although their use remains controversial.

Mannitol

Mannitol is an osmotic diuretic that is effective in reducing both cerebral oedema and raised intra-cranial pressure. It also has an attenuating action on oxygen free radicals, promotes vasoconstriction of cerebral arteries and suppresses cerebrospinal fluid production. There is a delay of 30–60 minutes before the effect on cerebral oedema is noted and it lasts for 2–4 hours. It is contraindicated in hypovolaemia and dehydration, and urine output should be monitored during therapy. Furosemide

therapy may be required during administration and electrolytes should be monitored and adjusted as required.

Antioxidants

The importance of oxygen free radicals as mediators of brain damage can not be over emphasised. One antioxidant drug that can be used is desferrioxamine mesilate, which has a primary indication for iron salts poisoning. It is an iron chelator that crosses the blood–brain barrier and inhibits iron-dependent oxygen free radical actions by forming an inert complex with iron released in haemoglobin breakdown. Administration of this drug must be slow, over 20 minutes, due to its strong hypotensive effects.

Lazaroids are methylprednisolone analogues which do not activate glucocorticoid receptors. Trilazad mesylate effectively inhibits lipid peroxidation and promotes the survival of tissue around the site of brain injury. It is useful in subarachnoid haemorrhage, CNS trauma and ischaemia.

Preparations for use in the subarachnoid space

Myelograms involve the administration of non-ionic water-soluble iodine contrast media such as omnipaque into the CSF. Figure 14.5 shows how the foramen magna can be located. The point of entry of the needle is in the centre of a triangle formed between the landmark bony prominences of the occipital crest and the wings of the atlas. Local anaesthetic agents, with or without the addition of an α-$_2$-agonist, or opioid, are administered into the spinal tissues either as an epidural (outside the dura mater) or a spinal block (subarachnoid administration).

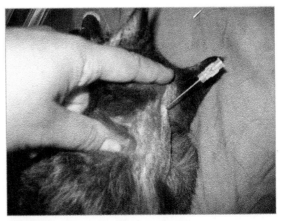

Fig. 14.5 Subarachnoid administration of medicines

Neuromuscular drugs

Drugs that affect skeletal muscle and nerve function fall into several therapeutic categories.

Anabolic steroids

These are compounds structurally related to testosterone that have anabolic effects on proteins and are therefore useful therapeutically in debilitated animals suffering from muscle atrophy. Potential side effects include increased libido in males, anoestrus, oedema due to water retention and jaundice. Nandrolone is the most commonly used example in this category.

Muscle relaxants and neuromuscular blocking drugs

Although some anaesthetic agents do produce muscle relaxation, there are situations where it is not profound enough and even drugs like the centrally acting muscle relaxants are unsuitable by themselves. Indications for relaxant use include:

- access to the abdominal cavity – easier when the skeletal muscles are relaxed
- thoracic surgery requiring intermittent positive pressure ventilation
- reduction of dislocated joints
- reducing laryngeal spasm during endotracheal intubation of cats
- ophthalmic surgery where movement of the patient and globe must be prevented
- may be indicated in the treatment of tetanus and in the capture of certain exotic species, e.g. crocodiles.

Neuromuscular blocking agents (NMBA) are quaternary ammonium compounds. Relaxants are unlikely to cross lipid membranes such as the blood–brain barrier, placenta or renal tubular epithelium to be reabsorbed after filtration into the urine, the major route of excretion. They have a similar chemical structure to acetylcholine and so are attracted to all cholinergic receptors. NMBA are of two types, the non-depolarising (or competitive) and the depolarising.

Non-depolarising agents occupy the receptor so that ACh can not act. The other group, depolarising agents (see below) act in a more complicated manner and initially cause depolarisation before blockage occurs. Figure 14.6 shows competitive inhibition, where the agent is of a similar structure to the ligand and non-competitive inhibition where the agent is structurally different and acts at another site to block the action.

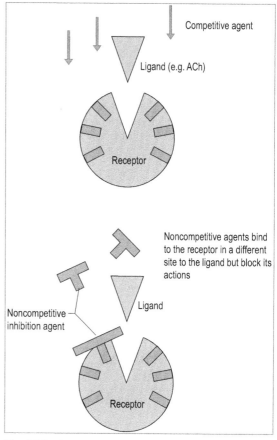

Fig. 14.6 Competitive and non-competitive inhibition

Non-depolarising agents are reversible. They interfere with the transmission of impulses from motor nerve endings to skeletal muscle by interfering with the effectiveness of the neurotransmitter ACh to activate nicotinic cholinergic receptors. They are therefore sometimes called competitive muscle relaxants. The clinically useful agents are:

- vecuronium – cardiovascularly stable
- atracurium – cardiovascularly stable and useful in hepatic and renal dysfunction
- pancuronium – causes tachycardia and increased arterial blood pressure due to catecholamine release
- rocuronium – rapid onset
- other examples are gallamine and alcuronium
- renal problems delay excretion of gallamine and pancuronium.

The skeletal muscle paralysis that ensues is not associated with depression of the CNS – the animal is fully conscious throughout the period of immobility. They do not gain entry into the brain and so no CNS depression is seen. This is because they are highly charged, lipophobic compounds and cross lipoprotein barriers poorly.

Reversal of non-depolarising agents can be achieved by the administration of anticholinesterases, as these drugs allow the ACh to persist at the neuromuscular junction and displace the NMBA from its receptors. ACh levels are increased everywhere, however, and anticholinergic drugs should be administered concurrently to avoid side effects such as bradycardia, bronchospasm, diarrhoea and salivation. Box 14.2 shows some of the drug interactions to be aware of.

Depolarising agents bind to the postsynaptic membrane and initially cause muscle contraction due to their similarity to ACh. Suxamethonium (also called succinylcholine) is an example of a depolarising agent. It works by interfering with ACh-mediated depolarisation of postsynaptic membranes. The relaxation produced is of 5 minutes duration in the cat and 20 minutes in the dog unless liver disease is present, when the effects are prolonged as the liver produces the enzyme responsible for the degradation of the drug.

Box 14.2

Drug interactions with muscle relaxants

- aminoglycoside antibiotics (streptomycin, neomycin, gentamicin) prolong the duration of action
- polymyxin antibiotics (tetracycline, lincomycin, clindamycin)
- local anaesthetics, barbiturates, procainamide, propranolol, phenytoin all potentiate the block
- calcium antagonists – used to treat cardiac arrhythmias
- diuretics – including furosemide
- corticosteroids – decrease the potency of the NMBA
- immunosuppressants (cyclophosphamide, chlorambucil) and organophosphates inhibit cholinesterase enzyme action

---

Questions for Chapter 14

State whether the following are TRUE or FALSE:

1. There are two kinds of synaptic transmission, chemical and electrical. Electrical synapses pass the message directly from neurone to neurone and the information can run both ways. In the CNS most synapses are chemically mediated by neurotransmitters.

2. There are three neurotransmitters: ACh, dopamine and serotonin.

3. Acetylcholine is a neurotransmitter that is released from vesicles at the presynaptic membrane and diffuses across the synapse before being hydrolysed by acetylcholinesterase. In the CNS the effects of ACh are due to its interaction with two types of receptor: muscarinic and nicotinic.

4. Dopamine is a major neurotransmitter in the CNS with a primarily stimulatory action.

5. Histamine is a neurotransmitter in the CNS.

6. The blood–brain barrier limits diffusion into the brain of hydrophilic substances and proteins and therefore causes problems with the administration of some drugs.

For answers go to page 243

Fifteen

CHAPTER 15

Pharmaceutical Preparations Used for the Treatment of Endocrine Disorders

Learning aims and objectives

After studying this chapter you should be able to:

1. Understand the homeostatic mechanisms of the body
2. Describe how drugs act on the adrenal gland
3. Describe how drugs act on the pituitary gland
4. Describe how drugs act on the thyroid gland
5. List the types of insulin
6. Describe how drugs act on the parathyroid gland.

Homeostatic regulation of the body

Homeostasis is the act of keeping the body functioning in the most efficient way possible by regulating all of the body's processes such as the immune and inflammatory responses. It is the science of maintaining a balance.

The buffering properties of the body fluids and the renal and respiratory adjustments to the presence of excess acid or alkali are examples of homeostatic mechanisms. Many operate on the principle of negative feedback – deviations from a given normal set point are detected by a sensor and signals from it trigger compensatory changes that continue until the set point is again reached.

Adenosine

Adenosine is a very active, important molecule with many actions involving the equilibrium of the body and is therefore termed a homeostatic molecule. The actions of adenosine include:

- Transporting and storing energy – adenosine helps to release energy where needed.
- Acts as a hormone to switch on and off receptors – the action depends on the site of the receptor. They have been found in the brain, heart, liver, skeletal muscle, pituitary gland, uterus and gonads. In the brain there are two types of receptor and those which result in suppression

of electrical activity dominate. Therefore adenosine may help with regulating epilepsy.

- Accentuating cell messages – adenosine inhibits phosphodiesterase, which breaks down cell messengers. By allowing this molecule to persist, the strength and duration of the cell action is increased.
- Alters transmission between neurons – it is anti-arrhythmic as it inhibits the sinoatrial and atrioventricular nodes in the heart.
- Acts as a neurotransmitter – one of the results is relaxation of smooth muscle in blood vessel walls and subsequent vasodilation, increasing tissue perfusion.

Renin-angiotensin (aldosterone) (RAS) system

Angiotensin II has many actions in the homeostatic control of the body, one of which is the promotion of aldosterone secretion. Aldosterone release is not regulated solely by angiotensin II but also by several other factors. Angiotensin II produces arteriolar vasoconstriction and elevates vascular resistance and blood pressure. It regulates the glomerular filtration rate and renal blood flow by constricting the efferent and afferent glomerular arterioles. Angiotensin II has multiple effects on cardiac tissue.

Angiotensinogen is the inactive precursor of several angiotensin peptides, including angiotensin II. Angiotensinogen is produced mainly in the liver and is cleaved in the circulation by rennin to release angiotensin I. Angiotensin converting enzymes (ACE) convert the inactive decapeptide to the active octapeptide angiotensin II.

The enzyme renin is synthesised in the juxta-glomerular cells of the kidney. Its release is regulated by renal baroreceptors, which are stimulated in response to reduced renal perfusion pressure. Additional regulation is provided by the macula densa, a group of cells in the distal tubules near the end of the loop of Henle and adjacent to the afferent arteriole. These cells respond to tubular sodium delivery.

Aldosterone is the major mineralocorticoid and has two important actions – it regulates extracellular fluid volume and is a major determinant of potassium homeostasis. Aldosterone acts mainly on the distal convoluted tubule, where it increases the re-absorption of sodium and the excretion of potassium. Three mechanisms control aldosterone release:
- the RAS – keeps blood volume constant
- potassium – hyperkalaemia stimulates aldosterone secretion
- ACTH – stimulates aldosterone secretion acutely but its effects are not long lived.

Endocrine systems

An endocrine gland is a ductless gland that releases a hormone directly into the bloodstream. Both over- and under-production of these hormones can cause disease in the body and there are many drugs that act to correct these conditions.

Adrenal glands

One gland is found next to each kidney. They have a cortex (which produces steroids, mineralocorticoids and sex hormones) and a medulla (produces epinephrine and norepinephrine).

Corticosteroids

A number of corticosteroids are produced within the body. These naturally occurring corticosteroids include cortisol, corticosterone and aldosterone – all synthesised from cholesterol by the adrenal glands.

They are described as being either glucocorticoids or mineralocorticoids. Mineralocorticoids affect electrolyte metabolism (retention of sodium, chloride and water and excretion of potassium, phosphorus and calcium); glucocorticoids affect carbohydrate and protein metabolism and have an anti-inflammatory effect. Most corticosteroids have both glucocorticoid and mineralocorticoid effects. Synthetic analogues have been designed in such a way that the mineralocorticoid effects are minimised, thus maximising their anti-inflammatory action whilst minimising any effect on electrolyte balance.

Corticosteroids produce a diuresis and a consequent polyuria and polydipsia.

Cortisol and prednisolone

Figure 15.1 shows the chemical structure of cortisol and prednisolone. The small change to the chemical structure (the addition of a double bond) increases the anti-inflammatory activity, decreases the salt retention by 20% but produces the side effects of polydipsia and polyuria.

Betamethasone and dexamethasone

The addition of a double bond, as in prednisolone, together with a methyl group and a fluoride atom gives these steroids:
- greatly increased glucocorticoid activity
- increased side effects of polydipsia and polyuria
- the ability to induce parturition and abortion.

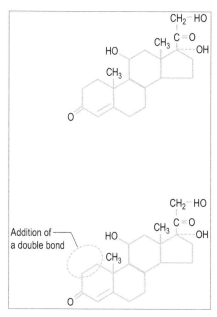

Fig. 15.1 The chemical structures of cortisol and prednisolone

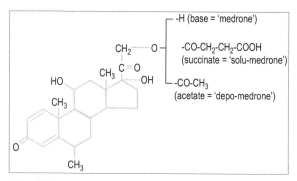

Fig. 15.2 Methylprednisolone can be modified to produce succinate and acetate salts

Methylprednisolone

The addition of a methyl group (CH_3) results in the compound methylprednisolone. This drug has 25% more anti-inflammatory activity than prednisolone, virtually no salt retention and decreased polydipsia and polyuria. Corticosteroids inhibit antidiuretic hormone (ADH) and increase glomerular filtration rate, leading to the increased thirst as the animal tries to compensate for increased urine output. It is thought that methylprednisolone has less of an effect on ADH and therefore less of a tendency to cause polyuria.

Methylprednisolone is available in three different salts, each with its own individual characteristics; Figure 15.2 illustrates the different chemical structures. These are marketed by Pharmacia and Upjohn as Medrone, Solu-medrone and Depo-medrone:

- Medrone – the straight methylprednisolone
  - 25% greater activity than prednisolone
  - reduced incidence of side effects, especially polyuria and polydipsia
  - short-acting, therefore suitable for alternate day therapy
- Solu-medrone – methylprednisolone as the succinate salt
  - a highly soluble form
  - distributed very quickly around the body
  - can be administered by i.v. injection to treat shock, for overwhelming infections/toxicity and for spinal cord compression.

- Depo-medrone – methylprednisolone as the acetate salt
  - an insoluble form
  - a slow-release, long-acting formulation
  - administered by i.m. or intrasynovial injection
  - used to treat inflammatory and allergic conditions such as dermal, ocular and otic inflammatory conditions, musculoskeletal and autoimmune disorders.

When an animal needs long-term corticosteroid therapy the risk of side effects can be minimised by the use of alternate-day therapy (Table 15.1, Box 15.1). This allows the animal's adrenal glands to function on the 'off day' while treatment on the 'on day' controls the symptoms. This type of dosing is only possible with those steroids with a short duration of action.

The pharmacologic effects of corticosteroids are as follows:

Energy metabolism

Glucocorticoids have an antagonistic effect to that of insulin, leading to increased glucose production from amino acids (gluconeogenesis) and reduced incorporation of amino acids into protein. Glucocorticoids enhance lipolysis, however glucocorticoid excess (as seen with steroidal therapy) results in redistribution of fat due to stimulation of appetite and lipogenesis.

Box 15.1

Dispensing tip

- Dogs should receive their steroid medication in the morning and cats in the evenings for the most natural effect as this is when their bodies produce their own steroids. This is because cats are nocturnal.

Table 15.1 Comparison of the steroids available in veterinary medicine

Steroid	Glucocorticoid potency (anti-inflammatory)	Mineralocorticoid potency (electrolyte disturbance)	Alternate day therapy
Hydrocortisone	1	1	No
Prednisolone	4	0.8	Yes
Methylprednisolone	5	0	Yes
Dexamethasone	30	0	No
Betamethasone	30	0	No

Water and electrolyte balance

The polyuria and subsequent polydipsia is caused by inhibition of ADH release. They also have some mineralocorticoid activity and therefore are responsible for salt retention and potassium loss.

Immune and haematological effects

The concentration, distribution and function of peripheral leucocytes are altered. They work by inhibiting arachidonic acid release, a mediator of inflammation that leads to both leukotriene and prostaglandin production. Glucocorticoids decrease formation of histamine and antagonise toxins and kinins which would usually cause inflammation. Cell-mediated immunity is suppressed but high doses of corticosteroids will also reduce antibody production (humoral immunity). Lymphocytes and eosinophils are reduced and virus-induced interferon synthesis is inhibited.

Cardiorespiratory effects

Glucocorticoids have positive chronotropic and inotropic actions on the heart. They act on capillaries to reduce their permeability, therefore reducing cell migration and protein transport into damaged areas and reducing inflammation. Because glucocorticoids are necessary for the capillaries to respond to catecholamines, they contribute to vascular tone.

Endocrine effects

Glucocorticoids can provoke diabetes mellitus and can have marked effects on the hypothalamus and pituitary function. Box 15.2 shows the hormones whose synthesis and secretion is suppressed. The anti-inflammatory dose of prednisolone is 0.5 mg/kg q12h orally, but even physiological doses of 0.22 mg/kg q24h orally will suppress the production of cortisol by the adrenal gland. In humans large doses of glucocorticoids stimulate excessive production of acid and pepsin in the stomach and may cause peptic ulcer (gastroduodenal ulceration). Glucocorticoids facilitate fat absorption and appear

> **Box 15.2**
>
> **Hormones whose synthesis and secretion is suppressed by glucocorticoids**
>
> - adrenocorticotrophic hormone (ACTH)
> - thyroid stimulating hormone (TSH)
> - follicle stimulating hormone (FSH)
> - growth hormone (GH)

to antagonise the effect of vitamin D on calcium absorption.

Toxicology

CNS effects

Induce a state of wellbeing, decrease seizure threshold; lethargy and panting may occur. Rapid withdrawal induces depression and irritability.

Musculoskeletal effects

Chronic administration induces catabolism and muscle atrophy. Bone growth is inhibited and animals become weak. Antagonism of vitamin D results in osteoporosis.

Dermatological effects

Glucocorticoids reduce collagen synthesis and therefore reduce wound healing. The skin becomes thin and more easily stretched and bruised due to increased capillary fragility. A bilaterally symmetrical alopecia may develop.

Immunologic effects

Any clinical disease or latent infection will be exacerbated due to the immune suppression. Animals on chronic glucocorticoid therapy have higher incidences of bacterial infections; in one study, 75% of dogs on glucocorticoids for allergic skin disease had clinical or subclinical urinary tract infections.

Reproductive effects

High doses induce parturition during the latter part of pregnancy in ruminants and horses. Dexamethasone has been linked to abortion in the dog. They have teratogenic effects and should be avoided in pregnancy.

Mineralocorticoids

Aldosterone was synthesised in the mid-1950s to treat Addison's disease (hypoadrenocorticism). It is the most potent regulator of electrolyte excretion and is essential for life but is not available for therapeutic use. The two available preparations are desoxycorticosterone pivalate (Percorten-V; Novartis) and fludrocortisone acetate (Florinef acetate; Squibb). Once the animal is stable, serum sodium and potassium measurement should be performed on a monthly basis. Side effects are rare but include hypokalaemia, hypernatraemia and muscle weakness.

The treatment of choice for initial stabilisation is hydrocortisone sodium succinate because it possesses both glucocorticoid and mineralocorticoid properties. Traditionally maintenance therapy consisted of a semi-selective mineralocorticoid (fludrocortisone) together with a semi-selective glucocorticoid (cortisone acetate or prednisolone).

Adrenolytic drugs and steroid synthesis inhibitors

Cushing's disease (hyperadrenocorticism) is characterised by excessive secretion of the glucocorticoid hormone cortisol. In 90% of cases the cause is excess ACTH production by the pituitary. Dopamine deficiency has been proposed as a cause, so one method of treatment is to use a drug that prevents the breakdown of dopamine by the enzyme monoamine oxidase (e.g. Selegiline). Other drugs that target the adrenal cortex include mitotane and ketoconazole.

Mitotane

Mitotane requires a SIC (previously special treatment authorisation) from the VMD. It is not licensed in the UK and has been superseded by the authorised (licensed) product trilostane.

The chemical is similar to the insecticide DDT and results in selective destruction of the adrenal gland cells that produce cortisol. It causes severe progressive necrosis of the cells of the adrenal cortex, namely the zona fasciculata and zona reticularis, thereby reducing the production of adrenal cortical hormones. Due to its cytotoxic nature, gloves must be worn when handling it. It is no longer the drug of choice for the treatment of Cushing's but is useful for both the pituitary-dependent type and adrenal tumours. Diabetic animals need careful monitoring as the decreased cortisol makes the animal more sensitive to insulin – insulin requirements can change rapidly during the early stages of therapy. Side effects generally arise as the result of a too rapid drop in cortisol levels; they include gastrointestinal problems, neurological problems and mild hypoglycaemia. Most importantly, it can cause mineralocorticoid and glucocorticoid deficiency and relapses are frequently seen.

Mitotane has been used to treat adrenal gland hyperplasia in ferrets as it is able to destroy the parts of the adrenal gland that produce sex hormones.

Ketoconazole

Ketoconazole is an imidazole antifungal drug that suppresses steroid synthesis, including cortisol, oestradiol and testosterone, through its action on cholesterol. It has been used effectively in the management of canine hyperadrenocorticism. It has a slow onset of action and in humans causes abdominal pain in some patients. It requires an acidic environment for dissolution of the drug and therefore can not be given with antacids. The main side effects are vomiting and anorexia. It is teratogenic and should not be used in pregnant animals.

Trilostane

Trilostane is a synthetic steroid with no inherent hormonal activity. It acts as a competitive, and therefore reversible, inhibitor of 3-β hydroxysteroid dehydrogenase enzyme system and, in doing so, blocks adrenal synthesis of glucocorticoids, mineralocorticoids and sex hormones. Serum levels of trilostane peak 1.5 h after oral dosing, with levels returning to normal in approximately 18 h. In view of the short-lived action of the drug it is possible that twice-daily dosing will be required to control clinical signs. The ACTH response test should be performed 4–6 h after trilostane administration. Excretion is via urine or faeces.

Adverse effects include mild increases in serum potassium, bilirubin and calcium. About 70% of dogs respond with improvement of clinical signs within the first 10–30 days of treatment. Skin changes resolve in about 60% of cases but can take up to 3 months to improve from the time when the ideal dose is identified. Around 10% of dogs with pituitary-dependent hyperadrenocorticism show poor clinical response. An initial period of decreased appetite and lethargy is seen in some dogs, especially toy breeds, soon after starting trilostane. A cortisol withdrawal syndrome may be responsible. Trilostane should be stopped for 4–6 days and then restarted on an alternate-day basis for the next 10 days.

Pituitary

Anterior pituitary hormones or their analogues are used in diagnostic tests. For example, tetracosactrin, an adrenocorticotrophin analogue, is used in ACTH stimulation tests to diagnose hyperadrenocorticism (Cushing's).

Cabergoline (Galastop)

Cabergoline is a potent anti-prolactin drug used in the management of pseudopregnancy. It is an ergoline derivative that causes vomiting in some patients but should not be given with metoclopramide, which antagonises the hypoprolactinaemic effects of cabergoline.

Desmopressin

This is an analogue of the posterior pituitary hormone vasopressin. It is used in the diagnosis and treatment of diabetes insipidus. It has greater potency and slower metabolism than the natural ADH molecule and one dose lasts from 10 to 27 hours. It can be administered orally, by injection, directly into the nasal passages or into the conjunctival sac. The conjunctival route, however, results in variable amounts of drug reaching the bloodstream and a variable duration of action. It has also been used for bleeding disorders (von Willebrand's disease and haemophilia A) as it increases plasma levels of factor VIII and von Willebrand factor and increases platelet adhesion.

Oxytocin

Oxytocin is commonly used to stimulate smooth muscle contraction in the oestrogen-sensitised uterus and is used to induce parturition when uterine inertia is present. It can also be used to promote let-down of milk. Low doses must be used initially as over-stimulation of the uterus can be damaging to both mother and fetus.

Thyroid

Methimazole (Felimazole)

Methimazole (MMI) is the only authorised drug for the treatment of feline hyperthyroidism. It interferes

Table 15.2 Adverse effects of methimazole

Adverse effect	Cats affected (5)
Anorexia	11.1
Vomiting	10.7
Lethargy	8.8
Excoriations (face and neck)	2.3
Bleeding	2.3
Hepatopathy	1.5
Thrombocytopenia	2.7
Agranulocytosis	1.5
Leucopenia	4.7
Eosinophilia	11.3
Lymphocytosis	7.2
Positive antinuclear antibodies	21.8
Positive direct antiglobulin test	1.9

with the synthesis of thyroid hormones by inhibiting the enzyme-driven reactions that oxidise iodine. It also prevents the iodination of thyroglobulin and the formation of T_3 and T_4. The administration of 5 mg q8h results in normal serum concentration within 3 weeks. Blood tests are then advised to adjust the dose – when stable the drug need only be given once a day, a major advantage for owner compliance. It is important not to miss doses, however, because even one missed day results in elevated serum T_4 levels.

Despite having a serum half life of 4–6 hours, it can be found in the thyroid gland, where it is needed, for up to 20 hours. Table 15.2 lists the adverse effects noted. It should also be noted that by treating the hyperthyroidism, the glomerular filtration rate is reduced and serum creatinine and urea levels should therefore be monitored to check for renal failure. In cats, 15% show some mild side effects but some of the GI effects mean treatment must be discontinued. The tablets must not be crushed or broken. As thiamazole is a suspected teratogen, women of child-bearing age should wear gloves when handling litters of treated animals.

Carbimazole

Carbimazole is a human authorised medicinal product and is a carbethoxy derivative of MMI. Figure 15.3 shows the difference in structures. Carbimazole is rapidly metabolised to the parent compound, which is responsible for the action of the drug. As it is a larger molecule, twice the dose is required but fewer side effects are reported with its use than are seen with MMI.

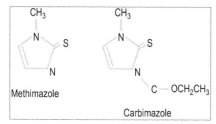

Fig. 15.3 Antithyroid drugs

Levothyroxine

Sodium levothyroxine is a synthetically prepared form of thyroxine (T_4) with authorisation for use, in the UK, for the treatment of canine hypothyroidism. There are a variety of dosage regimens recommended due to:

- the variation between animals in absorption and metabolism
- the variable degree of thyroid hormone secretion by the remaining glandular tissue of the thyroid
- possible circulating T_4 antibodies
- resistance to overdose by the methods stated above
- vague criteria by which clinical improvement is judged
- increased thyroid levels seem to be required during the colder months of winter
- older hypothyroid patients require lower doses of T_4.

It is better to treat with T_4 than T_3 for the following reasons:

- T_4 is the main secretory product of the thyroid gland
- the more potent T_3 is normally produced from T_4
- T_4 influences serum TSH levels more than T_3
- it is the only way to get both normal T_3 and T_4 levels
- the CNS and pituitary derive their T_3 from local deiodination of T_4
- T_4 is less expensive.

A number of synthetic T_3 products for thyroid hormone replacement therapy (THRT) exist in Europe. T_3 administration, however, circumvents the normal physiological process of T_4 deiodination to T_3. This may result in normal/therapeutic levels of total and free T_3, but will not normalise total and free T_4 levels.

Symptoms of over-dosage include tachycardia, excitability and excessive panting but are rare due to the ability of dogs and cats to clear thyroid hormone via biliary and faecal excretion. The mechanism of action of the thyroid hormones is shown in

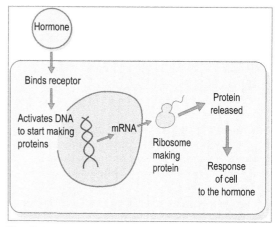

Fig. 15.4 Mechanism of action of steroid and thyroid hormones

Figure 15.4. Along with steroid hormones, they work by binding to their receptors inside cells which then activates the DNA, stimulating the production of new proteins which carry out the effects of the hormone.

Endocrine pancreas

Insulin

Insulin is used to treat insulin-dependent diabetes mellitus and as adjunct therapy in the management of hyperkalaemia. Insulin is the most potent physiological anabolic agent which acts by promoting the synthesis of glycogen, facilitating the uptake of glucose by cells and its metabolism. It also promotes the synthesis of protein and fat and the uptake of ions such as potassium into the cell. The structure of the insulin receptor is shown in Figure 15.5.

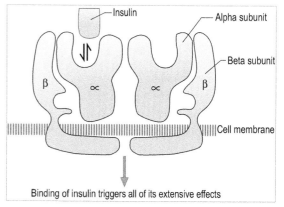

Fig. 15.5 Structure of the insulin receptor

It is made up of four units and insulin binds to the central two α units.

There are several types of insulin including:

- soluble (neutral) insulin – duration of up to 8 hours
- isophane that contains protamine to increase the duration of activity to 12 hours in the cat and up to 24 hours in the dog
- lente insulins that rely on the different concentrations of zinc to provide different durations of activity – the protamine zinc insulin (PZI) lasting up to 24 hours in both the cat and dog.

Bovine insulin is antigenic and is likely to stimulate the formation of anti-insulin antibodies. Pure porcine and human insulins do not appear to do this and are therefore preferred.

Treatment of diabetes mellitus requires injection of insulin, although trials of oral and nasal administration have been conducted. The short-acting regular insulin preparations can be injected i.v., i.m. and s.c., the intermediate and long-acting insulins are for s.c. use only. The preferred injection site should be the flank, where insulin uptake is most reliable. Fast-acting preparations are for treating complicated diabetics, i.e. those patients that can not take food orally, such as the vomiting ketoacidotic patient or the comatose animal.

The goal of therapy is to maintain a mild hyperglycaemic state, rather than the strict normoglycaemic state desirable in humans to prevent complications such as retinopathy and neuropathy. It is more important in animals to avoid hypoglycaemia. Box 15.3 lists the drug interactions to be aware of when using insulin. Sulphonylureas such as glipizide stimulate the pancreas to produce insulin. Most diabetic animals require insulin for treatment as their β cells can no longer secrete insulin and so sulphonylureas are not used much in veterinary medicine.

Diazoxide

This is a non-diuretic benzothiadiazine that inhibits insulin release from the β cells. It is used to manage hypoglycaemia caused by hyperinsulinism and is useful in the treatment of insulin-secreting tumours. It has many side effects including vomiting and diarrhoea and its efficacy diminishes over a period of months.

Streptozotocin

Streptozotocin is a nitrosourea alkylating agent that is cytotoxic to pancreatic β cells and has been used to treat humans with inoperable or metastatic insulinomas.

β-cell tumours, or insulinomas, secrete insulin along with other hormones such as somatostatin. Clinical signs are due to the hypoglycaemia and treatment includes glucocorticoids, which antagonise insulin, and diazoxide to inhibit the release of insulin. Streptozotocin (SZN) is a broad-spectrum antibiotic and anti-tumour agent that can be used to treat unresectable islet cell tumours. Toxic side effects include acute renal failure, bone marrow suppression, vomiting, anorexia, diarrhoea, transient hypoglycaemia and insulin-dependent diabetes mellitus. An aggressive saline diuresis protocol is used prior to and following the infusion of the chemotherapeutic agent to minimise the risks of renal problems. Butorphanol has been given in conjunction with streptozotocin because of its central anti-emetic action.

Sex hormones

Oestradiol (oestradiol benzoate) (Mesalin)

Oestradiol is an oestrogen used for the treatment of misalliance and hormonal urinary incontinence in bitches. It can also be used to treat anal adenomata and prostatic hyperplasia in male dogs. Oestradiol may be toxic to bone marrow and stilboestrol, another oestrogen hormone, can cause hepatic impairment, feminisation of males and arterial thrombosis.

Megoestrol acetate (Ovarid)

This is an oral progestogen, indicated for the prevention of oestrus in the bitch. Treatment should be

---

Box 15.3

Drugs and insulin

- Drugs that antagonise the hypoglycaemic effects of insulin
  - corticosteroids
  - thiazide diuretics
  - thyroid hormones
- Drugs that increase the effect of insulin
  - anabolic steroids
  - β-adrenergic blockers, e.g. propranolol
  - ethanol
  - phenylbutazone
  - salicylates
  - tetracycline

started during anoestrus. It can cause temperament changes and pyometra, as well as increasing the risk of mammary tumours.

Progestins such as proligestone (Delvosteron) given as injectable depot preparations (crystalline suspensions) are used to prevent oestrus in bitches, queens and jill ferrets and to control miliary dermatitis in cats. It has both central and peripheral progesterone-like effects with anti-oestrogenic and anti-androgenic activity. The use of progestins has recently been shown to induce the production of growth hormone from collections of cells in the mammary glands. These progestin-induced increases in growth hormone are also associated with increased levels of insulin-like growth factor 1. Administration of proligestone has been used to treat pituitary dwarfism in dogs and resulted in an increase in body weight and the development of an adult coat.

Danazol

Danazol is a synthetic androgen that has synergistic actions with corticosteroids in the treatment of immune-mediated thrombocytopenia and auto-immune haemolytic anaemia. Its onset of action is slow and it is teratogenic. Other side effects include hepatotoxicity and increased muscle mass.

Nandrolone (Laurabolin)

Nandrolone is a testosterone derivative with anabolic and anti-catabolic action. It is indicated wherever excessive tissue breakdown is occurring and is often used to treat the anaemia associated with chronic renal failure. It may be hepatotoxic and its use in immature animals may result in early closure of epiphyseal growth plates.

Parathyroid

Salcatonin is a synthetic salmon calcitonin. It is rarely used in veterinary medicine to manage hypercalcaemia. It inhibits bone resorption and intestinal resorption of calcium. It may also help to manage pain in patients with bone tumours.

Vitamin D formulations

Vitamin D activity is derived from a group of sterols of plant or animal origin that undergo transformation by ultraviolet light and subsequent modification by animal tissues to produce the active vitamin. Hormonal properties of vitamin D are essential to calcium and phosphorus metabolism.

Vitamin D is available as D_2 (ergocalciferol or calciferol), D_3 (cholecalciferol), dihydrotachysterol, alfacalcidol and calcitriol (1,25-dihydroxycholecalciferol). These different drugs have differing rates of onset and duration. The preferred forms of use are calcitriol and alfacalcidol as they have a rapid onset of action (1–4 days) and a short half-life of less than 1 day.

Delmadinone acetate (Tardak)

Delmadinone acetate is a progestin with anti-androgen and anti-oestrogen effects. It is used in the treatment of hypersexuality in the male dog and cat. It is also used in the treatment of prostatic hypertrophy, anal adenomas and hormonally driven canine aggression. Due to this drug's central calming effect, it can not be relied upon as an indicator of the effect of surgical castration on behavioural problems. It is often referred to as chemical castration.

Questions for Chapter 15

1. Describe the protocol for the ACTH stimulation test and what it is used for.

2. What is the TRH stimulation test used for?

3. What is the TSH stimulation test used for?

4. What are the therapeutic uses of ADH?

5. What are progestins and how do they function to inhibit oestrus?

6. What drugs interfere with thyroid hormone therapy and testing and why?

7. What potential side effects would you warn an owner of when commencing therapy with methimazole for hyperthyroidism in a cat?

8. What is the body's response to shock and how do steroids help?

9. How do cats respond to the available treatments for hyperadrenocorticism?

For answers go to page 243

Sixteen

Pharmaceutical Preparations Used in the Eye, Ear, Nose, Throat and Mouth

After studying this chapter you should be able to:

1. **State the methods of delivering drugs to the eye**
2. **Describe the treatments available for glaucoma**
3. **List the topical preparations available for ophthalmic use**
4. **State the range of therapies available for otitis externa**
5. **List drugs for oral diseases.**

Ophthalmic pharmacology

Drugs can be administered by topical, subconjunctival (Fig. 16.1), palpebral, retrobulbar or intraocular routes. Systemic administration is also used. Box 16.1 lists the factors affecting the choice of administration.

- Topical – solutions, suspensions, ointments or emulsions are incorporated within drug delivery systems. Dilution of the drug and washout by tears are the inevitable result of drug application. A small amount is taken up by the conjunctival circulation.
- Subconjunctival – injecting an aqueous solution or suspension under the bulbar conjunctiva results in a subconjunctival bleb of drug which is

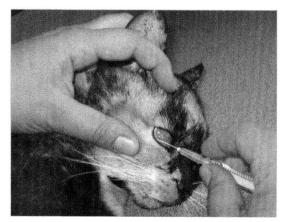

Fig. 16.1 Subconjunctival injection

Factors affecting choice of medication

- characteristics of the drug
  - solubility
  - available formulations
- the disease
  - severity
  - location
  - presence of normal ocular barriers
- patient factors
  - species
  - behaviour
- human factors
  - compliance with treatment instructions
  - cost of treatment

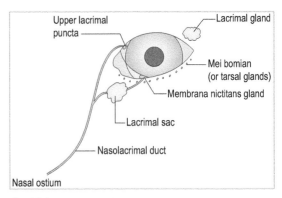

Fig. 16.2 The lacrimal system

slowly released from the site and diffuses across the sclera.

- Retrobulbar – this route is mostly used for regional anaesthesia of the orbit or face. The technique involves directing a needle through the eyelids and orbital fascia and depositing a drug behind the globe.
- Intracameral – placement of a drug into the anterior chamber. Drugs are either absorbed or metabolised locally and can be given this way to treat severe intraocular infection (endophthalmitis).
- Intravitreal – used to chemically destroy the ciliary epithelium in cases of chronic glaucoma. Needles are placed 3 mm behind the limbus and drugs enter the anterior chamber by diffusion.
- Systemic – drugs must cross the blood–aqueous and blood–retinal barriers.

Topical anaesthetics

Proparacaine and tetracaine are the most commonly used agents available as 0.5% solutions. Anaesthesia of the cornea takes 1 minute after application and lasts for 10–20 minutes. The conjunctiva requires 4–5 applications over 2–3 minutes to become anaesthetised. Tear production and the blink reflex are suppressed following the use of local anaesthesia and this will therefore affect Schirmer tear test readings.

Diagnostic agents

Fluorescein dye can be used to detect corneal ulceration and to check the patency of the nasolacrimal duct. Figure 16.2 shows the openings of the naso-

lacrimal duct in the upper and lower eyelids. In brachycephalic dogs and cats the nasolacrimal duct is short and wide, and often opens more caudally so that the fluorescein drains into the nasopharynx. It is important, therefore, to examine the tongue and pharynx when using the agent diagnostically.

Since the corneal stroma is hydrophilic, it will pick up water-soluble fluorescein. This positive staining is seen as yellow in white light but green under a cobalt blue filter or UV light. Rose-Bengal stains abnormal corneal cells deep red and so is useful to diagnose early keratoconjunctivitis sicca and feline herpes virus keratitis.

Topical corticosteroids

Prednisolone acetate penetrates the cornea well due to its lipid solubility. It is used to treat anterior uveitis and is a human authorised product. Treatment should be every 2–3 hours and combined with a mydriatic such as atropine 1% to reduce the pain from ciliary spasm that constricts the pupil. Combinations of gentamicin and betamethasone or neomycin and flumethasone are available as human authorised products.

Topical corticosteroids are contraindicated in the presence of ulceration as they delay corneal healing by impairing fibroblastic and keratocytic activity. They also predispose to infection and enhance the activity of degradative enzymes.

Ciclosporin

The immunosuppressive drug ciclosporin is used as a topical preparation to treat keratoconjunctivitis sicca (dry eye) in dogs. It acts through inhibition of T-cell lymphocytes and reduces both inflammation of lacrimal glands and ocular surface inflammation when administered topically. It can also be of benefit in mast cell mediated allergic conjunctivitis. Ciclosporin is available as a veterinary authorised product (Optimmune; Schering Plough).

Antimicrobial agents

In ulcerative keratitis where the corneal epithelial barrier is lost, corneal penetration becomes possible for drugs that would not usually cross.

- Topical gentamicin is the first choice if Gram-negative bacteria are suspected.
- Neomycin is often combined with bacitracin and polymyxin B to maximise the spectrum of antibacterial activity. It is a good first choice against acute, external ocular infections and is a human authorised product.
- Chloramphenicol is active against *Chlamydia* but unreliable as a treatment for ocular mycoplasmosis. It is a good first choice for treating intraocular infections due to its ability to penetrate the corneal and blood–aqueous barriers.
- The combination of trimethoprim-sulfadiazine is effective against ocular toxoplasmosis. Prolonged systemic therapy may, however, cause dry eye in the dog due to a direct toxic effect on the lacrimal gland.
- Fusidic acid or fusidin is a steroidal antibiotic chemically related to cephalosporin P. It is effective against Gram-positive organisms and some Gram-negatives. It is contained within a carbomer gel vehicle that provides lubrication and a sustained release of the active ingredient, making it suitable for once-daily application. The Veterinary Authorised Product is Fucithalmic Vet (Vet XX).
- Aciclovir (Zovirax) is an antiviral preparation used to treat ocular herpes virus infections. Feline herpes virus (FHV) can infect the superficial layers of the cornea causing a keratitis. Aciclovir inhibits the incorporation of one of the bases into viral DNA and is efficacious in the treatment of FHV keratitis if used early. This is a human authorised product.

Miscellaneous agents

Glaucoma can be managed with drugs such as the diuretic acetazolamide that reduces the proportion of bicarbonate in aqueous humour and the water secreted with it, thus lowering intraocular pressure. Additional drugs like pilocarpine are used to produce miosis within 10 minutes which lasts for 6–8 hours. Acetazolamide is not a diuretic per se, but rather a carbonic anhydrase inhibitor. It acts within the eye to reduce the proportion of bicarbonate in aqueous humour and the water secreted with it.

Carbonic anhydrase inhibitors act elsewhere in the body, producing side effects such as lethargy, GI disturbances and mild metabolic acidosis. Hypokalaemia occurs with long-term use and supple-mentation should be given. Topical therapy using a human authorised carbonic anhydrase inhibitor, e.g. dorzolamide (Trusopt), has also been effective but produces a burning sensation in people when applied to the eye.

Mydriatics such as atropine are drugs that dilate pupils. This is useful to relieve discomfort in some disorders and to open the pupil to allow examination of the retina. They are also used to diagnose autonomic dysfunction such as Horner's syndrome. The two mechanisms by which drugs produce papillary dilation are:

- paralysis of the iris sphincter muscle
- stimulation of the dilator muscle of the iris.

Atropine is the mydriatic of choice in treating anterior uveitis. Tropicamide is a short-acting agent with a greater mydriatic effect than atropine.

Osmotic agents are used for rapid reduction of intraocular pressure – mannitol is the most commonly used.

Lacrimomimetics or tear substitutes can be divided into aqueous solutions, mucinomimetics and lipid replacements. Methylcellulose is a semi-synthetic cellulose derivative in colloid form that is water soluble, viscous and virtually inert.

Therapeutic principles for otitis

Most products are a combination of antibiotics, antifungals, antiparasitics and corticosteroids. The use of a polypharmacy approach can lead the clinician to neglect the search for the primary cause of disease. The principles of therapy are shown in Box 16.2. Systemic therapy is indicated when there is rupture of the tympanic membrane, otitis media, general malaise, fever or anorexia. In some instances the inability of the owner to topically medicate the animal would also necessitate systemic therapy.

Figure 16.3 shows a dog undergoing retrograde (against the normal direction) flushing of the external ear canal. The technique, whereby a urinary catheter is placed into the ear canal and the ear is flushed out with saline or acetic acid, allows the debris at the base of the ear to be washed out more effectively. It is also a good method of delivering a drug to its desired site of action.

Systemic glucocorticoid therapy has several beneficial effects including:

- antipruritic
- anti-inflammatory
- reduces exudation, swelling, glandular secretion and proliferative changes
- promotes drainage and ventilation.

Principle aims of therapy for otitis

- cleaning products
  - ceruminolytics and detergents
  - avoid use if tympanic membrane is ruptured
- acidification
  - useful against Gram-negative bacteria
  - acetic acid (vinegar) can be used
- anti-inflammatory
  - relieves pain as well as reducing swelling and redness
  - topical glucocorticoids are very useful
- anti-bacterial
  - Gram-positive bacteria are the most common isolates
  - aminoglycosides are effective against Gram-negatives
- antifungal
  - *Malassesia pachydermatis* and *Candida albicans* are the most common isolates
- antiparasitic
  - must treat all animals in household

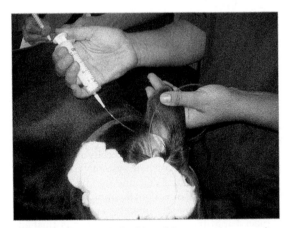

Fig. 16.3 Retrograde flushing of the external ear canal

Otitis interna

Also called labyrinthitis, this condition is a medical emergency and is usually caused by a spread from an otitis media or by haematological spread. Therapy should include:
- aggressive treatment with blood–brain barrier-penetrating antibiotics such as chloramphenicol or trimethoprim-sulfadiazine

- anti-inflammatory therapy using corticosteroids to reduce meningeal inflammation.

Drugs acting in the nose

Indications for decongestants include sinusitis of allergic or viral causes. Antihistamines such as chlorpheniramine and the sympathomimetic drugs, i.e. α-adrenergic agonists, can be used topically to reduce side effects. Stimulation of α receptors on the arterioles in the nose causes vasoconstriction and reduces blood flow to the mucosa. This decreases the excess extracellular fluid associated with a runny nose and reduces the mucosal volume, reducing congestion. Topical applications work within minutes but repeated use can cause ischaemic necrosis and mucosal damage due to lack of nutrients.

Topical corticosteroids are highly effective for the treatment of allergic rhinitis. The agents available include beclomethasone, fluticasone and flunisolide. They result in a reduction of sneezing and nasal itching within a few days but should only be used for short periods to reduce the risks of adrenal suppression.

Eucalyptus oil inhalation helps to decongest nasal mucosa.

Figure 16.4 shows a cat with a nasal catheter in place. This method can be utilised to deliver oxygen and certain aerosolised drugs in a concentrated form directly to the respiratory passages.

Drugs acting on the throat

Antitussives are agents that reduce coughing. The aim is to achieve this without impairing mucociliary

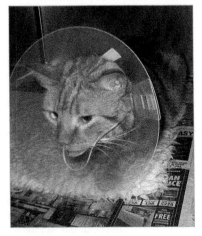

Fig. 16.4 Nasal cannula placement

defences. The cough reflex is stimulated by broncho-constriction – it can be blocked peripherally with mucolytics or expectorants or centrally at the cough centre in the medulla. Narcotics such as codeine and non-narcotics such as butorphanol are centrally active agents. Further information is provided in Chapter 10.

Drugs active against oral disease

- Chlorhexidine is a topical antiseptic found in dental products to control oral bacterial proliferation and halitosis. It is not inactivated by organic matter.

- Stomatitis and chronic gingivitis have been treated with aurothiomalate and auranofin. Both are gold salts used for the treatment or management of autoimmune diseases. Several months of therapy are required before results are seen. Pulse antibiotic therapy has also been advocated with metronidazole, 1 week on followed by a week off. Metronidazole has effects on the immune system through modulating cell-mediated immune responses.

- Lidocaine, a local anaesthetic, is available in both an oral spray solution and an oral viscous solution. The spray is used as a short-term topical anaesthetic and the gel can be applied to mouth ulcers for longer-lasting analgesia.

- Depo-medrone.

- Antivirals to boost immune defences in FeLV/FIV cats.

Questions for Chapter 16

1. Why should intranasal corticosteroid therapy be used only for seasonal allergic rhinitis and not for life-long control?
   a. prolonged use results in bronchospasm
   b. long-term use would predispose patients to hypoglycaemia
   c. to minimise adrenal suppression
   d. to prevent CNS depression

2. What is the term given to treatment of a condition using several different agents at once as in the topical otitis externa preparations?
   a. polymyxin
   b. polypharmacy
   c. multipharmaceuticals
   d. polytherapy

3. Prior to antihistamine therapy for allergic otitis externa or rhinitis, what should you check the patient's history for?
   a. hypertension, hyperthyroidism, diabetes mellitus, glaucoma, prostatic hyperplasia
   b. urinary retention, constipation, blurred vision
   c. glaucoma, prostatic hyperplasia, asthma, sedative drugs
   d. hypertension, hyperthyroidism, nasal decongestant use

4. Mouthwashes used to debride and cleanse minor oral lesions prior to oral surgery will contain:
   a. lidocaine
   b. chlorhexidine
   c. hydrogen peroxide
   d. atropine

For answers go to page 245

CHAPTER 17

Pharmaceutical Preparations Used in Dermatology

Learning aims and objectives

After studying this chapter you should be able to:

1. **State the advantages and disadvantages of topical therapy**
2. **List the topical antiseborrheics**
3. **State the pharmacological properties of the antihistamines**
4. **List suitable treatments for common skin disorders.**

Topical therapy

The epidermis forms an effective barrier for transdermal drug absorption (Fig. 17.1), but this can be overcome by several routes:

- through the stratum corneum via the intracellular route
- passive diffusion through the lipid layer (intercellular route) (Fig. 17.2)
- appendageal route.

Factors affecting the rate of absorption are shown in Box 17.1.

The advantages of topical therapy include:

- easily accessible target organ
- negligible systemic absorption, therefore few side effects (not true of corticosteroids and certain other drugs)
- maximum drug concentration at desired site of action.

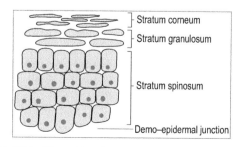

Fig. 17.1 The epidermis

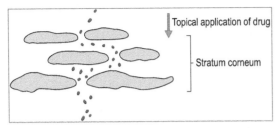

Fig. 17.2 Diffusion through the stratum corneum

Box 17.1

Factors affecting the rate of absorption

- drug factors
  - lipid solubility
  - molecular weight of the drug
  - contact time
  - the drug concentration in the vehicle
  - the release of the drug from the vehicle (penetration enhancers)
- patient factors
  - hydration
  - intact or broken skin
  - temperature
  - anatomical site
  - age

The disadvantages of topical therapy include:
- potential ingestion (especially in cats and other fastidious groomers)
- human exposure
- messy and laborious nature
- perceived simplicity by the owner of this approach.

Preparations contain 'active ingredients' and additives such as stabilisers, emulsifiers, preservatives, colour and fragrance, and a vehicle to carry the agent. Traditionally the drugs were delivered as solids, greases, aqueous or alcoholic solutions. Modern methods of delivery include wipes, liposomes, multilamellar micro- or nanocapsules, microparticles, spherulites and microemulsions for slow release of drugs. Chitosanide is an agent that is often added to preparations to help topical spreading. The dense hair coat poses a problem in some dogs and clipping can therefore be of benefit – allowing the application of topical products, as well as allowing the skin to 'breathe'. Topical medicines are classed as:
- shampoos (short duration)
- cream rinses (medium duration)

- leave-on sprays or conditioners (prolonged action).

The main application has been antibacterial, antifungal and antiparasitic, but the value of topical treatment to restore and maintain skin barrier function in cornification disorders and atopic dermatitis is being recognised.

The stratum corneum protects the body against drying out (desiccation) by regulating water loss and retention via its intercellular lipids and natural moisturising factor (NMF). NMF is very soluble and easily leached from cells by water. In healthy skin, the lipid bilayers surrounding the corneocytes act as a seal to prevent loss of NMF. If skin dries, the cells that are usually exfoliated remain connected and pile up on the surface, resulting in scaling and itching – moisturising alleviates this dysfunction. Water alone only transiently hydrates the skin, which then evaporates, leaving the skin even drier. A good moisturiser provides both humectants to compensate for the loss of NMF and lipids to replenish those lost from the intercellular lipid layers of the stratum corneum. Urea and glycerin are good moisturisers.

Topical antimicrobials

Iodine is widely used for its bactericidal, sporicidal, fungicidal, viricidal and protozoacidal activities. Due to its insolubility, iodine requires the addition of other agents to increase its solubility. Iodine does stain skin but the product povidone-iodine does not.

Chlorhexidine is highly bactericidal but not viricidal. It is not inactivated in the presence of necrotic tissue and has a sustained release action. When applied to skin, it binds to the protein portion of the stratum corneum. Systemic absorption and toxicity are minimal. It is available in the following concentrations:
- 7.5% solution
- 2% shampoo (Malaseb)
- 4% surgical scrub (Hibiscrub)
- 0.05% aqueous solution for ophthalmic use
- several oral cleansing solutions.

Antiseborrhoeics (keratolytics and keratoplastics)

These include:
- sulphur – non-irritating, antipruritic, antibacterial, antifungal and antiparasitic
- salicyclic acid – non-irritating, antipruritic, antibacterial
- coal tar – potentially irritating, mildly degreasing, toxic in cats

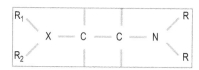

Fig. 17.3 General formula of most H_1 antihistamines

- benzoyl peroxide – antipruritic, follicular flushing, degreasing, antibacterial
- selenium sulphide – degreasing, antifungal
- ethyl lactate – antibacterial.

Antihistamines

These agents act on the histamine receptor to limit its accessibility to histamine and prevent it from causing its actions. Figure 17.3 shows the general formula of the antihistamines that act on the histamine receptor subtype 1. The nucleus of the structure is ethylamine, which is also present in histamine. The different chemical substitutions give the drugs their potencies and side effects.

The H_2 antihistamines differ from the H_1 blockers in their chemistry, pharmacokinetics and pharmacodynamics. The H_2 blockers are less lipid-soluble and do not effectively penetrate the blood–brain barrier. Hence the H_2 antagonists do not cause sedation – a side effect seen with H_1 blockers.

Effects on the body

- Histamine in excess can displace antihistamines which work better in preventing actions of histamine than in reversing them.
- H_1 antihistamines work well on bronchial, intestinal, uterine and vascular smooth muscle.
- They antagonise the vasoconstrictor effects of histamine and the more important vasodilator effects, as well as the increase in capillary permeability produced by histamine.
- They counteract urticaria, wheal formation and oedema, allergens, antigens or histamine-releasing drugs.
- H_1 antihistamines reduce itching associated with allergic reaction.
- H_1 antagonists do not block the stimulant effect of histamine on gastric secretion, which is an H_2-dependent function. H_2 antagonists are used extensively in the treatment of gastric ulceration.
- Side effects of the H_1 antagonists include sedation or CNS excitement, GI disturbance, parasympatholytic actions and teratogenic effects.

Common skin diseases and their therapies

Canine atopy

The aim of therapy is to reduce the level of pruritus to an acceptable level with as safe a treatment as possible. This is done by:
- Avoidance of the allergen
- Removal of allergens from the skin through regular washing
- Repair and maintenance of the skin barrier
- Interruption of the itch–scratch cycle. The use of antihistamines is controversial. The findings of 12 recently controlled trials are reported in Box 17.2
- The synergistic effect between antihistamines and essential fatty acids in the management of atopy
- Drug use – those most commonly reported to be effective in the control of atopy include hydroxyine, chlorpheniramine, diphenhydramine and clemastine
- Allergen specific immunotherapy – this is reported to have a 50–80% success rate in dogs but reliable evidence to support this is as yet unavailable
- Reduction of cutaneous inflammation – essential fatty acids modulate prostaglandin and leukotriene production and improve epidermal

---

Box 17.2

Antihistamine efficacy in controlling atopy

- low efficacy
  - chlorpheniramine
  - pheniramine
  - hydroxyzine
  - promethazineoxatomide
  - trimeprazine
  - astemizole
  - loratadine
  - cetirizine
- medium efficacy
  - clemastine
  - chlorpheniramine and hydroxyzine combined
  - terfenadine
  - oxatomide

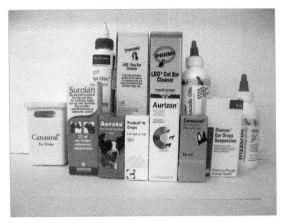

Fig. 17.4 Some of the available topical preparations used to manage otitis externa. Courtesy of G. Cousquer

barrier function. Gamma linoleic acid (GLA) or fish oil has been shown to be beneficial. Topical glucocorticoids (such as 0.015% triamcinolone acetonide spray) have high efficacy and low harmful effects with short-term use. Topical calcineurin inhibitors (tacrolimus) have been used with good success for localised lesions. Oral calcineurin inhibitors (ciclosporin) have good success rates with many dogs, reducing their pruritus by 50% within 6 weeks. The oral phosphodiesterase-4 inhibitor arofylline is as effective as prednisolone but there are marked GI side effects. The prostaglandin analogue misoprostol (Cytotec) also reduces pruritus. Secondary otitis externa is commonly seen in cases of atopy.

Some of the available topical preparations used to manage otitis externa are shown in Figure 17.4.

Flea bite hypersensitivity

Adult fleas are obligate ectoparasites and topical flea control is an essential part of the management of flea allergic dermatitis (FAD). Shampoos and washes are not particularly effective since they are rinsed off with little residual activity. The following are possible treatments:

- flea collars with good efficacy (such as those containing diazinon)
- aerosols containing organophosphates (dichlorovos and fenitrothion) or permethrin (beware toxicity in cats)
- fenthion exhibits good knockdown and has a residual efficacy of 95% 4 weeks after application
- microencapsulated clorpyriphos environmental spray results in adulticidal activity for 8–10 weeks

- topical washes or 'spot-on' with fipronil (a GABA antagonist) have a residual effect for 1–2 months after application
- imidocloprid as a 'spot-on' provides residual activity for 4 weeks
- systemic organophosphates, such as cythioate (oral administration) or fenthion (topical)
- insect growth regulators such as methoprene (environmental application) or lufenuron (oral application) act at specific immature stages, but have little effect on adult insects
- the potential for vaccination against the salivary proteins or concealed antigens within the flea gut is being researched.

Pyoderma

The term pyoderma means bacterial skin infection. The vast majority are associated with *Staphylococcus* species and many develop secondary to an underlying cause (Box 17.3). It is clear then that although antibiotics might contribute to the treatment, they are rarely effective alone in the management of surface pyodermas such as acute moist dermatitis.

Superficial pyodermas involve the epidermis (impetigo) or the hair follicle (folliculitis). With time, deep pyoderma may follow, with infection breaking into the surrounding dermis (furunculosis) and subcutaneous tissues (cellulitis).

Shampoos are usually beneficial (Box 17.4 shows the active ingredients), but any topical agent, especially containing benzoyl peroxide, has the potential to irritate the skin. Where superficial pyoderma becomes generalised and progresses to furunculosis and deep pyoderma, systemic treatment will often become indicated. The ideal contact time for shampoos is around 10 minutes and clipping the

---

Box 17.3

Examples of underlying causes of pyoderma

- cutaneous
  - allergic
  - keratinisation defects
  - follicular disorders
- metabolic
  - hypothyroidism
  - hyperadrenocorticism
  - diabetes mellitus
- immunological abnormality
  - hyperadrenocorticism

Shampoos and their active antimicrobial agents

- Etiderm: ethyl lactate
- Malaseb: chlorhexidine and miconazole
- Nolvasan: chlorhexidine
- Paxcutol: benzoyl peroxide
- Seleen: selenium sulphide
- Hexocil: hexitidine

hair may be beneficial in cases of deep pyoderma, especially in long-haired dogs.

Antibiotic therapy should be selected based on the likely effect on *S. intermedius* as this organism produces the enzyme β-lactamase, which renders some antibiotics ineffective. A bactericidal antibiotic should be selected if the dog is immunosuppressed. Box 17.5 lists the antibiotics likely to be effective. If the treatment is not successful within 2 weeks,

Antibiotics that may be effective treatments in pyoderma

- cephalosporins
  - cefadroxil
  - cephalexin
- potentiated amoxicillin
  - clavulanate-potentiated amoxicillin
- fluoroquinolones
  - difloxacin
  - enrofloxacin
  - ibafloxacin
  - marbofloxacin
- lincosamides and macrolides
  - clindamycin
  - lincomycin
  - erythromycin
- potentiated sulphonamides
  - trimethoprim and sulfadiazine
  - baquiloprim and sulfadimethoxine
- others
  - tylosin
  - mupirocin (exclusively for topical use)
  - rifampin

swabs for culture and sensitivity should be taken after a period of time without treatment. Some dermatologists advocate either pulse antibiotic therapy (one week on, one week off) for recurrent superficial folliculitis or suboptimal therapy (treating every other day) but these may encourage resistance. Immunomodulation with autogenous vaccines, levamisole and cimetidine, has been investigated but few cases resolved and the cost of cimetidine is very high.

Eosinophilic skin lesions in cats

These common problems in feline dermatology include:
- miliary dermatitis
- eosinophilic plaque
- eosinophilic granuloma
- indolent ulcer.

In addition to controlling underlying causes such as fleas, glucocorticoids are commonly used. Prednisolone or methylprednisolone acetate are both suitable but long-term use can cause iatrogenic hyperadrenocorticism and occult diabetes mellitus with urinary tract infections. These cats should be clinically monitored every 3–6 months and haematology, biochemistry and urinalysis performed at least once a year.

Antibiotic treatment is successful in some indolent ulcers but this does not imply a bacterial cause as some antibiotics have anti-inflammatory properties. Ciclosporin can induce remission of severe glucocorticoid-resistant lesions and both chlorambucil and gold salts have been used.

Megestrol acetate should be used with caution due to the range of commonly encountered side effects including:
- behavioural disorders
- polyphagia
- mammary hyperplasia
- pyometra
- diabetes mellitus
- hyperadrenocorticism.

Pemphigus foliaceus

Pemphigus foliaceus is the most common autoimmune skin condition in the dog and cat. There are three forms:
- spontaneous – seen especially in Akitas and Chow Chows
- drug-induced – Labrador Retrievers and Dobermanns may be predisposed
- associated with prior skin disease.

Effective drugs include:
- topical glucocorticoids in mild cases
- oral (methyl) prednisolone
- cats may respond better to dexamethasone by daily injection
- gold therapy (chrysotherapy)
- chlorambucil (Leukeran; Wellcome)
- azathioprine (Imuran; Wellcome)
- combination therapy.

Preventative medicine in veterinary dermatology

It is particularly important to advise owners travelling abroad with their dogs about hygiene, care and control of some of the dermatological conditions.
- Rabies vaccination – may cause cutaneous lesions in some animals, such as permanent alopecic patches (or injection site fibrosarcoma in cats).
- Prevention of sarcoptic and notoedric mange – once-monthly administration of spot-on selamectin. This will also protect against otodectic mange, fleas, cheyletiellosis and heartworm. Its efficacy against European ticks is controversial (the product is registered only for *Rhipicephalus sanguineus*) and it has no repellent activity against the sandfly vectors of Leishmaniasis.
- Prevention of Leishmaniasis – repellent deltamethrin collars protect animals from sandfly bites and prevent *Leishmania* infection. The use of a microencapsulated permethrin spray or spot-on once weekly to twice monthly may serve as a repellent for sandflies and a prevention for flea and tick infestation.
- Prevention of tick-transmitted diseases – microencapsulated permethrin sprays and amitraz collars are excellent tools for tick prevention.

Questions for Chapter 17

1. What is the most superficial layer of the epidermis called, which is the primary barrier to percutaneous absorption?
   a. stratum corneum
   b. stratum lucidum
   c. stratum granulosum
   d. stratum spinosum

2. What percentage of body weight does the skin make up?
   a. 1% in the puppy and 5% in the adult dog
   b. 24% in the puppy and 12% in the adult dog
   c. 52% in the puppy and 52% in the adult dog
   d. 75% in the puppy and 65% in the adult dog

3. Which of the following statements is true?
   a. histologically the skin can be divided into two units: the epidermis and the dermis
   b. the epidermis consists of columnar epithelium
   c. the thinnest skin is found on the foot pads and the planum nasale

   d. the stratum corneum allows free movement of water from the body to the surface of the skin

4. What are the differences between avian and mammalian skin? (More than one correct answer)
   a. birds have no melanocytes, the cells that impart colour to the skin
   b. birds have lipids in their epidermis but mammals do not
   c. avians possess no skin glands
   d. avians do not have a cutaneous blood supply

5. What has no effect on whether a drug can penetrate the skin?
   a. the vehicle the agent is in
   b. the hydration state of the stratum corneum
   c. the integrity of the stratum corneum
   d. the presence of pigment in melanocytes

6. What happens to the vehicle a drug is carried in after application to the skin?
   a. absorption of the vehicle through the stratum corneum

b. evaporation from the skin surface

c. physical removal (rubbing, licking, scratching)

d. all of the above

7. What is dimethylsulphoxide (DMSO) used for in topical therapy?

a. it is a penetration enhancer by disrupting the normally organised lipid layer of the stratum corneum

b. it causes vasodilation of the cutaneous vessels

c. it increases sebum production

d. it decreases sebum production

8. What is/are the disadvantage(s) of wound powders?

a. water-absorbing powders coalesce and occlude the skin's surface

b. those that contain starch or other carbohydrates give bacteria and fungi a source of energy allowing them to proliferate and cause skin infections

c. talc can cause severe granulomatous reactions in body cavities and abscesses

d. all of the above

9. What is the difference between keratolytics, keratoplastics and antiseborrheics?

a. keratoplastics function by loosening keratin which facilitates the loss of the dry top layer of the stratum corneum, keratolytics attempt to normalise keratinisation by slowing cell division through inhibition of DNA synthesis, and antiseborrheics modulate sebum production in the skin

b. keratolytics function by loosening keratin which facilitates the loss of the dry top layer of the stratum corneum, keratoplastics attempt to normalise keratinisation by slowing cell division through inhibition of DNA synthesis, and antiseborrheics modulate sebum production in the skin

c. keratolytics function by loosening keratin which facilitates the loss of the dry top layer of the stratum corneum, antiseborrheics attempt to normalise keratinisation by slowing cell division through inhibition of DNA synthesis, and keratoplastics modulate sebum production in the skin

d. antiseborrheics function by loosening keratin which facilitates the loss of the dry top layer of the stratum corneum, keratoplastics attempt to normalise keratinisation by slowing cell division through inhibition of DNA synthesis, and keratolytics modulate sebum production in the skin

10. Which agent is keratolytic, keratoplastic and antiseborrheic as well as being antibacterial and antipruritic with a mild follicular flushing action?

a. DMSO

b. clotrimazole

c. sulphur

d. chlorhexidine

For answers go to page 245

Eighteen

CHAPTER 18

Pharmaceutical Preparations Used for Malignant Disease and Immunosuppression

Learning aims and objectives

After studying this chapter you should be able to:

1. **Describe the unwanted effects of antineoplastic agents**
2. **List the mechanisms of action of cancer treatments**
3. **List the immunosuppressive agents available.**

The development of a tumour

Most cancers are believed to arise through a process called multi-step carcinogenesis. This theory is based on the fact that in the majority of cancers, at least two genetic changes have occurred prior to the induction of malignancy. There are three basic steps in multi-step carcinogenesis, which ultimately lead to the evolution of a cancer cell from a normal cell:

1. *Initiation*: Initiating agents induce a permanent and irreversible change in the DNA of the affected cell. In and of itself, the initiating event is not significant enough to induce neoplastic transformation. Initiated cells cannot be distinguished from other cells in the surrounding environment.
2. *Promotion*: Promoting agents cause reversible tissue and cellular changes. They can induce changes in cellular morphology, mitotic rate, and degree of terminal differentiation. Promotion serves to expand the initiated cell population and alter it in such a way as to increase the likelihood of another irreversible change occurring.
3. *Progression*: Progressing agents are able to convert an initiated cell, or a cell undergoing promotion, into a cell exhibiting malignancy, capable of developing into a mature neoplasm. The process of progression is irreversible.

In order for a tumour to result, the affected cell must be irreversibly altered at least twice. The cell is altered once in the initiation phase and once in the progression phase. The promotion phase changes the affected cell in a way to increase the likelihood that the cell changed by the initiation will be in a position to be changed by the progression phase.

Guidelines for chemotherapy

Several criteria must be met before chemotherapy is undertaken:

- a histological diagnosis is required
- the patient's health status must be established – history, physical examination and supporting data
- safe dosage schedules for the species being treated must be used
- monitoring of toxicosis to alter or limit treatment in the interests of the patient
- informed consent must be obtained from the owner; information on the side effects of therapy, prognosis and expectations should be provided.

Antineoplastic drugs

General clinical considerations

Cancer is the number one natural cause of death in geriatric cats and dogs, and it accounts for nearly 50% of deaths each year. Although cancer is the leading cause of death in geriatric patients, it is also the most treatable disease when compared with congestive heart failure, renal failure and diabetes mellitus.

Chemotherapy is the term used to describe the treatment of cancer using chemotherapeutic agents. Whilst surgery remains the treatment of choice for discrete solid tumours and whilst radiotherapy can be effective for localised disease, rapidly progressing or generalised disease is likely to require chemotherapy. Benefits of chemotherapy include:

- complete cure
- the ability to control generalised or rapidly progressing disease
- the prevention of spread of a neoplasm by controlling early, rapidly proliferating metastases, that are unlikely to contain resistant cells
- the ability to increase the disease-free interval following other modes of treatment
- the provision of symptomatic relief and temporary restoration of deteriorating function.

Clinically useful drugs achieve a degree of selectivity based on certain characteristics of cancer cells, e.g., rapid rate of malignant cell division and growth, and variations in the drug uptake and sensitivity

of different types of cells. The decision to use antineoplastic therapy depends on the type of tumour to be treated, the stage of malignancy and the condition of the animal. Chemotherapy is not a panacea for cancer – many malignant tumours are unresponsive to chemotherapy and, even where treatment is beneficial, it is rarely curative. Responses range from palliation (remission of secondary signs, generally without increase in survival time) to complete remission (in which clinically detectable tumour cells and all signs of malignancy are eliminated).

The effectiveness of chemotherapy depends on the ability to balance the killing of tumour cells against the inherent toxicity of many of these drugs to host cells. Because of their narrow therapeutic indices, dosages are calculated on body surface area rather than body mass – it is thought to be physiologically more accurate but this may not be true of all drugs. Antineoplastic agents are commonly administered in various combinations – referred to as protocols or combination chemotherapy. The use of a number of different drugs to attack different specific segments of the cell cycle increases the success rates of treatment. The fraction killed by one drug is independent of that killed by another. The main indications for chemotherapy as a first-line treatment are systemic diseases such as lympho-sarcoma, myeloma and certain forms of leukaemia. Cytotoxic drugs are also used as an adjunct to surgery or radiotherapy or to help prevent metastasis of solid tumours.

Mechanism of action

Most chemotherapeutic agents either bind directly to genetic material in the cell nucleus or affect a cell's ability to synthesise protein, which may damage growth and reproduction of normal cells as well. Both normal cells and cancer cells go through the same cell division cycle. However, most tumour cell populations are characterised by genetic instability, which can impact the effect of chemotherapy drugs. For instance, individual tumour cells can mutate and produce variant cells. These variant cells are genetically distinct from the tumour cell of origin. This genetic instability is an important concept because it can be linked to chemotherapy-resistant cells.

Chemotherapeutic agents are classified according to their pharmacological action, and the point in the cell cycle at which they interfere with cellular reproduction. Cell division is the pinnacle of the cell cycle which is shown in Figure 18.1. This involves a tightly regulated process whereby the DNA double helix separates and an identical copy of each strand is made (synthesis phase or S-phase). Either side of the S-phase in the cell cycle are two important phases known as G1 and G2. During each of these there

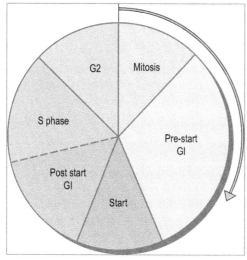

Fig. 18.1 Sequence of events during the cell cycle

is a frenzy of protein and RNA synthesis and other metabolic events (depending on the tissue type). M-phase is the time when the cell actually divides (mitosis phase). Drugs that are active only during a specific phase of the cell cycle are considered cell cycle phase-specific. Drugs that are active regardless of the cell cycle phase are called cell cycle phase-non-specific. The use of cell cycle phase-non-specific drugs appears to result in the death of both resting cells and cycling cells. Following cell death, resting cells are 'awakened' into the reproduction cycle and are then more susceptible to chemotherapeutic agents.

There are three potential targets for cytotoxic chemotherapy:
- DNA metabolism
- protein metabolism
- specific cellular functions.

Regardless of the specific mechanism of intracellular disruption, the cell will die as it attempts cell division (unless it is capable of repairing itself). The cell kill rate of various drugs is related to the concentration of the drug and to the degree of tumour cell exposure over time. Therefore, an apparent resistance due to inadequate blood levels can occur when a drug is poorly absorbed or when the drug is excreted or metabolised at an increased rate. There are more factors than this one – including the number of dividing cells (there is generally a greater number of dividing cells in a small population than in a large):
- the agent must reach the site of action
- the effective contact time (drug concentration × drug exposure time) (as described above – affected by route of administration and absorption, biotransformation, etc.)
- distribution of the drug.

Combining cytotoxic drugs is an important, effective strategy in chemotherapy. When drugs are used in combination, they often enhance the activities of each other. This synergistic action can occur by either sequential scheduling or by pharmacological mechanisms. Drugs are also combined to minimise their dose-limiting toxicities. Furthermore, combination chemotherapy helps reduce the development of tumour resistance, since cells resistant to one of the drugs in a combination regimen may be sensitive to another drug within that regimen.

Patterns of toxicity

Antineoplastic drugs that act primarily on rapidly dividing and growing cells produce several common patterns of toxicity including bone marrow suppression, gastrointestinal (GI) complications and immune suppression. These drugs act on rapidly dividing tissues as they pass through the cell cycle. Tissues that naturally demonstrate a high cell turnover, such as tissues of the gastrointestinal tract and haemolymphatic system, are therefore vulnerable to toxic effects. Some of the complications are:
- leucopenia leading to increased incidence of infection
- haemorrhage from thrombocytopenia
- anaemia
- nausea and vomiting, ulcerative enteritis, diarrhoea, stomatitis
- inhibition of spermatogenesis
- teratogenesis
- carcinogenesis
- alopecia
- tissue necrosis due to extravasation of certain drugs.

Adverse effects

Practically all anticancer drugs have side effects. However, their potential effect against the cancer generally outweighs the possible side effects. Although serious adverse effects can occur with any chemotherapy, there is a less than 5% chance that a patient will be hospitalised with side effects and a less than 1% chance of fatality. Below are listed some potential side effects of many chemotherapeutic agents.

Hair loss (alopecia)

When a person loses hair as a result of chemotherapy, it can be devastating. Pets rarely lose their hair, however; but if they do, they are not bothered by it as much as people are. In most pet animals, hair does not grow continually throughout life, therefore hair loss in pets is rare. Exceptions are certain breeds of dogs, such as poodles, Old English Sheepdogs and other breeds whose hair grows continually. In general, if a pet needs to visit a groomer periodically to be clipped, then the pet may experience some degree of hair loss as a result of chemotherapy. Wire-haired and curly coated breeds seem more likely than others to develop alopecia. Cats may be more prone to alopecia than dogs, however, and may lose all or most of their whiskers following administration of doxorubicin.

Reduction in the number of white blood cells (leucopenia)

There are various types of cells in the blood. The decrease in the number of infection-fighting white blood cells is known as neutropenia or leucopenia as both humoral and cell-mediated immunity are affected. Many chemotherapeutic agents impair the bone marrow's ability to produce cells. As a result, neutropenia may occur 7–10 days after chemotherapy. Neutropenia alone is not a danger to a patient. However, a patient's ability to fight off infection is impaired by neutropenia. All patients are given a complete clinical examination, and a blood test called a complete blood count (CBC) is performed prior to most chemotherapy administrations. Should the patient have a significant reduction in the number of white blood cells, it may be advisable to perform periodic blood tests, and/or have the veterinarian in charge of the case prescribe antibiotics to protect against infection.

Patterns of myelosuppression vary with the chemotherapeutic agent used, some are more profound and persistent than others. Regular CBCs should be performed regardless of the original findings – recommended leucocyte counts at which treatment should be postponed vary (4000/μl has been suggested, with 2500 granulocytes/μl) and will evolve as this field of veterinary medicine evolves.

Anaemia and thrombocytopenia must also be checked for throughout therapy.

Stomach or intestinal (gastrointestinal) discomfort

Many patients experience some form of stomach or intestinal discomfort 2–7 days after a chemotherapy treatment. Vets usually prescribe medication to try to prevent or treat the discomfort. Below are listed some steps that a client can take at home.

'Upset stomach' (nausea)
- If a pet begins to show any signs of upset stomach (drooling, 'smacking' lips) or loss of appetite, administer the medicine prescribed for nausea.
- Do not give any food for 12 hours, and offer ice cubes every few hours.

- After 12 hours, feed small, frequent meals instead of one large meal.

Vomiting
- Do not give any food or water for 12 hours.
- After 12 hours, offer ice cubes, then water, then small bland meals.

Loss of appetite
- If a pet begins to show any signs of upset stomach or loss of appetite, administer the medicine prescribed for nausea.
- Offer four small meals a day.
- Add warm broth, animal fats, and favourite foods to increase flavour and appeal.

Diarrhoea
- If a pet begins to show signs of diarrhoea, administer the medicine prescribed for diarrhoea.
- Keep water available at all times.
- If a pet is also not eating, offer chicken or beef broth.

Tissue damage

If some chemotherapy agents are accidentally given outside the vein, then severe tissue reactions can result. Therefore, chemotherapy agents are handled with the utmost care, and are only administered by highly trained technicians following established protocols. If irritation of the injection site develops in the form of pain or redness, apply ice packs for 15 minutes every 3 hours.

Allergic reactions

Allergic reaction to chemotherapeutic agents is rare, and not a problem the client will have to treat at home. Should a patient have an allergic reaction, it would develop upon administration and should be treated as for any other allergic anaphylaxis.

Heart damage

Some chemotherapeutic agents, in some rare cases, can irreversibly damage the heart muscle. The dose of these agents prescribed is below the dose that usually causes heart disease. Less than 10% of patients develop heart disease as a result of chemotherapy.

Drug administration

Intravenous injection is the most likely route of administration. A secure, pre-placed, over-the-needle catheter should always be used. Many drugs when injected extravascularly result in severe and extensive tissue necrosis requiring aggressive surgical reconstruction or limb amputation. A vein should not be used within 24 hours of a previous attempted catheterisation or venepuncture. Poor circulation in the chosen limb results in slow drug egress and increases the likelihood of local leakage. Regularly used veins can become difficult to catheterise and should be used in rotation and not for routine phlebotomy.

Chemical restraint should be considered for nervous patients or those requiring long infusions. An animal should never be left unattended whilst an infusion is taking place. Frequent drawing back and observation of the site is recommended. An attempt to dilute the extravasated drug should not be performed, but an experienced oncologist should be contacted for advice.

The catheter and giving set should be flushed with saline before they are removed as one unit to minimise the exposure to the operator. The greatest risk of self-injury is whilst recapping a needle – so it is recommended to dispose of the needle without recapping it or removing it from the syringe. Small-volume injectables, such as vincristine, can be given via a short extension set, such as a T-port, or into a free-running drip line – making the patient easier to restrain and therefore less likely to pull the catheter out. Injections should never be made against resistance. Catheters should be flushed with non-heparinised saline immediately prior to drug administration to ensure patency and to remove any traces of heparin, which may cause precipitation of certain drugs.

Drug categories

The drugs can be grouped by biochemical mechanism of action into the following categories; Table 18.1 gives examples of each group.

Alkylating agents

Alkylating agents (e.g. cyclophosphamide) have an alkyl radical substituted for a hydrogen atom. Alkylation causes breaks in the DNA molecule and cross-linking of the broken strands. This then interferes with DNA replication and RNA transcription. Alkylating agents are used to treat haemolymphatic neoplasms, sarcomas, lung and mammary carcinomas and mast cell tumours. Side effects include nausea, vomiting and alopecia. They are cycle specific and act at all phases of the cell cycle. They are frequently called radiomimetic drugs because their action in causing DNA-strand breaks resembles that of radiation. Cyclophosphamide is the most widely used alkylating agent in veterinary practice. A range of side effects may be seen. Haemorrhagic cystitis may be seen and is likely to limit prolonged use.

Antimetabolites

Antimetabolites (e.g. folic acid) are structural analogues of normal metabolites that are required for cell replication and function. These drugs can mimic basic building blocks of nucleic acids and either interfere with the enzymatic process or actually become incorporated into a non-functional nucleotide polymer. They are predominantly S-phase specific – the time in the cycle when DNA is synthesised. Side effects include leucopenia, nausea, and delayed hepatotoxicity. The antimetabolites do not have a major role in chemotherapy due to their non-specific toxicity and their S-phase specificity. The half life of cytosine arabinose is about 8 minutes – during this time less than 5% of dividing cells will be in S-phase and susceptible. Therefore to be effective this drug needs to be given as a continuous infusion over 24 hours. These drugs are used to treat Sertoli cell tumours and osteosarcomas.

Table 18.1 Classes of antineoplastic agents

Class	Mode of action	Examples
Alkylating agent	Adds to DNA, causes breaks in the DNA (see text)	Cyclophosphamide Chlorambucil Melphalan Cisplatinum Carboplatin
Antimetabolites	Interferes with nucleotide or 5-fluorouracil DNA synthesis	Cystosine arabinose Methotrexate
Spindle poisons	Prevents mitosis	Vincristine Vinblastine
Spindle synthesis	Prevents mitosis	Taxanes
Protein synthesis	Cellular functions	L-asparaginase
Biological modifiers, e.g. hormones	Various, modify cell function	Corticosteroids

Vinca alkaloids/spindle poisons

The vinca alkaloids are plant alkaloids derived from *Vinca rosea*. They act specifically in M phase by interfering with chromosomal separation, poisoning the spindle and preventing it from functioning. Taxanes (expensive for routine use) prevent the formation of the spindle in the first place. Both vincristine and vinblastine are given intravenously and can cause sloughing and ulceration, exposing underlying tendons and bone. They are used to treat a variety of cancers including mast cell tumours, carcinomas, sarcomas and transmissible venereal tumours.

Antineoplastic antibiotics (anthracyclines)

The antitumour antibiotics are products of the soil fungus *Streptomyces* and include doxorubicin. Toxicities can be acute (e.g. vomiting, transient ECG changes and arrhythmias) or delayed (e.g. cardiac toxicity). A wide range of soft tissue and bone sarcomas can be treated with doxorubicin. In contrast to the alkylating agents, anti-tumour antibiotics appear to have some selectivity for cancer cells over normal cells. Doxorubicin is a non-specific DNA intercalating agent, i.e. it binds between the two strands of DNA. In addition to generally interfering with transcription and other processes that involve DNA, doxorubicin is an inhibitor of the enzyme topoisomerase II (responsible for untangling the DNA). Without this enzyme the DNA strands do not get put back together properly. Doxorubicin also has other actions, not least of which is direct oxidative damage to DNA. It is not untypical for a cytotoxic agent to have more than one mode of action – indeed, this may increase its overall efficacy.

Hormonal agents

Hormonal agents are not primarily cytotoxic and are therefore more selective in their actions than other cytotoxic drugs. Hormonal agents used in chemotherapeutic protocols include corticosteroids and sex hormones.

Adrenal corticosteroids can have anti-tumour as well as anti-inflammatory effects. The cell lysis associated with corticosteroid-induced cell death may arise through dissolution of the cell membrane and activation of endonucleases.

The anti-tumour effects are related to the agents' lympholytic properties. They can inhibit mitosis and protein synthesis in sensitive lymphocytes. Toxic effects of steroid treatment include gastric ulceration, glucose intolerance, polydipsia and polyuria, immunosuppression, cataracts, Cushing's and osteoporosis. Dexamethasone, prednisolone and prednisone are especially useful in the treatment of leukaemias and lymphomas of the CNS since they readily cross the blood–brain barrier and enter the CSF. The major effect of these drugs on brain tumours is due to a reduction in local inflammation and oedema.

Prednisolone is often part of chemotherapy protocols and even when used alone it can have very good effects. Without therapy, the average survival time for dogs with leukaemia is 6–8 weeks, but with prednisolone therapy this is extended to 3 months. Hormones play an important role in the regulation of normal cells and the growth of certain tumours may be hormone-dependent and can be blocked by specific antagonists. Sex hormones have proved useful in the treatment of hormone-dependent tumours of mammary, prostatic or perianal gland origin. Perineal adenoma is almost exclusively seen in entire male dogs and is dependent on testosterone for growth. This growth promotion can be blocked by the drug delmadinone acetate, an androgen antagonist.

Non-steroidal anti-inflammatory drugs

Regular use of NSAIDs has been shown to reduce the risk of colorectal neoplasia by up to 50% in human studies; a reduced risk of malignant transformation of benign rectal adenomata to adenocarcinomata has also been demonstrated. Piroxicam has been shown to reduce the incidence of both the above-mentioned rectal tumours and slows the progression of transitional cell carcinoma of the canine urinary tract. The antineoplastic effects of NSAIDs may be due to inhibition of prostaglandin E_2 production, resulting in enhanced local immune responses and stimulation of cytoprotective prostaglandin production.

Miscellaneous antineoplastic agents

Three drugs commonly used as antineoplastics in veterinary medicine that do not fall into any of the above categories are L-asparaginase, cisplatin and mitotane. L-asparaginase is used to treat lymphoreticular neoplasms but can cause hypersensitivity reactions resulting in anaphylactic shock. It is an enzyme of bacterial origin that degrades the amino acid asparagine. By depleting the stocks of this essential amino acid, protein synthesis is disrupted and can lead to cell death. Cisplatin is ototoxic and can cause a peripheral neuropathy but is useful in the treatment of osteosarcoma. Mitotane causes atrophy of the inner zones of the adrenal cortex and so is useful in the treatment of hyperadrenocorticism (Cushing's).

Bisphosphonates are a group of drugs that inhibit osteoclasts and are postulated to induce tumour cell death. They are used in human medicine to treat postmenopausal osteoporosis and metastatic bone cancer. Use of the bisphosphonate alendronate in dogs with osteosarcoma has shown promising results. It should be given in the morning on an empty stomach and at least 30 minutes prior to feeding. It should not be given concurrently with NSAIDs.

Carboplatin is less nephrotoxic than many other agents and may be useful in the management of osteosarcoma, melanoma and various carcinomas in dogs.

The challenges of chemotherapy

It has been estimated that a 20 kg child with acute lymphoblastic leukaemia has 10^{10} cancer cells when clinical signs lead to diagnosis, 10^9 when declared to be in remission (i.e. the cancer can no longer be clinically detected) and 10^{12} at death. One gram of tumour contains 10^9 cells. An antitumour agent that killed 99.9% of the cells in a patient with 10^{12} cells would leave 10^9 cells behind. To kill the remaining cells would require additional courses of therapy, but would require spacing to allow recovery of the bone marrow and gut epithelium – to avoid the patient dying from drug toxicity. Clinically successful chemotherapy requires that there be a significant difference between the proportion of cancerous and normal cells killed and that normal cells rebound more rapidly from the therapy. Resistance to chemotherapy can be attributed to three factors:

- low concentration of drug in the tumour
- small fraction of cells in a susceptible state
- biochemical resistance of the tumour cells to the drug.

Blood flow to the tumour is often the limiting factor in tumour growth. The centre of a tumour is often ischaemic and necrotic due to lack of nutrients and oxygen, and a build up of toxic waste products – drug delivery is therefore obviously impaired. Also, chemotherapeutics are most effective against rapidly dividing cells, which occurs in small, young tumours. By the time a tumour has become large enough to be detected, the cell turnover has often subsided and cytotoxic therapy is far less effective or ineffective.

Cytotoxic drugs

Cytotoxic drugs are those that kill actively dividing cells. They are used in the treatment of certain cancers as discussed above. It is important to remember that they have a narrow therapeutic index and should be handled with care. Cyclophosphamide is an example of a potent cytotoxic drug. Intravenous preparations should be prepared and handled only by trained personnel and reconstitution or transfer to syringes should be carried out in designated areas. Pregnant women should not handle cytotoxic agents.

Patients excrete potentially harmful drugs and their metabolites in urine, faeces, vomit, saliva and sweat for variable periods of time following administration of injectable or oral cytotoxic drugs. Such excretions can potentially contribute to the exposure of veterinary personnel and owners. Table 18.2 shows the suggested precautionary periods for handling urine/faeces following cessation of treatment with commonly used cytotoxic drugs.

Photodynamic therapy

Photodynamic therapy (PDT) is a method of cancer treatment utilising the interaction between a photosensitive agent, light and oxygen. The photosensitive agent is preferentially taken up or retained in tumour cells at a higher concentration than in normal tissues, leading to selective toxicity. After a period of time the lesion is exposed to light of a wavelength which corresponds to one of the absorption maxima of the photosensitiser. This then produces free radicals which damage cell membranes (mitochondrial membranes, endoplasmic reticulum and lysosomal, nuclear and plasma membranes) culminating in cell death. Release of inflammatory mediators from damaged cells causes vasoconstriction, platelet aggregation and blood stasis, leading to coagulation necrosis and tumour cell death.

An example of a photosensitising agent is 5-aminolaevulinic acid, used as a topical agent with

Table 18.2 Precautionary periods for handling urine/faeces following cessation of treatment

Drug	Route	Urine	Faeces
Doxorubicin	i.v.	6 days	7 days
Vinca alkaloids	i.v.	4 days	7 days
Cyclophosphamide	any	3 days	5 days
Cisplatin	i.v.	7 days	unknown

a red light-emitting diode to treat squamous cell carcinomas of the nose and pinnae in cats. In one study, 85% of lesions responded completely after just one treatment, although 63% of lesions reoccurred within 6 months.

Immunosuppressive and immunostimulating drugs

Immunosuppressants are of use in immune-based joint disease such as rheumatoid arthritis and autoimmune skin conditions like the pemphigus complex. All of the following drugs fall into this category.

- Aurofin and aurothiomalate are gold salts whose toxic effects include diarrhoea, renal tubule damage and bleeding mucous membranes.
- Azathioprine suppresses cell-mediated hypersensitivities and alters antibody production. It has been used in the management of immune-mediated thrombocytopenia (IMT) but toxic effects include bone marrow suppression.
- Chlorambucil and cyclophosphamide are antineoplastic immunosuppressive drugs that can cause anorexia and nausea.
- Danazol is a synthetic androgen used to manage IMT and autoimmune haemolytic anaemia.
- Melphalan is used to treat myeloma and lymphosarcoma.
- Prednisolone is commonly used as an immunosuppressant. Its side effects include polydipsia, polyuria, polyphagia, GI ulceration, impaired wound healing and susceptibility to infections.
- Vincristine sulphate is used to treat neoplasias and IMT. Severe irritation occurs if injected extravascularly.

Ciclosporin

Ciclosporin is a potent immunosuppressive drug that inhibits T cell activation and suppresses cell-mediated immune responses. It acts by binding to the intracellular receptor cyclophilin and inhibiting calcineurin, which is believed to be involved in the transcription of cytokines. It also inhibits alpha interferon, which is responsible for multiplication of macrophages and monocytes. It is highly bound to plasma proteins and is metabolised in the liver. Ciclosporin treatment for anal furunculosis in dogs is effective at resolving lesions in most dogs as the condition has an immune-mediated component. Residual or recurrent lesions remain a potential problem – surgical resection or long-term therapy may be necessary. Around 58% of dogs show side effects including diarrhoea, hair loss, vomiting, lethargy and hind-limb lameness.

Ciclosporin A and ketoconazole can be used as a combined therapy for the treatment of anal furunculosis as there is an interaction between the two agents – improving the success of treatment. The use of ketoconazole reduces the quantity of ciclosporin required – with a reduction in side effects and costs. Ketoconazole affects the biotransformation pathway of ciclosporin by competitive inhibition, causing the serum half-life to double in dogs. Using doses of ketoconazole at 7.5 mg/kg q12h and ciclosporin at 0.5 mg/kg q12h provides a cost reduction of approximately 70% over the use of ciclosporin alone at 5 mg/kg q12h.

Ciclosporin has been specifically implicated in an increased risk of developing lymphoma in humans and cases have been reported following its use in dogs. It may be because immunodeficiency leads to suboptimal surveillance for cancer cells by the body and they are allowed to proliferate rather than being destroyed by the immune system.

Levamisole

This is an example of a drug that stimulates the immune system. It is a broad-spectrum anthelmintic, but it also acts to stimulate T-cell differentiation and the response to allergens, e.g. increasing phagocytic activity in macrophages and neutrophils. It works best when there is depressed T cell function and has little or no effect on the immune system of healthy animals.

Questions for Chapter 18

1. What is the term applied when all clinical evidence of cancer has disappeared but microscopic foci of cancer cells may remain?
   a. cured
   b. relieved
   c. remission
   d. regeneration

2. What is defined as the application of drugs to kill or inhibit the growth of viruses or foreign cells such as bacteria in the body without any surgical intervention?
   a. neoadjuvant therapy
   b. adjuvant therapy
   c. chemotherapy
   d. palliative treatment

3. When a cell divides, how long does mitosis typically take?
   a. 1 hour
   b. 1 day
   c. 1 week
   d. 1 month

4. What group of chemotherapeutics are said to be non cell-cycle-specific? i.e. they are toxic to all cells whether dividing or not.
   a. vincristine
   b. dactinomycin
   c. doxorubicin
   d. alkylating agents

5. Anticancer drugs are frequently dosed on the basis of surface area rather than body weight (BW). What is the formula to convert weight to surface area?
   a. surface area $= BW^4 \times K/10^4$ where K is a constant with the value of 10.0 and 10.1 for cats and dogs respectively
   b. surface area $= BW^{0.67} \times K/10^4$ where K is a constant with the value of 10.0 and 10.1 for cats and dogs respectively
   c. surface area $= BW^{0.67} \times K/10^{0.67}$ where K is a constant with the value of 10.0 and 10.1 for cats and dogs respectively
   d. surface area $= BW \times K/10$ where K is a constant with the value of 10.0 and 10.1 for cats and dogs respectively

For answers go to page 245

CHAPTER 19

Pharmaceutical Preparations used to Treat Poisoning Cases

Learning aims and objectives

After studying this chapter you should be able to:

1. **Describe how substances counteract poisons**
2. **List the antidotes to common poisonings**
3. **State the methods of nursing poisoning cases.**

Antidotes

A substance given to counteract a poison is called an antidote. Mechanisms of action include:

- some form complexes with the toxicant (e.g. the oximes bind with organophosphates, EDTA chelates lead and other divalent heavy metals; Fig. 19.1)
- others block or compete for receptor sites (e.g. vitamin K competes with the receptor for coumarin anticoagulants)
- a few affect metabolism of the toxicant (e.g. nitrite and thiosulphate ions release and bind cyanide).

A few of the common toxicities and their antidotes are listed in Table 19.1. Poisoning is not a common cause of illness. Although some poisons produce specific signs, the majority does not and unless there is evidence of exposure, the exact cause is often

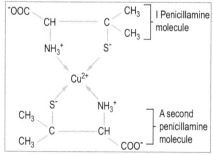

Fig. 19.1 Chelation of toxic metals (copper) by a chelating agent, penicillamine

183

Table 19.1   A few of the more common toxicities and their antidotes

Toxic agent	Example	Antidote
Anticoagulant rodenticides	Warfarin	Vitamin K
Organophosphate/carbamate insecticides	Vet Kem overdose	Atropine sulphate
Cholecalciferol (Vitamin D)		Calcitonin
Ethylene glycol	Antifreeze	Ethanol 20%
Lead, arsenic		Succimer/dimercaptosuccinic acid (DMSA)
Lead, zinc	Paint	$CaNa_2.EDTA$

unknown. Some of the more common toxicities are described below (with the main clinical sign in **bold** where appropriate). The incidence of poisoning depends very much on the population of animals and location being considered. Rural areas – where large amounts of pesticides, rodenticides, herbicides and other chemicals are used – are likely to experience a higher incidence of poisonings.

Ethylene glycol

Sources

Antifreeze and coolant from motor vehicles. Access possible following spillages in garages and workshops. It is palatable to dogs and cats and therefore commonly ingested.

Clinical effects

Ethylene glycol toxicosis can be divided into three clinical phases. The initial phase is manifested by excitement, ataxia, tachypnoea, polyuria/polydipsia and tachycardia. The second phase occurs 4–6 hours after ingestion and coincides with the onset of metabolic acidosis provoked by glycolic acid, a metabolite of ethylene glycol. Clinical signs include vomiting, anorexia, depression, miosis and hypothermia. Delayed effects cause deposition of calcium oxalate crystals in the kidney tubules, acidosis, haematuria and albuminuria. This third phase is characterised by oliguric **renal failure** and occurs 1–3 days after ingestion.

Treatment

Specific antidotes include ethanol and 4-methylpyrazole (Fomepizole), both of which prevent the metabolism of ethylene glycol to its toxic metabolites by inhibiting alcohol dehydrogenase. Ethylene glycol is metabolised very fast; in order to be effective, treatment must therefore be given as soon as possible after ingestion. Maintenance of urine output is critical. Oral administration of activated charcoal may be of use.

The acidosis is treated with sodium bicarbonate, aiming to keep urine pH at about 7.5–8.0. If blood gases are not available, 0.5–1 mmol/kg should be administered i.v. slowly over 30 minutes. Peritoneal dialysis is recommended in acidotic dogs with oliguria. Fluid therapy is essential, but central venous pressure and urine output should be monitored in dogs with renal dysfunction to prevent the development of pulmonary oedema.

Metaldehyde

Sources

Slug bait or dead snails and slugs killed by this agent. Slug bait is often mixed with palatable food items such as peanuts and illegally used to poison wildlife.

Clinical effects

Incoordination, unconsciousness, hyperthermia, hyperaesthesia, **convulsions**, cyanosis, nystagmus, salivation, mydriasis, opisthotonos. It is thought that these neurological signs result from the depletion of GABA within the CNS, resulting in loss of its central inhibitory action. There is sometimes hyperaemia of the liver, kidneys and lungs and haemorrhages in the intestines.

Treatment

Emesis or gastric lavage and administration of liquid paraffin. Barbiturates or diazepam to control the convulsions.

Organophosphates and cholinesterase-inhibiting insecticides

Sources

Organophosphates and carbamates are used for flea and tick control in dogs. These chemicals are also found in pesticides and flame-retardants.

Clinical effects

Organophosphates and carbamates inhibit cholin-esterase enzymes, including acetylcholinesterase, which is responsible for breaking down acetyl-choline. Clinical signs (as the result of overstimula-tion of parasympathetic muscarinic receptors) include diarrhoea, GI hypermotility, vomiting, salivation, sweating, excessive lacrimation, dyspnoea, bronchospasm progressing to cyanosis, miosis and bradycardia. There can be muscular twitching, weakness and CNS depression that may progress to convulsions.

Treatment

Following exposure, the priority centres on decon-tamination to prevent further absorption. The skin may be washed. If the patient is showing symptoms of poisoning, atropine should be administered before decontamination, as it blocks muscarinic receptors and at high doses can provide immediate but temporary relief. It must be re-administered if signs of poisoning reappear. Atropine sulphate is given by slow i.v. injection and is usually administered to effect, doses may therefore vary.

Paraquat

Sources

Herbicides, illegal baits.

Clinical effects

Paraquat is thought to produce its toxic action through the production of free radicals and the subsequent damage to lipid membranes. Paraquat is concentrated in alveolar cells and initial clinical signs include mucosal irritation, stomatitis, depres-sion, vomiting, diarrhoea, hyperexcitability and ataxia. The characteristic pulmonary oedema and congestion is usually seen several days after exposure and results in considerable respiratory distress.

Treatment

Decontamination with Fuller's earth or bentonite is recommended. These two adsorbants bind para-quat better than activated charcoal. Supportive and symptomatic care is essential. Treatment with superoxide dismutase and N-acetylcysteine is recommended.

Phenol

Sources

Phenols are found in pine oil disinfectants. TCP antiseptic contains a mix of phenols, chlorinated phenols and iodinated phenols. It may be used by clients to disinfect and treat wounds on their pets. Ingestion of the phenols then readily occurs during grooming activities.

Clinical effects

Gastritis, vomiting and diarrhoea are commonly seen. They may be followed by depression and a range of neurological symptoms – muscular convulsions, mild seizures and unconsciousness.

Treatment

Demulcents and gastric lavage.

Bleach (sodium hypochlorite)

Sources

Household disinfectant – may be contacted when falling into buckets, drains or toilet bowls. Chlorine gas may be released if the bleach is mixed with an acid solution.

Clinical effects

Burning and irritation of the skin as well as the oral and ocular mucous membranes may be seen. Oral ingestion results in irritation with oedema of the pharynx, glottis, stomach, larynx and lungs. The severity of the symptoms shown depends on the concentration of the bleach solution – a dilute solution may only provoke mild gastric irritation.

Treatment

Liberal washing/flushing of all surfaces to remove the irritant. Occlusive creams should never be applied. If the chemical was swallowed, vomiting should not be induced as it is likely to cause further burning. The administration of water or milk can help to dilute and neutralise the sodium hypochlorite.

Non-steroidal anti-inflammatory drugs (NSAIDs)

Sources

Human and veterinary authorised medicines may be administered to or consumed by pets. Poisonings due to paracetamol, salicylic acid and ibuprofen are not uncommon.

Clinical effects

NSAIDs act by inhibiting prostaglandin synthesis. The toxicity varies considerably but cats are gene-rally more sensitive than dogs. The most commonly seen adverse effects include erosive gastritis, peptic ulceration and haemorrhage, vomiting and epigastric pain. Anaemia and hypoproteinaemia may be seen subsequent to gastrointestinal ulceration and blood loss. Nephrotoxicity may also be seen and is manifested by acute interstitial nephritis, acute papillary necrosis, nephrotic syndrome and acute and chronic renal failure.

Treatments

Gastrointestinal decontamination and supportive care are appropriate in acute cases. Repeated doses of activated charcoal are indicated. Gastrointestinal ulceration can be treated with cimetidine or ranitidine, together with sucralfate. Fluid therapy is the most important element in the treatment of acute renal failure. The use of furosemide, mannitol or low-dose dopamine may be required to promote diuresis.

Warfarin/anticoagulant rodenticides

Sources

Anticoagulant rodenticides are commonly used to control pest species such as mice and rats. Table 19.2 shows the estimated fatal doses of the commonly used agents.

Clinical effects

Anticoagulant rodenticides competitively inhibit the enzyme vitamin K reductase that is responsible for converting vitamin K epoxide to its active form. The active form of vitamin K is responsible for the final activation of a number of clotting factors. The supply of these clotting factors is generally exhausted 1–3 days after ingestion of a toxic dose, resulting in the appearance of coagulopathies. Signs of coagulopathy (**haematuria, melaena, petechial haemorrhages**) are seen within a couple of days following ingestion and haemorrhages can be massive and acute, or slow and sustained.

Table 19.2 Anticoagulants and their lethal dose

Anticoagulant	Fatal dose
Brodifacoum	5 g bait/kg body weight
Bromadiolone	126 g bait/kg body weight
Chlorphacinone	1 kg bait/kg body weight
Coumatetralyl	700 g bait/kg body weight
Difenacoum	1 kg bait/kg body weight
Diphacinone	20 g bait/kg body weight
Flocoumafen	1.5 g bait/kg body weight

Treatment

Apomorphine, or another emetic, may be used following recent ingestion. Vitamin K can be injected subcutaneously. Doses will vary depending on the specific compound ingested – higher doses are indicated for the newer anticoagulants such as brofidacoum. Intramuscular injections are not recommended due to the risk of haemorrhages – treatment can be continued orally. The oral bioavailability of vitamin K is increased if it is fed with a fatty meal. Blood transfusions may be necessary if the clinical signs are severe.

The one-stage prothrombin time (OSPT) is a useful indicator as the test measures Factor VII, the clotting factor with the shortest half-life of those that are affected by the anticoagulants. A normal PT at 48–72 hours would indicate that poisoning has probably not occurred. As a general rule, vitamin K can be withheld completely unless the OSPT elevates. Vitamin K should start to reverse any hypoprothrombinaemia within an hour or so of administration, with full effect being noticed in 4–6 hours. Daily parenteral vitamin K should be given until the OSPT is normal and then the animal should continue to receive vitamin K orally for up to 4 weeks, depending on the rodenticide consumed. The dose should be reduced by 50% each week.

Poisoning in small animals from commonly ingested plants

About 12% of inquiries received by the veterinary poisons information service concern plant ingestions. Box 19.1 lists some of those not covered in more detail below.

Daffodil

One bulb can cause serious toxicity in small animals and 15 g of bulbs can be fatal in a dog. Clinical signs are rapid in onset and include vomiting, diarrhoea, abdominal tenderness, anorexia, salivation, lethargy and pale mucous membranes. Severe cases show signs of collapse, hypotension and hyperglycaemia. Emetics should be given within 2 hours and rehydration commenced.

Honeysuckle

Low toxicity – mild gastroenteritis follows ingestion. Treatment is supportive.

Ivy

English ivy (*Hedera helix*) contains hederagenin, a triterpenoid saponin. All parts are toxic and poisoning

Some of the plants known to be toxic

- Garden plants
  - Yew
  - Acorns
  - Ragwort
  - Bracken
  - Rhododendron
  - Azalea
  - Brassicas
  - Laburnum
  - Water dropwort
  - Mycotoxins
  - Cotoneaster species
  - Blue green algae
- House plants
  - Leopard lily
  - Easter and Tiger Lilies
  - Marijuana
  - Christmas or winter cherry

occurs from eating the berries or other plant parts. Small quantities result in mild GI signs. Ingestion of larger quantities can cause muscle twitching and paralysis. The use of sedatives and ventilation may be required.

Horse chestnuts/conkers

Bark, fruit and leaves are all toxic, however, young growth, sprouts and mature nuts are most dangerous. Do not confuse with edible chestnuts. The toxic principal is a glycosidic saponin called aesculin. Clinical signs occur within 6 hours and include abdominal tenderness, severe GI signs, ataxia, pyrexia and rigidity. Treatment includes emesis. The use of adsorbents such as activated charcoal is contraindicated as it may exacerbate obstruction, a potential problem with this toxicity.

Holly

Although the plant contains glycosides, saponins, triterpenes and a compound with digitalis-like activity, mild GI signs are the usual result – requiring antiemetics and fluid therapy.

Mistletoe

The plant is potentially highly toxic as it contains viscotoxins and alkaloids. GI upset is the main sign – gastric decontamination is required.

General management of the poisoned animal

Treatment must be urgent and vigorous. The general first aid principles are:
- stabilise the cardiovascular and respiratory systems
- get a good history and perform a full clinical examination
- prevent further absorption/increase the speed of elimination of the drug
- administer an antidote if available
- monitoring and supportive therapy.

Convulsions can be treated with barbiturates. Diazepam is also useful but may need topping up at regular intervals. If respiratory depression occurs, doxapram can be administered and intubation performed. Oxygen administration is essential and positive pressure ventilation may be required. Dehydration or circulatory collapse may require correction with intravenous saline. The acid–base balance, PCV and electrolyte balances should be monitored.

Large doses of soluble corticosteroid may be useful in cases of shock. The animal's body temperature should be maintained in normal limits. Hyperthermia should be treated with ice packs and cold-water baths. Pain can be relieved with pethidine in most species.

Nursing care of the poisoned small animal

Prevention of further absorption

Remove the patient from the source of the toxin and establish a priority list. Where there are no other clinical priorities, residues should be washed from the skin with water. Detergents can increase the absorption of some poisons and are best avoided. If the poison has been ingested gastrointestinal decontamination (GID) is useful. GID consists of gastric evacuation, administration of an adsorbent and catharsis.

Emetics should not be given where there are convulsions or the poisoning is due to barbiturates, paraffin or corrosive substances. Vomiting can be induced with washing soda crystals placed on the back of the tongue, salt water, mustard and water, syrup of ipecacuanha, 1% copper sulphate or hydrogen peroxide. Apomorphine is the emetic of choice in dogs but should not be used in cats. Xylazine can be used in either species but may cause sedation.

Gastric lavage requires general anaesthesia and the establishment of a secure airway. A stomach tube can then be passed and the stomach lavaged. Warm water should always be used to avoid chilling the patient – this is particularly important in small patients. The body should be angled in such a way as to allow the efflux to drain from the mouth. It may be appropriate to collect and save material for analysis. Water, saline or activated charcoal (5–10 ml/kg) is introduced and allowed to drain under gravity or is aspirated.

In human medicine whole bowel irrigation is now performed, this involves the oral administration of large volumes of an electrolyte-balanced solution until a clear rectal effluent is obtained. A polyethylene glycol GI cleanser is used for this purpose. This technique may be appropriate in animals – particularly where the ingested poison is poorly taken up by activated charcoal or likely to provide sustained release of a toxin.

Activated charcoal is used to absorb organic materials and repeated doses are effective in stopping enterohepatic recycling of several poisons. Cathartics such as saline, sorbitol and magnesium or sodium sulphate hasten excretion of the poison.

Enhancing elimination via the urinary tract is useful for several toxicities. For example, alkalinisation of the urine to a pH above 7.0 with sodium bicarbonate enhances the elimination of weak acids such as ethylene glycol, salicylates and phenobarbital.

Occlusive creams should never be applied to the skin over a chemical burn as they are likely to trap chemical agents on the skin, causing further burning.

Fluid therapy

The perfusion status of the animal should be assessed using mucous membrane colour, CRT and peripheral pulse quality. The hydration status can be assessed by the moistness of the gums, skin turgor and perfusion parameters. If a patient requires fluid therapy, a choice must be made as to whether to use crystalloids, colloids or blood products. Intravascular crystalloid equilibrates with the interstitial space and only 20–25% of the infused volume remains within the intravascular space 1 hour following infusion. Hypertonic saline draws water from the tissues and produces a rapid expansion of intravascular volume – however it should not be used in dehydrated animals.

The induction of diuresis is perhaps indicated in all patients as there will always be some metabolites or waste products requiring elimination.

Nutritional support

Poisoned animals may need nutritional support due to ulceration of the mouth, vomiting and diarrhoea, or many other debilitating conditions preventing normal feeding. Enteral feeding is always preferable, as the intestinal epithelium requires glutamine and regular access to nutrients to maintain the health of the enterocytes. Methods of enteral feeding include assisted feeding, chemical stimulation of the appetite and infusion of nutrients via feeding tubes within the GI tract. Parenteral nutrition is supplied by the intravenous route and is indicated in all patients whose needs are not met by enteral feeding. Monitoring of nutritional support in the critically ill patient involves full clinical examinations, twice-daily weight checks, total protein and blood urea nitrogen and PCV measurement.

The cause of any intoxication may be difficult to determine. Good history taking is important. The owner should always be asked to bring a sample, labelled if possible, of the item they believe may have been ingested to the surgery for identification. In many situations advice and further information should be sought from the Veterinary Poisons Information Service.

Questions for Chapter 19

1. Which of the following is not a treatment for heavy metal toxicosis?
   a. sodium calcium edetate
   b. penicillin
   c. dimercaprol
   d. penicillamine

2. Which of the following is indicated in the treatment of organophosphate poisoning?
   a. epinephrine
   b. atipamezole
   c. atropine
   d. azathioprine

3. What is the role of a cathartic in the treatment of poisoning?
   a. to induce vomiting
   b. to hasten gut transit time and the evacuation of the poison
   c. to absorb the poison
   d. to hydrate the patient

4. Vomiting can be induced by the administration of
   a. washing soda crystals
   b. apomorphine
   c. xylazine
   d. all of the above

For answers go to page 245

Twenty

CHAPTER 20

Pharmaceutical Preparations Used for Nutrition and Fluid Balance

Learning aims and objectives

After studying this chapter you should be able to:

1. **Describe the benefits of the disease-modifying anti-osteoarthritis drugs (DMAOD)**
2. **List the minerals used in treating clinical conditions**
3. **State the benefits of vitamins**
4. **State the contents of the different fluids available for therapy.**

Introduction

A large number of nutritional (and medicinal) supplements are available for the treatment of a wide range of conditions. In the UK, where the product is 'medicinal by function' it will require a marketing authorisation as a veterinary medicine. A product is medicinal by function if it possesses recognised properties for treating or preventing disease in animals, or if it may be administered to animals with a view to restoring, correcting or modifying a physiological function. Products may also be considered medicinal by function due to their route of administration. A vitamin supplement administered by injection, for example, would be considered medicinal by function, as would any eye-drop applied directly to the eye.

This chapter will present a range of supplements indicated for, and used in, the management of conditions such as osteoarthritis, liver disease and hypovitaminoses. A discussion of the quality, reliability and labelling of nutraceuticals will highlight some of the issues that nurses should be aware of when advising and educating pet owners.

Disease-modifying anti-osteoarthritis drugs

Pentosan polysulphate sodium

Pentosan polysulphate (PPS) is a semi-synthetic polymer with anti-inflammatory activity and the ability to promote the regeneration of cartilage. It has been shown to correct many of the metabolic imbalances that exist in osteoarthritic joints. The sodium derivative of PPS (Cartrophen; Arthropharm) is an authorised veterinary medicinal product in the UK with an indication for the management of lameness and pain of osteoarthritis in the dog. It is administered as a course of four s.c. doses of 3 mg/kg at 5–7-day intervals. The drug targets the pathology of arthritic cartilage, periarticular tissues and blood vessels. Sodium PPS possesses mild anticoagulant properties and should not, therefore, be used together with drugs such as aspirin that may potentiate this anticoagulant effect. Its use should also be avoided where there is haemorrhaging from tumours or where there has been a history of trauma or uncontrolled bleeding.

Glucosamine

Glucosamine is available in three forms – glucosamine sulphate, glucosamine hydrochloride and N-acetyl glucosamine – which are the building blocks of glycosaminoglycans (GAG) and proteoglycans.

- These large polysaccharides are used in the production of many tissues including connective tissues, joints and mucous membranes.
- GAGs include the chondroitin sulphates and hyaluronic acid, which combine with collagen to form the extracellular matrix.
- They are also present in the protective mucous membrane layer in the digestive, respiratory and genitourinary tracts.
- A deficiency of N-acetyl glucosamine leads to an inability of the body to replace the cells in joints and the GI tract and supplementation seems to be protective and restorative, leading to less pain and inflammation.
- Several products have been used for the prevention of cystitis in cats prone to reoccurrence of the condition with good success in the right patient.
- Glucosamine is a major component of joint cartilage and, like chondroitin, helps cartilage absorb water and keeps the joint lubricated.

Supplements are derived from the shells of shellfish such as shrimp, lobster and crab. It is available over the counter as a nutraceutical product. Glucosamine supplementation provides the natural building blocks for growth, repair and maintenance of cartilage; it is supposed to slow deterioration of cartilage, relieve the pain associated with osteoarthritis and improve joint mobility.

The scientific evidence of efficacy for glucosamine in the treatment of osteoarthritis is sufficient to cause the Arthritis Foundation to state that 'The notion that glucosamine and chondroitin might have disease-modifying effects in OA is highly appealing and supported by preliminary data'. Studies on glucosamine in humans are promising. A review of two studies, each of which analysed more than a dozen glucosamine studies, found this supplement to significantly and consistently improve pain and joint function, as well as or better than conventional drug therapy (NSAIDs). In humans it has been shown through radiolabelling studies that the bioavailability of glucosamine hydrochloride is 84%. By contrast, the bioavailability of the sulphate salt is only 47%, indicating that less than half of the oral dose of this salt reaches the systemic circulation. This means that the oral dose of the sulphate salt should be double that of the hydrochloride salt. Extrapolation of these data to animal patients should be undertaken cautiously. Selection of a good-quality supplement is very important and clients should be provided with advice on the most suitable supplement for their pets.

Chondroitin

Chondroitin is another component of human cartilage, bone and tendon. It is believed to enhance the shock-absorbing properties of collagen and block enzymes that break down cartilage. In supplements, chondroitin sulphate usually comes from bovine trachea or pork by-products. It is supposed to reduce pain and inflammation, improve joint function and slow disease progression. It is often supplied together with glucosamine but there is no convincing evidence that glucosamine and chondroitin together are more effective than each one individually or alone.

Turmeric

Turmeric is a yellow-coloured powder ground from the roots of the lily-like turmeric plant. It is a common ingredient in curry powder. Turmeric is traditionally used in Chinese and Indian Ayurvedic medicine to treat arthritis; the active ingredient in turmeric is curcumin. Turmeric is found together with glucosamine and chondroitin in some preparations.

Saturated and unsaturated fatty acids

Injectable fatty acids are available on the Continent and provide relief from arthritic symptoms within 3–4 days of injection, lasting up to 2–3 months.

Minerals

Various minerals are used in disease treatment:

- Calcium borogluconate is used to treat hypocalcaemia. It may be administered intravenously to avoid tissue irritation or it can be administered subcutaneously. Other calcium salts used in the treatment of hypocalcaemia include calcium gluconate and calcium hydroxide.
- Calcium carbonate is used as an intestinal phosphate binder to reduce phosphate absorption in renal failure. Long-term calcium supplementation has been linked with the development of various bone and joint diseases in young dogs.
- Iron is used to treat iron-deficiency anaemia associated with GI haemorrhage. The oral route should be used but may cause nausea and diarrhoea.
- Magnesium sulphate is used to treat arrhythmias.
- Magnesium chloride is often added to calcium preparations and is indicated in the treatment of parturient paresis in cattle and sheep where there is a requirement for increased blood magnesium.
- Sodium bicarbonate is used in metabolic acidosis and to alkalinise urine. Excessive use can lead to heart failure.
- Zinc sulphate has been used to inhibit collagen production in liver disease by inhibiting enzymes involved in collagen synthesis. Adverse effects include vomiting, diarrhoea and abdominal discomfort.
- Phosphate, in the form of sodium hexametaphosphate, has been found to inhibit dental calculus formation in dogs. As calculi are calcium carbonate with small amounts of calcium phosphate, by substituting the hexametaphosphate, the plaque can not calcify – due to the formation of soluble calcium complexes. When added as a surface coating to dry dog food, the drug reduced calculus by 81% over 4 weeks without any adverse side effects.
- Potassium therapy is available in the following formats:
  - potassium chloride
  - potassium carbonate
  - potassium bicarbonate
  - potassium citrate
  - potassium gluconate
  - potassium monohydrogen
  - dihydrogen phosphate.

Potassium can be administered as an aqueous solution or in lactated Ringer's solution (Hartmann's). Care must be taken when administering the potassium salt because rapid increases in blood potassium can be cardiotoxic.

Enteral nutritional products

Examples of this group are the essential fatty acid (EFA) drugs. Lipid emulsions are available for those patients receiving nutritional support. EFA preparations are used to help manage poor coats; medium-chain triglycerides are used as energy sources in animals requiring low-fat diets.

Antioxidants

Cognitive performance can be improved with a diet supplemented with a broad spectrum of antioxidants, which are believed to mop up free radicals – the damaging molecules produced as a result of energy production in mitochondria. Antioxidants prevent the damage to neurones and promote recovery in neurones showing signs of neuropathy. Therefore commercially available diets (such as Hills b/d) or nutritional supplements (such as Activait) offer another option in the treatment of age-related behavioural disorders. Table 20.1 lists some nutrients and herbal supplements that are used as cognitive enhancers.

Glutamine

Glutamine is a primary energy source for GI tract mucosal cells. Diseases of this system increase the requirements for glutamine as the body replaces damaged cells. Supplementation has been of benefit in inflammatory bowel disease and to reduce loss of muscle mass in times of stress or injury.

Coenzyme Q_{10}

This is a lipid-soluble benzoquinone that is produced naturally in mammals. It is an essential component of mitochondria and controls the flow of oxygen within a cell. This has made it of use in the management of ischaemia in heart diseases such as myocardial ischaemia and in cardiomyopathies. Other potential indications include:

- periodontal disease – decreases inflammation and bleeding
- immune dysfunction
- decreased physical performance.

Table 20.1 Nutrients and herbal supplements used as cognitive enhancers

Substance	Comments
Nutrients	
Acetyl L carnitine choline	Precursor to ACh, found in eggs and meat
Cytidine-5-diphosphate choline L-alpha-glycerylphosphorylcholine-2-dimethylaminoethanol (DMAE)	Found in the brain and in sardines; appears to increase ACh production
Phospatidylserine	Found on the surface of nerve membranes and at the synapse
Other substances and herbs	
BR-16A	A herb from India
Ginkgo biloba	Increases cerebral circulation, increases glucose utilisation by the brain and increases choline reuptake
Ma-huang	A herb from China
Oxymethacil	Reduces oxidation of molecules in the brain
Pyritinol	Similar to vitamin B6, increases cerebral blood flow

Shark and bovine cartilage

Early indications for these were for potential use against cancer. Shark cartilage especially was found to contain an angiogenesis inhibitor (prevents the growth of new blood vessels). Inflammation and pain are reduced in patients who suffer from osteoarthritis and rheumatoid arthritis.

Green-lipped mussel

Perna canaliculus is a New Zealand marine bivalve used to treat degenerative joint disorders; 10% of its carbohydrates are GAG products. It contains an inhibitor of prostaglandin synthesis – which may explain its anti-inflammatory effects. Other areas of treatment interest include inflammatory skin conditions, reversing some ageing processes and increasing sperm motility.

Probiotics

Illness, injury and stress can alter the normal commensal bacterial flora within the gut. *Lactobacillus bulgaris* and *L. acidophilus* were the first recognised microbials used in nutritional therapy. Beneficial bacteria aid the host by:
- supplying nutrients to the host
- aiding digestion
- producing better food conversion
- neutralising toxins produced by pathogenic bacteria
- producing B vitamins and enzymes beneficial to the host.

Vitamins

Vitamins have an important role in treatment:
- Ascorbic acid/vitamin C supplementation is often used in hepatic disease. It is used to treat methaemoglobinaemia associated with acetaminophen toxicity.
- Cyanocobalamin/vitamin B12 is indicated in patients presenting with small intestinal overgrowth and exocrine pancreatic insufficiency as these conditions may give rise to a vitamin B12 deficiency.
- Thiamine/vitamin B1 supplementation is required in animals fed fish-based diets. It is used to treat vitamin B1 deficiencies and the associated cerebrocortical necrosis.
- Vitamin A supplementation is used in some skin disorders such as sebaceous adenitis, seborrhoea and keratinisation disorders.
- Vitamin D is a general term used to describe a range of compounds that influence calcium and phosphorous metabolism.
- Vitamin K is used in the management of vitamin K deficiencies arising due to fat malabsorption or the ingestion of rodenticides.

Nutraceuticals

The term nutraceutical is not a legal term; it was coined in the 1980s by a physician referring to oral compounds that were neither nutrients nor pharmaceuticals. Where a product claims to have veterinary medicinal properties, it will require a marketing authorisation as a veterinary medicinal product. Where no such claims are made, the product can be marketed as a supplement. Unfortunately there are, as yet, no mechanisms in place to hold a manufacturer accountable for the labelling and content of such non-medicinal products. There can be considerable differences in the quality of products. Many chondroitin sulphate supplements, for example, have been found to be seriously deficient. In contrast, glucosamine is much more likely to be accurately labelled with regard to content.

Clients should be advised clearly how to establish the quality of any product they are considering purchasing and should be encouraged to purchase veterinary medicinal products. They should also be advised that nutraceutical use is often no substitute for veterinary medication and should be directed to reliable sources of information. The arthritis foundation web site, for example, is a good source of information on alternative remedies for the treatment of osteoarthritis (http://www.arthritis.org/conditions/supplementguide/).

A list of supplements considered to have veterinary medicinal properties is available from the Veterinary Medicines Directorate. Essential fatty acids are not included in the list of medicinal products but could be if they were claimed to be antipruritic. Some important supplements with medicinal properties include:

- adenosylmethionine (aka SAMe) – used in the treatment of liver disease, depression, behavioural problems and osteoarthritis
- taurine – used in the treatment of heart disease
- milk thistle – used in the treatment of liver disease.

Fluid therapy

Fluid therapy is indicated where there is a requirement for water and electrolytes. Such a requirement arises following excessive fluid losses and may be seen in patients presenting with vomiting, diarrhoea, haemorrhaging, blood loss or heat stroke. If a patient is judged to be excessively hypovolaemic or vasoconstricted, blood volume restoration therapy should be instituted and continued until the patient is out of danger. Life-threatening hyperkalaemia, metabolic acidosis, hypoxaemia and hypoventilation should be dealt with at this time as well.

The goal of fluid therapy should be to restore the volume and composition of body fluids to normal and, once this has been achieved, to maintain fluid and electrolyte balance so that input by treatment matches ongoing fluid losses. The choice of fluids should be based on the degree of volume depletion and the nature of the fluid losses. For animals in shock, replacement fluids are preferred. Crystalloids are generally indicated where shock is due to water and sodium depletion. Where plasma volume depletion is secondary to haemorrhage, immunologically compatible whole blood is the best replacement fluid. Where this is not available, and the loss of plasma proteins has dropped the plasma oncotic pressure, the use of plasma expanders is indicated.

Crystalloids

Conventional crystalloids are fluids that contain a combination of water and electrolytes. Isotonic solutions do not cause lysis of red blood cells and include:

- normal saline 0.9%
- Hartmann's (also know as lactated Ringer's)
- dextrose 4%, saline 0.18%
- dextrose 5%.

Normal saline consists of 9 g of NaCl per litre of water. It contains 154 mmol/L of sodium and 154 mmol/L of chloride, giving it an osmolality of 308 mosm/L. The main potential problem of fluid therapy with normal saline is the risk of hyperchloraemic metabolic acidosis; this is most likely with renal insufficiency. Normal saline has a sodium concentration similar to that of the ECF – this limits the distribution of the fluid to the ECF. Within the ECF, the fluid is distributed between the interstitial fluid (ISF) ($^3/_4$) and the intravascular fluid (IVF) ($^1/_4$) in proportion to their contribution to ECF volume.

Hartmann's solution contains 131 mmol/L of sodium, 111 mmol/L of chloride, 29 mmol/L of lactate, 2 mmol/L of calcium and 5 mmol/l of potassium – giving it an osmolality of 279 mosm/L. It is indicated as a water/electrolyte replacement fluid, particularly if metabolic acidosis is present. The main potential problem associated with its use is the risk of potassium accumulation.

Crystalloid fluids may need to be given in quantities of 40–90 ml/kg or more in order to achieve adequate blood volume restoration. The cat has a smaller blood volume than the dog (50–55 ml/kg compared with 80–90 ml/kg) and should receive a proportionally smaller dose of fluids.

The end-point of fluid administration is determined by improvement(s) in the perfusion of and/or supply of blood to peripheral tissues, the return of an acceptable pulse quality and return of urine output. Objective measurements of the adequacy of blood volume restoration and preload to the heart can be valuable when external signs are hidden. Central venous pressure should be returned to a high normal level (8–10 cmH$_2$O). Further therapy might include a β-agonist if contractility is thought too low, or a vasodilator/constrictor if systemic vasomotor tone is thought to be too high/low.

Fluid administration should be conservative in animals that have pre-existing pulmonary oedema, cerebral oedema or congestive heart failure. Fluid therapy should be sufficient to achieve adequate but not complete blood volume restoration. Colloidal solutions may be more effective in restoring blood volume while minimising the exaggeration of the interstitial oedema situation.

Only about 20% of a crystalloid fluid remains in the vascular fluid compartment 30 minutes following its administration. The remainder readily diffuses across the endothelial membrane and is redistributed into the interstitial fluid compartment. The volume restoration achieved by crystalloid fluids may be fleeting and if hypotension or vasoconstriction re-occur, further fluid administration may be indicated.

Excessive haemodilution is a common limitation to crystalloid fluid administration. This is defined as a PCV below 15–25%.

Hypertonic saline

In some situations it may be difficult to administer sufficient volumes of fluids rapidly enough to resuscitate the patient. In these situations, achieving the greatest cardiovascular benefit with the least volume of infused fluids is desirable. Hypertonic saline provides better volume expansion and higher cardiac output, blood pressure and tissue perfusion. Hypertonic saline also causes vasodilation.

The deleterious effects are an increase in sodium and chloride concentration and osmolality and a decrease in potassium and bicarbonate concentration. Changes are moderate and of minimal clinical importance, unless the patient has pre-existing electrolyte abnormalities or if repeated doses are administered. Arrhythmias might be a problem if more hypertonic solutions are administered close to the heart and haemolysis might occur if administered into small peripheral veins. The commonly recommended dose of 7.5% hypertonic saline is 4–6 ml/kg.

Colloid therapy

If the total protein is low, or is likely to be reduced with crystalloid therapy, plasma or a plasma substitute (dextran, hetastarch) should be administered as part of a fluid therapy programme. The colloids are more effective blood-volume expanders than are the crystalloid fluids and should be considered when the patient does not seem to be responding to the crystalloid fluid infusion or when oedema develops prior to adequate blood volume restoration. Colloids, although more expensive than crystalloids, provide a better blood-volume expansion effect and less interstitial expansion compared with crystalloids. They maintain a higher colloid oncotic pressure so are cost effective. Despite these obvious theoretical advantages, there is continuing debate over the merits of colloid versus crystalloid therapy.

Colloids of a molecular weight less than 50 kDa are rapidly excreted in the urine and exhibit a short duration of action (2–4 hours). The remaining colloids are equally efficacious with regard to their plasma-volume expansion when administered in equivalent concentrations of similar-sized molecules. Preferences between products tend to be based on cost and the incidence of complications such as coagulopathies and immunological reactions.

Albumin

Albumin comprises about 50% of the total plasma protein and 80% of the plasma colloid oncotic pressure. There are approximately 5 grams of albumin per kilogram of body weight in the extracellular fluid – 40% in the intravascular space, 60% in the interstitial space. Albumin synthesis is regulated by osmoreceptors in the hepatic interstitial space; other intravascular colloids (hypergammaglobulinaemia and artificial colloid administration) may decrease albumin synthesis. Albumin maintains intravascular colloid oncotic pressure. It is strongly negatively charged and is an important carrier of certain drugs, hormones and chemicals and toxins such as cations, anions, toxic oxygen radicals and toxic inflammatory substances.

Hetastarch/pentastarch

Hetastarch (HES) is a modified amylopectin – a branched glucose polymer. Hydroxylation makes it more resistant to degradation by serum amylase. Several different HES solutions are available with varying degrees of hydroxylation (the greater the hydroxylation, the slower the metabolism). Half-life is dependent on hydroxylation and molecular size. Starches are metabolised by plasma and interstitial alpha-amylase.

Pentastarch has a smaller, more homogeneous particle size with less hydroxyethyl substitution. It has a colloid oncotic pressure of 40 mmHg (hyperoncotic) and therefore causes a greater initial blood volume expansion – 1.5× the amount administered.

These products are rarely required when shock is due to water and sodium depletion.

Dextran

Dextrans are mixtures of polysaccharides produced by the bacteria *Leuconostoc mesenteroides* or lactobacilli grown on sucrose media. Different molecular weights can be produced by acid hydrolysis of macromolecules. Molecular weights of less than 50 kDa are rapidly filtered at the glomerulus, while molecular weights above 50 kDa are widely distributed in the body and are metabolised by dextrinases at the rate of 70 mg/kg of body weight/day.

Dextran is hyperoncotic and causes a greater initial blood volume expansion, 1.5× the amount administered, but the duration of this effect is only 1.5–3 hours. Dextran 40 lowers blood viscosity but has been associated with renal failure. It is rapidly filtered by the glomerulus and may be associated with an osmotic diuresis. In states of active tubular resorption of sodium and water, the dextran concentrates in the tubular lumen, increasing the viscosity of the filtrate and perhaps precipitating out and plugging the tubules.

Dextrans produce a dose-related defect of primary haemostasis which is greater than that produced by simple dilution. When administered in large volumes, dextrans can induce a von Willebrand's-like syndrome. Prolongation of activated prothrombin time (APTT) is attributed to a reduction of factor VIII:C activity. Prolonged bleeding time and decreased platelet adhesiveness is attributed to inhibition of the von Willebrand factor activity. While it is not expected that even large doses will cause bleeding in normal patients, dextrans should be used conservatively in patients with bleeding tendencies.

In humans, naturally occurring dextran antibodies exist in the general population, resulting from exposure to dietary and gastrointestinal tract bacteria-produced dextrans. The incidence of allergic reactions is low, 0.03–5%, however the BSAVA Formulary states that anaphylactic reactions may develop.

Whole blood

If the PCV falls below 15–25% or is likely to be reduced with crystalloid fluid therapy, packed red cells or whole blood should be administered as part of the fluid therapy regime. The blood can be collected into an anticoagulant such as heparin (1 unit heparin/ml of whole blood). This is appropriate if the blood is to be immediately re-transfused. Alternatively acid citrate-dextrose (ACD) or citrate-phosphate-dextrose (CPD) (0.15 ml of solution/ml whole blood) may be used. CPD should be used if the blood is to be stored. Red cells are 70% viable for up to 4 weeks. After this time the plasma can be separated and stored frozen for at least a year – the red cells should be discarded.

Administration of fluids

Subcutaneous

A useful technique for rehydration of cats both at home and in the surgery is to attach a giving set and allow 50–100 ml of normal saline or Hartmann's to gravity feed every 24 hours. This supplements the oral intake well in chronic renal failure patients.

Intraosseous

Bone marrow access sites for the administration of fluids include:
- trochanteric fossa of the proximal femur (Fig. 20.1)
- the flat medial aspect of the proximal tibia distal to the tibial tuberosity and the proximal tibial growth plate
- cranial aspect of the mid diaphyseal ulna
- cranial aspect of the greater tubercle of the humerus.

A new site and needle should be chosen every 72 hours and when not in use the needle should be flushed every 6 hours with heparinised saline. Complications include:
- infection – skin should be prepared aseptically and the intraosseous system should be managed in a similar manner to an intravenous catheter
- fat embolisation
- damage to growth plates as the needle penetrates
- interfascial and subcutaneous leakage of fluids if the needle is incorrectly placed.

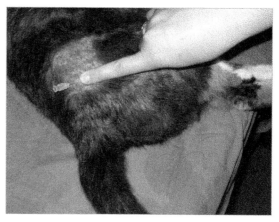

Fig. 20.1 Intraosseous administration of fluids

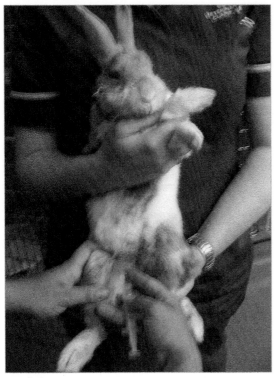

Fig. 20.2 Intraperitoneal administration of fluids

Intraperitoneal

- A useful technique when peripheral veins are inaccessible and cost prohibits alternative methods.
- Small mammals often receive their fluids via this route. Figure 20.2 shows the approach in a rabbit. The needle should enter either of the ventral quadrants to avoid the bladder lying midline.
- The peritoneal membrane is a large surface area for the uptake of fluids and drugs and so euthanasia is often performed this way by the administration of a barbiturate anaesthetic.

Antihaemorrhagic drugs

Etamsylate is a synthetic drug that stimulates platelet aggregation, reduces capillary permeability and can reduce bleeding times by up to 40%. It is available in France as Hémoced (Schering-Plough). N-butanol is a systemic coagulant that is able to stop traumatic and surgical haemorrhaging. It acts locally within the wounds, restoring tissue pH – it is available in France as Hémostat (Virbac).

Questions for Chapter 20

1. Which of the following nutraceuticals is not indicated in the treatment of osteoarthritis?
   a. glucosamine sulphate
   b. pentosan polysulphate
   c. turmeric
   d. vitamin A

2. Which of the following may show symptoms of cerebrocortical necrosis?
   a. sheep eating bracken
   b. snakes eating frozen fish
   c. cats fed a diet of frozen fish
   d. all of the above

3. Which of the following is isotonic?
   a. dextrose 4%, saline 0.18%
   b. saline 7.2%
   c. dextrose 10%
   d. all of the above

4. Which of the following is not likely to require a marketing authorisation as a veterinary medicine?
   a. topical eye ointment
   b. injectable vitamin
   c. a herbal medicine for the treatment of liver disease
   d. a herbal medicine that may boost the immune system

For answers go to page 245

CHAPTER 21

Twenty One

Premedicants and Local and General Anaesthesia

Learning aims and objectives

After studying this chapter you should be able to:

1. **Describe the method of action of sedative drugs**
2. **Understand the rationale behind the selection of a suitable premedicant**
3. **List the agents used in intravenous anaesthesia**
4. **Describe factors affecting the action of local anaesthetics**
5. **State the different properties of the inhalational anaesthetics.**

Premedicants

Premedicants are administered to a patient prior to the induction of general anaesthesia in order to improve the quality of anaesthesia. When used appropriately, they minimise stress and the deleterious side effects associated with many anaesthetic agents. The aims of premedication will be discussed first before focussing on the four main categories of pre-anaesthetic medications, namely:

- anticholinergics
- phenothiazine and butyrophenone tranquillisers
- α2 agonist(s)/tranquilliser(s) and opioid drug combinations
- opioids.

The aims of premedication are to:

1. Sedate and/or calm the patient – the tranquillised patient is generally easier to work with.
2. Reduce stress. The sedated patient is less likely to become stressed. Stress raises the levels of circulating adrenaline and this is undesirable where the heart may be sensitised to catecholamines by certain anaesthetic agents such as halothane. Consequently, there is generally a lower incidence of cardiac arrhythmias in premedicated patients.
3. Provide safe and uncomplicated induction of, maintenance of, and recovery from anaesthesia.
4. Eliminate or minimise pain. Pre-emptive analgesia is administered prior to any painful procedure and is recognised to be the most efficient way of managing pain.

5. Decrease the amount of potentially more dangerous drugs administered for general anaesthesia, sedation and muscle relaxation to be achieved. In the case of general anaesthetic agents, both induction and maintenance doses are reduced. Acepromazine (ACP) reduces the maintenance dose of anaesthetic agent by 33%, whilst medetomidine can reduce the maintenance dose by as much as 50%.

6. Provide muscle relaxation. Ketamine provides poor muscle relaxation when used on its own; premedication with an α2 agonist provides superior muscle relaxation and a better quality of anaesthesia.

7. Reduce unwanted autonomic side effects (whether of sympathetic or parasympathetic origin) – atropine is used to counteract the bradycardia caused through the parasympathetic nervous system and to reduce salivation and airway secretions.

8. Suppress or reduce vomiting and nausea – ACP is a good anti-emetic.

9. Promote smooth recovery – useful for methohexitone and alphadolone/alphaxalone (Saffan) where stormy recoveries can be seen.

Individual premedications should be selected for each procedure depending on the following:
- patient signalment (species, breed, age, sex)
- physical status
- medical history
- known allergies/previous reactions
- disposition
- surgical procedure and anticipated duration
- inpatient or outpatient surgery
- elective or emergency surgery
- familiarity with agents.

Box 21.1 lists the common pre-anaesthetic drugs.

Anticholinergics

Anticholinergic drugs are also called parasympathetic antagonists, antimuscarinics and parasympatholytics.

Box 21.1

Common premedicant drug groups

- anticholinergics
- phenothiazines
- benzodiazepines
- opioids
- α_2-agonists

Box 21.2

Doses of anticholinergics depend on the route of administration

- atropine sulphate
  0.02–0.04 mg/kg s.c. or i.m.
  0.01–0.02 mg/kg i.v.
- glycopyrrolate
  0.01–0.02 mg/kg s.c. or i.m.
  0.005–0.01 mg/kg i.v.

Their mechanism of action is to block acetylcholine at postganglionic cholinergic receptors in the autonomic parasympathetic nervous system. Box 21.2 shows how the dose varies with the route of administration. The main indications for use are:
- Primarily used to decrease salivary secretions and to inhibit the bradycardic effects of vagal stimulation.
- Reduce glandular secretions of the respiratory tract, gastrointestinal tract, oral and nasal cavities. Decrease salivation and decrease/thin respiratory secretions – especially useful in cats, small patients and brachycephalics (boxers, pugs and bulldogs) as these have a greater degree of vagal tone and have small airways which can easily block. They are also of use following ketamine anaesthesia, which can increase salivation in some patients. Figure 21.1 shows how atropine stops salivation by inhibition of the parasympathetic nervous system.
- These drugs counteract vagally mediated bradycardia. Various gaseous anaesthetic agents can enhance parasympathetic effects by suppressing sympathetic tone. Although most modern inhalational anaesthetics increase heart rate, halothane can increase vagal tone and therefore slow the heart rate (parasympathetic effect).
- Surgery of the eye and larynx. Eliminates the oculovagal reflex. Bradycardia can arise through reflex increases in vagal tone (oculovagal, laryngovagal and vagovagal reflexes arising through traction on viscera).

Atropine and glycopyrrolate are the two most commonly used parasympatholytics. Other effects of anticholinergics:
- dilation of bronchi
- increase respiratory dead space through bronchodilation
- decrease motor and secretory activity in the intestines

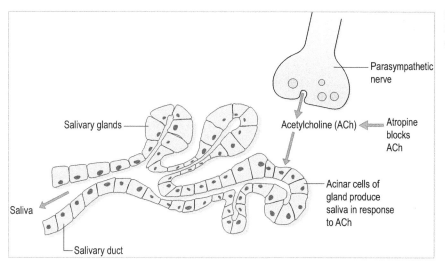

Fig. 21.1 How atropine blocks the neural control of salivation

- mydriasis – relaxes the iris muscle causing pupillary dilation in vertebrates with smooth muscle in their irises (i.e. not birds)
- reduces tear formation.

Box 21.3 shows some drug interactions that occur with atropine.

There are a number of differences between atropine and glycopyrrolate:

- glycopyrrolate is more expensive
- glycopyrrolate has a longer duration of action
- glycopyrrolate is less arrhythmogenic
- less pupillary dilation
- more potent anti-sialogue
- glycopyrrolate does not cross the blood–brain barrier and does not therefore produce the centrally mediated drowsiness seen with atropine and scopolamine.

Box 21.3

Drug interactions with atropine

- drugs that enhance atropine activity
  - antihistamines
  - benzodiazepines
  - procainamide
- drugs that can not be mixed with atropine in a syringe, i.v. tubing or cannula
  - norepinephrine
  - methohexitone
  - sodium bicarbonate
- drugs whose effects are antagonised by atropine
  - metoclopramide

Box 21.4

Tranquillisers and sedatives

- phenothiazines
  - acepromazine maleate 0.02–0.075 mg/kg s.c. or i.m.; max dose 3 mg
  - chlorpromazine (mainly used as an anti-emetic) 0.05–1.1 mg/kg i.m.
  - trimeprazine (antihistamine, sedative, antitussive, antipruritic)
- benzodiazepines
  - diazepam 0.1–0.6 mg/kg i.v. in dogs; 0.05–0.4 mg/kg i.v. in cats
  - midazolam 0.07–0.22 mg/kg i.m. or i.v.
  - zolazepam (combined with the dissociative drug tiletamine)
- butyrophenones
  - droperidol (combined with the opioid fentanyl)
  - fluanisone (can be combined with fentanyl)

Tranquillisers and sedatives are a large family of drugs including the phenothiazines, butyrophenones, benzodiazepines and α2 agonists. Box 21.4 lists some drugs that fall into this group.

Phenothiazines and butyrophenones

Both phenothiazines (e.g. acepromazine and promazine) and butyrophenones (e.g. droperidol and azaperone) have a similar mode of action – their calming and neurological effects appear to be mediated by depression of the reticular activating system and anti-dopaminergic effects in the CNS. Acepromazine (ACP) provides tranquillisation at lower doses and sedation at higher dose rates – although if low doses are ineffective, increasing the dose will have little effect on the drowsiness, whilst increasing the side effects. Phenothiazines produce mental calming and decreased motor activity, as well as increasing the threshold for responding to external stimuli. The other useful effects are:

- anti-arrhythmic
- antihistamine (useful pre-Saffan anaesthesia)
- anti-emetic effect mediated by anti-dopaminergic interaction in the CTZ
- antispasmodic (increases gut transit time).
  The unwanted effects include:
- hypotension (due to vasodilation)
- may lower the seizure threshold (phenothiazines lower the seizure threshold in animals with epilepsy, butyrophenones do not)
- hypothermia (central effect on hypothalamus and due to peripheral vasodilation)
- decreases heart and respiratory rate
- decreases packed cell volume by as much as 50%
- erection/priapism (penile prolapse, usually temporary but can be permanent, in stallions).

Box 21.5 shows the breeds that are particularly sensitive to acepromazine. ACP provides no analgesia but improves analgesic effect of analgesics.

α2 agonists and other tranquillisers

These two groups of drugs are often used in conjunction with opioids to provide neuroleptanalgesia. Neuroleptanalgesia is a state of CNS depression and analgesia produced by the combination of a tranquilliser and an analgesic drug. The benzodiazepines and α2 agonists are commonly used as the tranquillising component, with the analgesia being provided by an opioid drug.

Box 21.5

Breeds of dog sensitive to acepromazine

- Giant breeds, e.g. Great Danes and Bull Mastiffs
- Deep-chested breeds, e.g. Greyhounds and Setters
- Boxers – some collapse but the drug can be safely used if given with an antimuscarinic

---

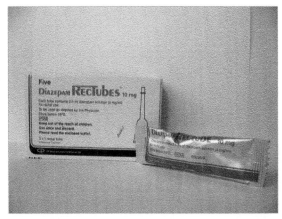

Fig. 21.2 Rectal administration of diazepam. Courtesy of G. Cousquer

Benzodiazepines

Benzodiazepines are sometimes referred to as minor tranquillisers and include diazepam and midazolam. This group of drugs exerts their effect by enhancing the activity of CNS inhibitory neurotransmitters (GABA and glycine), together with a hyperpolarising effect on cell membranes mediated via CNS benzodiazepine receptors and chloride channels. Depression of the limbic system, thalamus and hypothalamus result in a mild calming effect. They reduce polysynaptic reflex activity, resulting in muscle relaxation and produce anticonvulsant effects in most mammals. The calming effects are observed in sick, depressed or debilitated animals, whereas minimal or no calming effects are seen in normal animals.

The physical properties of diazepam differ from those of midazolam. Midazolam is water-soluble, whereas diazepam is not. Diazepam is solubilised by mixing with 40% propylene glycol, ethyl alcohol, sodium benzoate or benzoic acid. Propylene glycol is a cardiovascular depressant; rapid i.v. injection may produce bradycardia, hypotension, cardiac arrhythmias and even apnoea. Diazepam should only be given i.v., orally or rectally using an enema product like the one in Figure 21.2. Diazepam should not be given i.m. because it is painful.

Diazepam is also taken up by and interacts with plastic and should not be drawn up before it is required. Appetite is stimulated in some animals, especially cats. Diazepam can produce paradoxical increases in anxiety and fear responses in some animals. Phenothiazines are likely to provoke excitement and apparent involuntary extrapyramidal musculoskeletal effects.

As midazolam is water soluble it is therefore suitable for use i.m. (where it is rapidly absorbed) as well as i.v. It is twice as potent as diazepam. Equal

Safety tip when using benzodiazepines

The benzodiazepines can be reversed (antagonised) by the drug flumazenil 0.1 mg/kg i.v. hourly as required. Effects are seen within 2–5 minutes after administration

volumes of midazolam and ketamine are recommended by many authors, reportedly compatible when mixed in a syringe, and the important point is that they provide a relatively safe sedative combination. This can be given to effect in high-risk respiratory cases due to their minimal effects on the cardiac and respiratory centres.

Antagonists (e.g. flumazenil) are used to reverse the effects in human medicine, but *have not found use* (see Box 21.6) in veterinary medicine yet.

α2 agonists

α2 agonists include xylazine, medetomidine, detomidine and romifidine. This group of drugs produces CNS depression by binding to and stimulating presynaptic α2 adrenoceptors in the CNS and peripherally. The resulting reduction in norepinephrine release results in a decrease in CNS sympathetic outflow. A sleep-like state is produced that is comparable to, but more pronounced than, that produced by the phenothiazines. Analgesia is produced as a result of α2 receptor stimulation in the CNS. Muscle relaxation is seen and is produced centrally.

Medetomidine is a good alternative choice for the treatment of patients presenting in status epilepticus. The major effects are:

- depresses cardiac function
  - slows heart rate due to reduced CNS sympathetic outflow
  - increases peripheral vascular resistance
  - reduces cardiac output by 30–50% as a result of the reduced heart rate and increased vascular resistance
- biphasic effect on blood pressure – initial hypertension (due to increased PVR produced by peripheral α1 and α2 stimulatory effect) followed by prolonged hypotension (due to reduced CNS sympathetic outflow)
- mild depressant effect on ventilation due, in part, to a reduction in respiratory centre sensitivity; reductions in tidal volume and respiratory rate are seen
- peripheral vasoconstriction
- hypothermia is a common side effect.

Other side effects include:

- cyanosis due to the peripheral vasoconstriction and sludging of the blood is seen – however, perfusion to key organs is maintained
- vomiting in dogs and cats
- decreased intestinal motility
- muscle tremor
- increased uterine tone
- diuresis – increased urine production due to a decrease in antidiuretic hormone
- stimulates α2 receptors in the pancreas, thus suppressing insulin release
- second-degree heart block and bradyarrhythmias
- sweating in horses.

Atipamezole is an α_2 antagonist capable of abolishing the sedative and analgesic effects of medetomidine but there is incomplete reversal of the adverse cardiopulmonary effects. Yohimbine hydrochloride is an old drug alleged to have aphrodisiac characteristics. It is found in rauwolfia root and is a competitive α2 antagonist. It disappeared from clinical use years ago, but is now used as an α2 blocking agent.

Use of opioid drugs together with a tranquilliser

The only commercially available neuroleptanalgesic in the UK is a combination of the butyrophenone fluanisone with the very potent synthetic opioid fentanyl (Hypnorm). It is licensed for use in rabbits, in which it produces good-quality anaesthesia of some 20 minutes' duration. Other combinations are available as separate drugs but licensed for use together, these include:

- medetomidine and butorphanol
- xylazine and butorphanol
- iromifidine and butorphanol.

Other commonly used, but unlicensed, combinations include:

- acepromazine and buprenorphine
- acepromazine and butorphanol
- acepromazine and morphine
- diazepam/midazolam and morphine
- diazepam/midazolam and buprenorphine/butorphanol
- medetomidine and pethidine.

Including opioids with an α2 agonist such as medetomidine lowers the dose of α2 agonist required to achieve a given level of sedation. While α2 agonist/opioid combinations are safer than α2 agonists alone, it is recommended that they only be used in healthy animals. The use of a benzodiazepine instead of an α2 agonist is recommended in critically ill animals. The opioid component is generally given first and is followed by the benzodiazepine some 20 minutes later.

Opioids

These will be discussed further under analgesia.

Local anaesthetics

These agents cause a temporary peripheral blockade of sensory nerves. They are used topically on mucous membranes and conjunctiva, injected into the tissue around nerves (Box 21.7), injected into the epidural space or into a vein distal to a tourniquet to produce regional analgesia for minor surgery. Local anaesthetics provide desensitisation and analgesia of epidermal, epithelial and conjunctival tissues (topical anaesthesia), local tissues (local anaesthesia produced through infiltration and field blocks) and regional structures (regional anaesthesia produced by conduction and intravenous anaesthesia). Figure 21.3 illustrates the sites of nerve blocks on the head.

The mechanism of action is by prevention of the rapid influx of sodium into the axons which produces the action potential (nerve impulse). Local anaesthetic techniques are an alternative or adjunct to intravenous and inhalational anaesthesia in high-risk patients.

Vasoconstrictors such as epinephrine are sometimes added to the anaesthetic agent to cause vasoconstriction and keep the drug in the tissues for longer. There is, however, a risk of ischaemic damage when using epinephrine and it should not be used

> **Box 21.7**
>
> **Local anaesthesia nerve blocks**
>
> - easy to administer
>   - intercostal blocks for a thoracotomy
>   - alveolar mandibular nerve block for a mandibulectomy
>   - regional anaesthesia of the head – infraorbital, maxillary, ophthalmic, mental nerves
> - technically demanding
>   - brachial plexus blocks to stop phantom limb pain after amputation of a forelimb (nerves blocked include the radial, median, ulnar, musculocutaneous and axillary)

in ring blocks around areas of limited blood supply such as teats or digits. There are about 50 agents in clinical use, some of which are listed below:

- procaine – prototype of all local anaesthetics and used for comparison of anaesthetic effects. Good analgesia, weak tissue penetration, more tissue irritation.
- lidocaine – (old name lignocaine) excellent analgesia, good tissue penetration compared with procaine with effects evident in one-third of the time, no tissue damage or irritation, rapid onset of action (reflects tissue penetration), short-acting (1–1.5 hours – lasts 1.5× longer than procaine), low toxicity, licensed (in UK). Most stable drug in LA group.

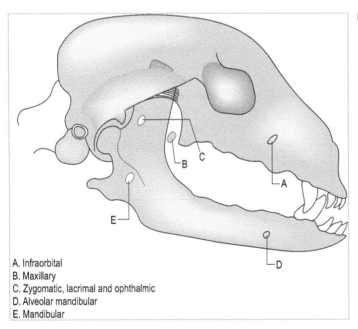

Fig. 21.3 Nerve blocks on the head

A. Infraorbital
B. Maxillary
C. Zygomatic, lacrimal and ophthalmic
D. Alveolar mandibular
E. Mandibular

- proxymetacaine – topical solution for ophthalmic use, rapid onset, short duration (15 minutes).
- prilocaine – slow onset of analgesia as slow spread throughout tissues.
- bupivacaine – 4× as potent as lidocaine, slow (intermediate) onset of action (15 minutes), no tissue irritation, long duration of action (4–6 h).
- mepivacaine – less tissue irritation than lidocaine, expensive, used in equine nerve blocks due to length of action and the reduced pain response upon injection.
- ropivacaine – similar to bupivacaine, long duration of action.
- EMLA cream – eutectic mixture of local anaesthetics, combination of lidocaine and prilocaine in a cream, used for cannulae placement 45 minutes prior to catheterisation.

The first clinically significant local anaesthetic to be used was cocaine hydrochloride. It was derived from the leaves of *Erythroxylon coca*, the coca tree, found in Chile and Peru. It was first used in 1884, when it was utilised to anaesthetise the eye. Spinal anaesthesia was first achieved (following injection into the subarachnoid space) in a dog and not until 15 years later was it accomplished in humans.

Pharmacokinetics of local anaesthetics

The pharmacokinetics of the various local anaesthetic agents differs; these differences must be appreciated in order to make an appropriate choice for any given clinical situation. The salt of the anaesthetic base is an ionisable quarternary amine with poor lipid solubility and therefore little or no anaesthetic properties of its own. The anaesthetic base is liberated in alkaline tissues and is then absorbed at the outer lipid nerve membrane. This is important as the tissue pH is lower in inflamed and infected tissues, little free base dissociates from the anaesthetic salt – resulting in poor local anaesthesia of these tissues. The way a drug is absorbed, distributed, metabolised and excreted has great importance as it determines the systemic disposition of the drug and its potential for toxicity.

- The absorption is influenced by:
  - the dosage (volume and concentration)
  - site of injection
  - presence of a vasoconstrictor, e.g. epinephrine.
- The distribution is influenced by:
  - whether it is classified as an ester (e.g. procaine) or an amide (e.g. lidocaine) as amides are widely distributed and esters are rapidly broken down
  - protein binding as it influences the free drug available for both activity and clearance by the liver.
- The metabolism and excretion of local anaesthetics is influenced by:
  - whether they are broken down in the plasma or the liver; the lungs and the liver are the major sites for plasma clearance of local anaesthetics
  - pregnancy reduces the clearance of the ester of local anaesthetics and increases their potential for toxicity
  - renal function and urine pH – in general, excretion is greater in acid urine
  - hepatic function and hepatic blood flow (reductions in which can be seen with the hypotension accompanying general anaesthesia).

Pharmacodynamics of local anaesthetics

Local anaesthetics are capable of blocking all nerves, hence their action is not limited to the usually desired loss of sensation – motor loss also occurs. The presence or absence of myelination affects the susceptibility of the nerve fibre to blockade. The priority of blockade is as follows: B-fibres, C-fibres, A_d fibres, A_a fibres. Nervous function is lost in the following order:

1. pain
2. cold/warmth
3. touch
4. deep pressure
5. motor function.

This suggests that sensory nerve fibres are more quickly blocked than the larger motor fibres, i.e. unmyelinated C fibres (those that transmit pain and temperature) are blocked first.

Clinical pharmacology

- *Anaesthetic potency* – affected by both (a) lipid solubility (hydrophobicity) – this determines how quickly the LA can penetrate a nerve fibre and (b) water solubility (hydrophilicity) – this is important for diffusion of the drug to the site of action. Figure 21.4 shows the basic molecular structure which most of the agents share. Most are weakly basic tertiary amines. Some, such as benzocaine, do not have the hydrophilic part and thus can not be injected as they are insoluble in water, but can be used topically. Other drugs with similar structures, such as antihistamines, also show weak local anaesthetic effects.

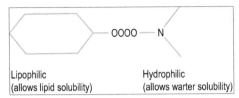

Fig. 21.4 Basic molecular structure of local anaesthetics

- *Onset of action* – related to the dose and concentration of agent administered. The addition of bicarbonate to raise the pH, together with the addition of the enzyme hyaluronidase to increase the diffusion to the site of action, both result in a faster onset of action.
- *Duration of action* – the site of injection affects how long local anaesthesia will last. Intrathecal injection is cleared rapidly compared with a peripheral nerve block. The strength of binding to the axonal protein also affects how long the agent's activity persists.

Anaesthetic agents

These can be divided into injectable (usually intravenous) and inhalation agents. Injectable agents have a rapid onset of action and are commonly used as induction agents to effect rapid passage through the light planes of anaesthesia, during which the patient may struggle. The drugs are eliminated by metabolism and excretion so there is often no way of increasing the rate of removal from the body to compensate for overdosage. One exception to this is to alter urinary pH to treat barbiturate poisoning. Another is that glomerular filtration rate can be increased to promote the renal excretion of drugs such as ketamine.

Injectable agents

Injectable agents can cause respiratory depression and periods of apnoea. Other effects include hypotension and tachycardia. The injectable agents can be grouped as follows:

Barbiturates

- Categorised according to their duration of action:
  - long (8–12 h) and intermediate (2–6 h)
  - short (45–75 min) and ultra-short (5–15 min)
- Barbiturates are respiratory depressants:
  - depress respiratory centre in the medulla
  - degree of depression related to dose and rate of administration
  - apnoea is associated with rapid i.v. injection

- Significant cardiovascular depression
- Sensitises the heart to epinephrine
- Short-acting barbiturates require 5–10 min to produce maximal CNS effect; ultra-short-acting barbiturates require 30 seconds
- Eliminated by renal excretion and/or destruction by hepatic oxidative processes
- Redistribution of ultra-short-acting barbiturates to lean body tissues (muscle) dictates their duration of action; emergence from sleep thus depends on the drug leaving the brain tissues and passing into lean body tissues
- Doses should be based on lean body weight
- Obesity delays drug elimination because of the high lipid solubility of barbiturates
- Possess anticonvulsant properties.

Thiopental is an ultra-short-acting barbiturate with an alkaline pH of over 12. It is therefore very irritating if injected extravascularly in concentrations of greater than 2.5%. The solution is unstable and, once prepared, should be stored in the refrigerator or for 3 days at room temperature. It rapidly distributes to the brain and then to muscles and lipid tissue but 85% of the drug is bound to plasma albumin – meaning only 15% is free to cross into the brain and exert an effect. Note that in disease states, where there is a reduction in protein levels (hypoalbuminaemia), there may be more free drug and the dose of thiopental will need to be reduced. The liver is the site of metabolism. Another notable effect is splenic enlargement; this may be significant clinically in splenectomies and in cases of diaphragmatic rupture where the spleen is in the thorax.

Thiopental causes a decrease in packed cell volume (PCV) and leucocyte numbers. The fall in PCV is thought to be due to splenic sequestration of red blood cells. Thiopental can also cause hypotension due to reduced myocardial contractility and peripheral vasodilation. In addition, it can cause cardiac arrhythmias as it sensitises the myocardium to catecholamines. Post-induction apnoea is common. The lethal dose is twice the anaesthetic dose and overdosed animals die from respiratory failure.

Methohexitone sodium (Brietal) is less irritant than thiopental because it is used at a lower concentration (1%) and has a pH of 11. It is metabolised more quickly by the liver so it is more suitable for dogs with low body fat stores, such as sighthounds. It is twice as potent as thiopental and has a rapid onset and fast recovery (5–10 minutes compared with the 10–30 minutes seen with thiopental).

Pentobarbitone is not very lipid soluble so it takes more time to cross the blood–brain barrier and hence has a slower onset of action and is metabolised more slowly. Recovery is also prolonged.

Propofol (Rapinovet)

This agent is an alkylphenol that is poorly soluble in water. It is therefore solubilised in a soybean oil and lecithin emulsion. Propofol gives a smooth induction and recovery and is non-irritant. It is rapidly metabolised both in the liver and in the lungs. Apnoea on induction is common and the formulation is capable of supporting bacterial growth – so the drug should be withdrawn aseptically from vials, using clean needles and after swabbing the rubber septum with alcohol. It is recommended that open vials and penetrated rubber-sealed bottles be thrown away after 8 hours. The drug is rapidly cleared from the body by hepatic and extra-hepatic metabolism. Maintenance of anaesthesia (in dogs) can be achieved either by continuous infusion at 0.2–0.4 mg/kg/min (useful for the control of seizures) or repeated bolus administration at 0.5–2 mg/kg. Cats often sneeze on recovery.

Both blood pressure and cardiac output decrease after administration but the heart rate is usually unchanged. Propofol decreases cerebral blood flow and cerebral oxygen consumption and increases cerebral vascular resistance – so, like the barbiturates, it is indicated where anaesthesia is required in patients with head trauma and cerebral oedema. Propofol has anticonvulsant properties and is indicated in patients with uncontrolled seizures.

Propofol is more likely to be associated with bradycardia than other injectable anaesthetic agents. When propofol is administered with other agents that increase vagal tone or for procedures where vagal tone may be increased, anticholinergics should be administered prophylactically. In humans, the risk of bradycardia despite prophylactic anticholinergics may still be considerable and several reports suggest an inadequate response of propofol-induced bradycardia to atropine. For this reason, propofol should be avoided in patients with conduction abnormalities or in patients taking β-blockers.

Propofol may cause myoclonic muscle twitching, has no analgesic properties and decreases intraocular pressure. Some animals show pain on injection although it is not irritating extravascularly. Induction may be associated with a transient lipaemia. It is not suitable for maintenance anaesthesia or repeated day use in cats as the feline liver is much slower at metabolising the drug. In cats it causes oxidative injury to red blood cells and when given over several days causes Heinz body formation, anorexia, malaise and diarrhoea.

Steroid anaesthetics

Alphaxalone and alphadolone acetate (Saffan) are steroid-based anaesthetics that are non-irritant and are rapidly metabolised by the liver. They should not be used in dogs, which may show an anaphylactic response. Histamine release is also seen in some cats, resulting in oedematous paws, ears and larynx – this can be reduced by premedication with acepromazine. It is viscous (due to the castor oil it is formulated in) and can be given by both the i.m. and i.v. routes. Muscle relaxation and analgesia are good and respiratory depression is minimal but it does cause some hypotension. Recovery is due to redistribution and hepatic metabolism but recoveries are often stormy.

Dissociative anaesthetics

Ketamine and tiletamine are cyclohexamine derivatives. They provide profound somatic, but little visceral, analgesia. There is pain on extravascular injection due to its pH of 4. It should be used with an α_2 agonist, e.g. medetomidine (Domitor), to avoid convulsions in dogs and to provide muscle relaxation. Onset of anaesthesia is slow, taking up to 1 minute to exert its effects on the CNS. Eyes remain open and palpebral, conjunctival, corneal and swallowing reflexes persist. It may precipitate seizures in epileptic patients and its use should be avoided. Another contraindication is in head trauma patients as ketamine induces significant increases in cerebral blood flow, which raises intracranial pressure. Apneustic breathing occurs, which is slow inspiration, a pause, then rapid expiration. This does not seem to affect blood gas values.

Ketamine increases heart rate and blood pressure, causes hypersalivation and increases in respiratory secretions, and may require anticholinergic drugs. There is rapid redistribution from the CNS to the other tissues resulting in a rapid recovery. Dogs metabolise the agent in the liver but the majority of the drug is excreted unchanged in the cat through the kidney. Low doses only should be given to animals with renal and hepatic dysfunction.

Etomidate

This common human anaesthetic agent is not licensed for veterinary use but is a useful agent for animals with severe trauma, advanced cardiovascular or hepatic disease, intracranial lesions or caesarean sections as it produces minimal cardiorespiratory depression and does not cause histamine release. It does, however, inhibit steroid production by the adrenal glands for up to 3 hours and may precipitate an Addisonian crisis if given over a long period.

Analgesia provided by injectable anaesthetic agents

Thiopental, etomidate and propofol do not block autonomic responses to noxious stimuli and thus painful procedures should not be carried out under these agents alone. Small doses (0.6–1.5 mg/kg) of thiopental can cause an increased sensitivity to somatic pain. Following induction with thiopental, anti-analgesia may be present for up to 5 hours in the recovery period. The hyperalgesic properties of sub-hypnotic concentrations of anaesthetics have also been reported for propofol. Only ketamine has been reported to possess analgesic properties. Induction with ketamine or addition of ketamine to general anaesthesia before surgical stimulation decreases postoperative pain and leads to better pain control. It appears that ketamine's analgesic properties reduce sensitisation of pain pathways and extend into the postoperative period. Low-dose infusion of ketamine has been advocated to provide postoperative analgesia.

Inhalational anaesthetics

The inhalational anaesthetics currently used in veterinary medicine are halothane, nitrous oxide, enflurane, isoflurane and sevoflurane. Ether, now largely obsolete, is still used in some parts of the world. Chloroform is also obsolete, due to the hepatotoxicity associated with free radical formation in liver cells. Inhalational anaesthetics are either gases or volatile liquids and are all organic compounds except nitrous oxide (N_2O). Figure 21.5 shows the chemical structures of some available agents. Understanding how the chemical structure of these agents affects their properties, helps you to make informed choices when using these agents.

The ideal agent should be:
- non-reactive, non-irritant and non-toxic
- potent with low blood gas solubility providing pleasant, rapid induction and rapid recovery
- safe – potentially reversible or easily controlled
- non-toxic to the patient and operators
- non-flammable, stable on storage and compatible with soda lime
- provide good analgesia, muscle relaxation and minimal cardiovascular depression
- excreted without being metabolised.

Modern agents are either aliphatic hydrocarbons or ethers. Adding halogens to an agent alters its properties as follows:
- chlorine and bromine increase potency
- substituting fluorine in the place of chlorine or bromine improves stability but reduces potency and solubility.

Vaporisers volatise liquid anaesthetics and deliver accurate, clinically useful, concentrations of anaesthetic vapour to the common gas outlet. Movement of a gaseous anaesthetic occurs between three key compartments – the alveoli, the blood and the central

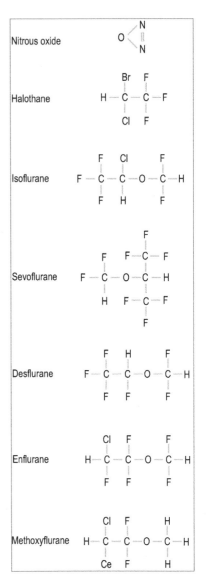

Fig. 21.5 Chemical structures of inhalant anaesthetics

nervous system. Movement of anaesthetic between the alveolar compartment and the blood compartment is a function of the blood-gas coefficient of the anaesthetic gas.

The depth of anaesthesia can be rapidly altered. Figure 21.6 shows the journey inhalational anaesthetics must take to reach their target tissue – the brain. The alveolar pulmonary membrane and the blood–brain barrier pose little problem as most agents are very lipid soluble. As can be seen in Table 21.1, methoxyflurane is the most lipophilic of the agents and is also the most potent. The extent to which a gas will dissolve in a solvent is expressed in terms of its solubility coefficient.

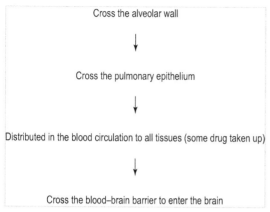

Cross the alveolar wall

↓

Cross the pulmonary epithelium

↓

Distributed in the blood circulation to all tissues (some drug taken up)

↓

Cross the blood–brain barrier to enter the brain

Fig. 21.6 The journey an inhalational agent takes from lungs to brain

Table 21.1 Comparing MAC values and blood-gas solubility coefficients of the inhalational agents

Inhalational agent	MAC value (%)	Blood-gas solubility coefficient
Nitrous oxide	~200	0.47
Halothane	0.87	2.5
Isoflurane	1.28	1.5
Sevoflurane	2.36	0.68
Desflurane	7.2	0.42
Enflurane	2.2	2.0
Methoxyflurane	0.23	15.0

Another way of comparing the properties of the agents is in terms of their minimum alveolar concentration (MAC). This is the concentration at which 50% of patients will not show a response to a stimuli. The higher the MAC, the lower the potency as more agent is required to produce the right depth of anaesthesia.

Elimination of the inhalational anaesthetics occurs when the agent leaves the blood and re-enters the alveoli. This then causes the agent to leave the brain and the patient regains consciousness. All the agents undergo some metabolism, which is important in toxicity as it is the metabolites that cause problems, not the agent itself. The free fluoride ions released from metabolism of methoxyflurane cause direct damage to the renal tubules and can cause renal failure. All of the volatile anaesthetics reduce renal blood flow and glomerular filtration rate in a dose-related manner. During anaesthesia, therefore, even healthy animals produce small amounts of concentrated urine and a transient increase in serum urea nitrogen, creatinine and phosphate is seen. In most cases the effects of inhalational anaesthesia on renal function are rapidly reversed after anaesthesia.

All inhalational agents are capable of causing hepatocellular injury by reducing liver blood flow. Halothane produces the most damage due to reactive compounds from its biotransformation causing some autoimmune reaction.

Nitrous oxide

Nitrous oxide is an inorganic gas that is a weak anaesthetic agent and must be delivered in concentrations of over 50% to have any effect on the patient. It has a rapid uptake, distribution and elimination and undergoes minimal metabolism. The second gas effect means it enhances the uptake of other agents administered with it and it has minimal effects on the cardiovascular and respiratory systems. These two properties combined mean it is a useful agent for allowing a reduction in dose rates of other, more cardiorespiratory depressant, agents. Because it quickly diffuses into air-filled spaces it can increase the volume of gas in dilated loops of bowl, increase the volume of a pneumothorax or cause increased pressure in the middle ear – occasionally causing a ruptured eardrum.

Halothane

Halothane is a colourless, volatile liquid that is non-inflammable and has a high potency and low blood solubility. Hypotension due to a fall in cardiac output is seen because halothane has a depressant effect on the myocardium. Dysrhythmias are not uncommon and the respiratory system is often depressed. It is stored in brown bottles because it breaks down in light and it contains a preservative, thymol, which causes damage to the vaporiser over time that requires it to be cleaned and recalibrated. As with all the inhalational agents (except for nitrous oxide), halothane is a poor analgesic and only a moderate amount of muscle relaxation occurs.

Isoflurane

Isoflurane, a halogenated ether, is a colourless liquid, stable in light, that gives rapid induction and recovery without less myocardial depression than the others. It does not contain a preservative. Isoflurane produces a decrease in tidal volume and an increase in respiratory rate. As with all inhalational anaesthetics, there is a negative inotropic effect on the myocardium, resulting in decreased contractility, but the heart rate increases to compensate maintaining the cardiac output. There is marked peripheral vasodilation and so hypotension is seen – as with halothane, but due to a different mechanism. Isoflurane produces more muscle relaxation than halothane.

Sevoflurane

Sevoflurane is a halogenated ether which allows rapid alterations in depth of anaesthesia due to its low blood gas solubility. It provides a rapid induction and recovery and no irritation to the respiratory tract – which gives it an advantage over isoflurane and desflurane. It is minimally metabolised (3%) and current information suggests that sevoflurane or its degradation products do not produce hepatic or renal injury. Unlike other contemporary inhalational anaesthetics, sevoflurane is degraded in the presence of soda lime, a commonly used carbon dioxide absorbent in anaesthetic delivery circuits. Except for causing a higher heart rate, sevoflurane's action on the circulatory and respiratory systems are similar to isoflurane. Sevoflurane does not increase the arrhythmogenicity of the heart.

Desflurane

Desflurane is a halogenated ether with a low blood gas solubility and therefore allows rapid induction and recovery. Its use is limited due to its expense, the special vaporiser required and the irritation it causes to the respiratory tract.

Methoxyflurane

Methoxyflurane is a good analgesic and provides good muscle relaxation but gives a slow induction due to its low volatility. It has been withdrawn from the market due to its nephrotoxicity.

Enflurane

Enflurane, a structural isomer of isoflurane, is another volatile liquid that is a potent anaesthetic agent. It causes myocardial depression and ECG changes that last for weeks and occasionally causes seizures which have resulted in its use being limited.

Ether

Ether is a colourless, volatile liquid that is flammable and explosive in oxygen. It has a high margin of safety, but is a slow induction agent with extended recovery periods due to its high blood solubility. Nausea and vomiting often occur postoperatively.

The inhalational agents can be ranked as follows:
1. Apnoeic and cardiac arrest therapeutic thresholds

isoflurane > methoxyflurane ≥ halothane > enflurane

2. Myocardial depression

enflurane > halothane ≥ methoxyflurane > isoflurane

3. Reduction in cardiac output

enflurane > halothane ≥ methoxyflurane > isoflurane

4. Reductions in systemic vascular resistance

isoflurane > enflurane > methoxyflurane ≥ halothane

5. Hypotension

enflurane > isoflurane > halothane ≥ methoxyflurane

6. Impaired tissue oxygenation

enflurane > isoflurane = halothane = methoxyflurane

7. Respiratory depression

enflurane > isoflurane > methoxyflurane > halothane

Questions for Chapter 21

State whether the agents would increase (I) or decrease (D) the following:

1. ACP
   - gastric fluid volume and acidity
   - vomiting and regurgitation
   - anaesthetic requirements
   - heart rate
   - intestinal peristalsis
   - muscle tone

2. Atropine
   - airway secretions
   - heart rate
   - hypersialism
   - bronchoconstrictive disease
   - sinoatrial arrest
   - the signs of organophosphate poisoning

3. Saffan
   - analgesia
   - respiratory rate
   - muscle tone
   - likelihood of laryngeal oedema
   - depth of narcosis

4. Fluanisone
   - sedation
   - opioid-induced vomiting

- heart rate
- defecation
- responsiveness to auditory stimuli
- hypotension

5. Why do sighthounds take longer to recover from thiopental anaesthesia?

6. List the differences between isoflurane and halothane.

7. The enzyme responsible for the breakdown of suxamethonium is produced by the liver and carried by plasma proteins in the plasma. What disease states or conditions would reduce the plasma levels of the enzyme?

8. What are the factors that determine speed of induction using an inhalant anaesthetic?

9. Compare mask induction with sevoflurane and isoflurane.

For answers go to page 245

CHAPTER 22

Analgesics

Learning aims and objectives

After studying this chapter you should be able to:

1. **State the methods to chemically alleviate pain**
2. **State the mechanism of action of the opioid drugs**
3. **Describe the method of action of the NSAIDs**
4. **List the potential side effects of NSAIDs**
5. **State the properties of the $\alpha 2$ receptor agonists.**

Introduction

Pain serves a number of useful functions – it can limit the extent of an injury, encourage rest and healing and ensure that an individual learns to avoid noxious stimuli in the future. Ongoing pain is undesirable, however, for it has no benefit and considerable disadvantages – in animals it is likely to result in stress, discomfort, depressed food intake and impaired breathing. It causes sensitisation of the central nervous system and can also lead to self-mutilation. Analgesia is the term used to describe the abolition of pain and its importance in veterinary medicine is increasingly recognised.

Analgesics are drugs that suppress pain or induce analgesia. The response to the agent varies with the individual. The drugs used and mechanisms of action are:

- non-steroidal anti-inflammatory drugs (NSAIDs) – inhibit mediators of pain both centrally and peripherally
- α_2 agonists – activate pain inhibition pathways
- opioid analgesics – reduce afferent pain pathways, both centrally and peripherally
- dissociative anaesthetics (e.g. ketamine) – produce antihyperalgesic actions
- local anaesthetics – block sensory nerve impulse transmission when used locally as a nerve block.

Tissue damage causes the release of inflammatory mediators, mainly prostaglandins, which excite the pain receptors – nociceptors. The information is taken to the spinal cord in sensory afferent nerves and processed in the brain. If tissue damage is severe, changes may occur in the spinal cord that result in a hypersensitivity state producing chronic pain after the tissue damage has healed. This explains why pre-emptive analgesia lessens the pain experienced.

Peripheral tissue nociceptors detect a range of pain stimuli and permit transmission of the nociceptive signal via primary afferent nerve fibres to higher centres of the central nervous system. There are four types of peripheral nociceptors:

- low- and high-threshold mechanoreceptors
- thermoreceptors
- polymodal nociceptors.

A range of stimuli, inflammatory mediators and processes can all stimulate nociceptors. Dilation and swelling can produce mechanical stimulation, burns can produce thermal stimulation and ischaemic necrosis can release inflammatory mediators, such as prostaglandins, that stimulate nociceptors.

It is important to make a distinction between the prevention of sensitisation of the CNS and the alleviation of pain that has already been inflicted. Sensitisation changes the excitability of the CNS such that normal inputs will produce exaggerated responses, leading to pain hypersensitivity. Pre-emptive analgesia may block the development of sensitisation but cannot eliminate postoperative pain. Thus, additional measures are required to ensure a comfortable recovery.

Opioids

Opioid drugs provide analgesia by inhibiting the pain fibres in the dorsal root (sensory afferent nerves), activating descending inhibitory pathways and producing a sense of euphoria. They work because all vertebrates and many invertebrates have endogenous opioids which are split into three types:

- β endorphin
- encephalins
- dynorphin.

Four opioid receptors have been cloned to date – OP1 (delta δ), OP2 (kappa κ), OP3 (mu μ) and ORL1 (the orphan opioid receptor that appears to be linked to the endogenous peptide, nociceptin). Most opioids used clinically are selective for the μ receptor and mimic the effects of endogenous opioids in the CNS. They may also have an action in inflamed peripheral tissues. Box 22.1 classifies the opioids into groups depending on the effect they have on the receptor. Figure 22.1 shows the general structure of the opiate analgesics.

In the CNS, opiate analgesics bind to specific opioid receptors and act as partial or full agonists. They mimic the effects of the endogenous opioids

---

Box 22.1

How some of the common opioids affect the receptors

- agonists
  - morphine
  - pethidine
  - fentanyl
  - methadone
- partial agonists
  - butorphanol
  - buprenorphine
- antagonists
  - naloxone

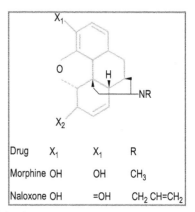

Drug	X_1	X_1	R
Morphine	OH	OH	CH_3
Naloxone	OH	=OH	CH_2 CH=CH_2

Fig. 22.1   General structure of the opiate analgesics

that normally bind to these receptors – this results in a variety of effects depending on the area of the brain affected. In addition to the desired effects of analgesia produced by binding in the spinal cord and periventricular grey matter a number of other effects can be seen, some of which may be undesirable:

- nausea and vomiting
- pupillary constriction – this is seen particularly in cats and can make the assessment of neurological status difficult
- drowsiness and sleep
- euphoria/excitement in high doses
- respiratory depression and suppression of the cough reflex
- mood change – usually euphoria but occasionally dysphoria
- decreased sympathetic outflow, urinary retention and constipation
- lowering of temperature
- cough suppression.

All of the above are due to action in the CNS. The peripheral effects of the opiate analgesics are also mediated by their effects on opioid receptors. These include a decrease in gastrointestinal motility and increased pressure within the biliary tract leading to biliary colic. Morphine can also cause vasodilation, an action that may be due to its ability to release histamine and suppress sympathetic outflow. Peripheral receptors develop at sites of inflammation and so intra-articular use has been advocated during joint surgery.

Morphine sulphate – pharmacological actions

Brain and spinal cord

Early changes include behavioural changes, depression in the dog and excitement in the cat and horse. Controversy exists as to whether morphine should be used in the cat because of its inability to consistently produce sedation; however, it remains the analgesic of choice for severe pain in cats. It is effective in reducing pain and the excitatory response frequently seen may be the effect of overdosage. The excitatory effects are seen less if the morphine is given to an animal in pain rather than pre-emptively. (*Note* – the poor reputation of morphine in cats is due to the work of Joel & Arndts in 1925 who used a dose of 20 mg/kg and overdosed their subjects.)

Emetic centre

Cats require considerably higher doses of morphine than dogs to induce vomiting.

Cough centre

This is more sensitive to morphine than other medullary centres. Morphine is an excellent cough suppressant and would be the drug of choice if it were not for its addictive properties.

Thermoregulation

Hypothermia is seen in dogs and rabbits, whereas hyperthermia usually occurs in cats and horses. In guinea pigs, rats and mice, low doses elicit a hyperthermia, while higher doses induce hypothermia. Morphine accelerates the release of 5-hydroxytryptamine (serotonin) from the hypothalamus. This stimulates heat dissipation responses and depresses the heat production responses – resulting in a drop in body temperature.

Eye

Morphine causes mydriasis in the cat and horse and miosis in dogs, rats and rabbits. The iris of the bird is not affected because it contains non-responsive skeletal muscles. This response is mediated via stimulation of the oculomotor nucleus, not via a direct action on skeletal muscle.

Respiratory system

This is initially stimulated in the dog and panting is seen due partly to the rise in body temperature. As body temperature declines and CNS depression increases, respiratory activity is depressed and respirations become shallower and slower. In normal healthy dogs, the respiratory minute volume and oxygen consumption are not decreased by more than 10%.

Cardiovascular system

Morphine induces coronary vasoconstriction and a reduction in coronary blood flow. There is a transient drop in arterial blood pressure and an increase in heart rate.

Urinary tract

Initially causes urination but then decreases urine production to 10% of normal by liberating an excess of the antidiuretic hormone from the posterior pituitary gland.

GI tract

Emptying the tract is the first response but then there is inhibition of tract motility. Since embryologically all peptide-hormone-producing cells are derived from neural ectoderm, it is not surprising to find opioid receptors in the GI tract. Morphine has a spasmogenic effect on the intestines, partly by a direct action and partly by a histaminergic mechanism. This causes an increase in sphincter muscle tone which, combined with the increased water resorption from the ingesta, can result in constipation.

Endocrine system

Opiates exert an important modulating effect on the hypothalamus; additional effects may occur at the pituitary and other organs. Opiate-induced endocrine actions appear to be mediated through dopaminergic and/or serotoninergic mechanisms. Endogenous opioids appear to be important in the physiological regulation of ACTH and gonadotrophin release. The inhibitory release of ACTH in Cushing's disease suggests a potential use of specific and long-acting opiate antagonists in the treatment of this condition.

Immune system

Immune and neuroendocrine systems have the capability of signalling to each other through common or related peptide hormones and receptors. Encephalins and endorphins can be considered immuno-modulators and modifiers of the physiologic response and may have important application in immunotherapy.

Absorption, fate and excretion

Morphine is a weak acid that is about 20–40% protein bound with an elimination half life of 2–4 hours. It is absorbed from the small intestine and some from the stomach but is not absorbed through intact skin. The liver is responsible for the biotransformation of the drug to its excretable form, 50% of which occurs through the urine.

Toxicity

Newborn animals are more sensitive to morphine than adults. This is because the blood–brain barrier, which usually prevents the drug from reaching the brain, develops with maturity. Convulsive seizures occur following high doses of morphine in most species.

Contraindications

Morphine should be used with care in uraemic and toxaemic dogs. It should not be administered to dogs suffering from shock because of its hypotensive effects. Opioids increase intracranial pressure and so should not be used in head traumas.

The effects of the other opioids are generally similar to those of morphine.

Codeine

Codeine is produced semi-synthetically from morphine and is rapidly metabolised and excreted in the urine a few minutes after injection. It is widely used to depress the cough reflex but does possess some of the constipating action of morphine. The analgesic action of codeine is less than morphine.

Methadone

This full agonist is similar in effect to morphine but with a longer duration of action and without some of the addictive properties. It is not licensed for use in animals but is useful when emesis is to be avoided. It does not cause the vomiting seen with morphine at a dose of 0.1–0.5 mg/kg i.m. in dogs. In cats the excitement seen limits its use.

Fentanyl

This rapidly acting agonist has 1000× the potency of morphine but a shorter duration of action, approximately 20 minutes, due to its high lipid solubility. It has a high abuse potential and is therefore a Schedule 2 controlled drug. Fentanyl is available in a transdermal delivery system, consisting of a small reservoir with a semipermeable membrane that is applied over the skin in a hairless area. The dose most commonly used in dogs and cats is 2–4 µg/kg/h and the patches can be half covered to reduce the absorption if the patch size is unsuitable.

Pethidine

This drug only has a tenth of the potency of morphine but is a good spasmolytic agent with sedative and analgesic properties. Pethidine is a pure (µ selective) agonist with a fast onset (10–15 minutes) and a short duration of action (30–45 minutes). It is best administered i.m. as s.c. injections cause local irritation and pain. It is administered as a premedicant to reduce the amount of anaesthetic required but, as with all opioids, the depressant effect varies with the individual. Its spasmolytic properties are due to the fact it possesses an atropine-like structure.

Papaveretum

This is a mixture of 50% morphine and 50% other alkaloids of opium. It causes less vomiting than morphine.

Alfentanyl

Due to its very high lipid solubility, this agent is very rapid acting and has a short duration of about 5 minutes. This allows it to be used intraoperatively as an infusion. It is a pure agonist with 10× the potency of morphine but less than fentanyl.

Remifentanil

Remifentanil is the newest synthetic opioid. It is 30× more potent than alfentanyl with a large therapeutic index and extremely short half life. It has the advantage over the other opioids of being broken down by the plasma enzymes and tissue esterases and does not require liver metabolism and urinary excretion. The pharmacokinetic and pharmaco-dynamic properties of the agent render it ideal for combination with propofol for total intravenous anaesthesia. The therapeutic advantages proposed for anaesthesia with remifentanil include the rapid control of the depth of anaesthesia, a predictable pharmacokinetic recovery profile and a lack of dependence on the liver and kidney.

In common with other opioids, it has minimal depression of the cardiovascular system, however, the respiratory depressant effects of remifentanil mean that IPPV is essential during anaesthesia. Due to its rapid metabolism, the analgesic effects do not persist into the recovery period and alternative analgesia must be given in conjunction. The administration of an anticholinergic drug, such as atropine premedication, is also recommended to reduce the marked vagomimetic effects of remifentanil. This is a human authorised medicinal product.

Buprenorphine

This Schedule 3 controlled drug is a partial μ agonist. It has 30–100× the potency of morphine and is highly lipophilic. It is slow to associate and dissociate from opioid receptors, resulting in a slow onset of action (approx 45 minutes). These properties mean that it must be administered at least 45 minutes before the analgesic effect is required, has a long duration of action (max of 8 h) and can not be displaced by other opioid drugs or opioid antagonists. It is licensed for use in dogs by the i.m. route, but can be administered via the i.m., i.v. and s.c. routes. Buprenorphine is also commonly used in cats.

Butorphanol

This partial agonist is not controlled currently in the UK and although it is licensed as an analgesic in the dog and cat it has very short-lived action (1 hour) and is considered to be a better sedative than analgesic. In addition to being a partial μ agonist, butorphanol is also a κ agonist. It is suggested that this makes it the opioid of choice in certain avian patients due to species differences in receptors.

Pentazocine

This is a weak opioid used for short-term management of mild pain in dogs. It has little sedative effect and only small effects on the GI tract. Unlike most opioids, it increases the heart rate. It was developed hoping it would not have the addictive effects of morphine. It is classed in Schedule 3 of the controlled drugs.

Naloxone

This opioid antagonist reverses the effects of both pure and partial agonists. It increases myocardial contractile forces as it releases catecholamines.

Opioids and spinal analgesia

These agents can be administered into the epidural or intrathecal space to provide analgesia without some of the side effects typical of opioid use. They interact with opioid receptors in the spinal cord as well as having some systemic effects. Epidural use of the more lipophilic opioids has little advantage over systemic use as they are taken up into the vasculature quickly and the short duration of action means repeated administration or continuous infusion is necessary.

Non-steroidal anti-inflammatory drugs

Any infection or physical injury to tissue results in inflammation, the signs of which include heat, redness, pain, swelling and loss of function. This protective process is designed to destroy the injurious agent. If the stimulus persists, the inflammation becomes chronic, resulting in tissue destruction and fibrous tissue formation. NSAIDs suppress inflammatory reactions, thereby providing symptomatic relief. Despite widely differing chemical structures, most NSAIDs share three basic properties:

- anti-inflammatory by their local actions
- antipyretic
- analgesic by their effects on the CNS.

The potency for each property varies from drug to drug.

White blood cells are attracted to a site of inflammation by substances called leukotrienes (LTs) and prostaglandins (PGs). LTs also cause vasodilation and an increase in vascular permeability, thereby increasing leucocyte migration into the tissues. PGs are particularly important because they create the sensation of pain when applied to nerve endings. PG production (Fig. 22.2) is catalysed by the enzyme cyclo-oxygenase (COX) and most NSAIDs work by inhibiting these COX enzymes. Certain prostaglandins have beneficial effects on gut wall function including the maintenance of gastric blood flow and mucus secretion. Inhibition by NSAIDs can lead to gastric ulceration and other side effects. NSAIDs also promote thrombocyte and leucocyte adhesion to the intima of gastric blood vessels and thereby diminish gastric blood flow.

There are two forms of the COX enzyme: a COX-1 responsible for the housekeeping functions such as reno- and gastro-protection, and a COX-2 responsible for the signs of inflammation. Carprofen and meloxicam have a prostaglandin-sparing effect, reducing adverse side effects, as they preferentially inhibit COX-2. As with all NSAIDs they should be used with care in patients with renal, cardiac or hepatic impairment. The mechanism of action of carprofen is unclear.

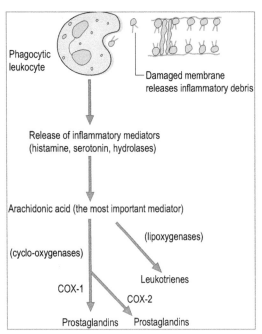

Fig. 22.2 Tissue damage leading to the production of prostaglandins

Structurally, NSAIDs can be classified into salicylate or carboxylic acid derivatives, including the indoles, propionic acids (ibuprofen and naproxen), fenamates (meclofenamic acid), oxicams (piroxicam) or the pyrazolones or enolic acids (phenylbutazone).

Aspirin

Aspirin is not veterinary licensed. In addition to inhibition of the COX enzymes, aspirin (the salicylic ester of acetic acid), inhibits the formation and release of kinins, stabilises lysosomes and removes the energy necessary for inflammation. Aspirin undergoes rapid metabolism and is about 50% albumin bound in the plasma. This means that hypoalbuminaemia results in increases in plasma drug concentrations with adverse effects. Toxic effects include depression, vomiting, hyperthermia, electrolyte imbalances, convulsions, coma and death. It is a COX1 inhibitor and can be used to control mild to moderate pain, as well as having a role in the prevention of arterial thromboembolisation.

Carprofen

Carprofen (Rimadyl) is an authorised veterinary medicinal product and is PG sparing. The mechanism of action appears to involve specific inhibition of COX-2 and although its effects are weak on the enzyme, it is a potent anti-inflammatory agent with good analgesic properties. The physiologic or protective actions of prostaglandins appear to be minimally inhibited with no loss of anti-inflammatory efficacy. It has been suggested that the actual mechanism of action may be inhibition of phospholipase and impaired release of arachidonic acid. Like other NSAIDs, carprofen is highly protein-bound. It is used commonly to treat osteoarthritis in dogs and the effects on cartilage synthesis appear to be concentration dependent. At higher doses, carprofen inhibits polysulphated glycosaminoglycan synthesis and protein synthesis. Cats and dogs do not tolerate long-term therapy with carprofen. The weak to moderate inhibition of both COX isoforms produced by clinical doses of carprofen in most species may explain its wide safety margin in comparison with most NSAIDs.

Flunixin meglumine

Flunixin meglumine (Finadyne) is an authorised veterinary medicinal product. Very potent, it helps with endotoxaemia as it has anti-endotoxin effects at doses below that which produce anti-inflammatory effects. It is a nicotinic acid derivative, which is particularly useful for visceral pain. Adverse effects are dose-related and reflect the changes expected with COX-1 inhibition and therefore the reduction in prostaglandin synthesis. Toxicity, most commonly manifesting as GI upset, limits the use of this drug in dogs to 2–3 days.

Ketoprofen

Ketoprofen is an authorised veterinary medicinal product. It is a propionic acid NSAID which is a strong inhibitor of COX1, with powerful anti-inflammatory, analgesic and anti-pyretic properties. Some of its efficacy may be attributable to its ability to inhibit some lipoxygenases and thus the formation of leukotrienes. Both the injectable and tablet preparations are licensed for use in cats as well as dogs.

Meloxicam

Meloxicam (Metacam) is an authorised veterinary medicinal product. It is PG sparing as it is a relative COX-2 selective inhibitor. It has a high safety profile but should not be administered to pregnant animals. Meloxicam, along with most other NSAIDs, is eliminated as glucuronide conjugates. Cats have a deficiency of bilirubin-glucuronoside glucuronosyltransferase enzyme and therefore the drug should only be administered for short courses – the suggested dose is a loading dose of 0.3 mg/kg followed by a dose of 0.1 mg/kg every day for four further days.

Paracetamol

Do not use paracetamol in cats as they lack glucuronyl transferase enzymes required to metabolise it and may therefore develop hepatotoxicity. It is mainly used for its antipyretic and analgesic properties; it is, however, considered a poor anti-inflammatory. The mechanism of action does not appear to involve inhibition of COX, instead it appears to modulate the concentration of prostaglandin intermediates.

Phenylbutazone

Phenylbutazone is an authorised veterinary medicinal product. It is a weakly acidic, lipophilic NSAID which is metabolised in the liver, with less than 2% being excreted in the urine. Bioavailability following i.m. injection is less than that following oral administration due to precipitation in the neutral pH of muscle. Box 22.2 shows some of the adverse effects and contraindications of use. Phenylbutazone may cause false low T3 and T4 values and it may displace a variety of protein-bound drugs including anaesthetics, thereby prolonging their effects.

Piroxicam

Piroxicam is not licensed; it is used to reduce the size of bladder carcinomas. This may be due to immuno-modulation but is more likely to be due to decreased inflammation at the tumour site. It is a potent anti-inflammatory in musculoskeletal conditions and oral absorption is rapid, with 100% bioavailability.

Box 22.2

Adverse effects and contraindications of phenylbutazone

- gastrointestinal irritation and ulceration
- renal papillary necrosis (renal failure)
- bone marrow suppression (including aplastic anaemia)
- nausea, vomiting, diarrhoea
- hepatotoxicity (cholestasis and parenchymal damage)
- fluid retention which may cause cardiac failure

Ibuprofen

Ibuprofen is a propionic acid derivative which has been used in dogs. It is a less effective analgesic than aspirin, possibly due to the different method of binding to the COX enzymes (reversible for ibuprofen and irreversible for aspirin). It is popular in human medicine due to the low incidence of GI side effects, but GI erosions consistently occur in dogs receiving therapeutic doses for 2–6 weeks and gastric lesions occur at doses less than those necessary to achieve therapeutic concentrations. It should be emphasised that this is an authorised human medicinal product, not a veterinary one.

Tolfenamic acid

Tolfenamic acid is authorised in both cats and dogs for short courses.

α_2 receptor agonists

α_2 receptor agonists such as medetomidine (Domitor; Pfizer) and xylazine (Rompun; Bayer) bind to α_2 receptors in the central and peripheral nervous system, producing sedation and analgesia. However, they have marked effects on the cardiovascular system and therefore are predominantly used in healthy patients. It is thought that analgesia occurs at lower doses than those which have adverse effects and their use as analgesics is growing.

Medetomidine is lipophilic, rapidly eliminated and induces sedation from which animals can become suddenly aroused. Higher doses do not increase sedation but do increase the duration of effect. Vomiting may occur following s.c. or i.m. injection in cats, less commonly in dogs and not in rabbits. Diuresis is observed with even low doses. Atropine premedication offsets the bradycardia but may exacerbate the initial hypertension medetomidine causes. Combination with ketamine enhances both sedation and analgesia and also counteracts the bradycardic effects.

Romifidine is a new agent that is an effective i.m. sedative in dogs, with a longer duration of action than xylazine.

Atipamazole is an α_2 receptor antagonist that reverses the effects of medetomidine. Severe hypotension and tachycardia can occur following the rapid intravenous injection of atipamazole, however, reactions to the agent when given appropriately are extremely rare.

Questions for Chapter 22

True or false

State whether the following are TRUE or FALSE:

1. Opioid analgesics and derivatives decrease peristaltic activity in the GI tract.

2. Specific opioid receptors are present not only in the CNS but also within the myenteric plexuses in the intestinal wall.

3. Opioids decrease the tone of the anal sphincter by blocking acetylcholine release.

4. Opiates can be used clinically as anti-emetics.

5. Opioids are locally acting antitussives which coat and soothe inflamed mucosae

6. Some of the adverse GI effects seen with NSAID use can be reduced by taking the drugs with or just after food.

7. NSAIDs can be used to treat ulcerative inflammatory bowel disease.

8. NSAID use can cause fluid retention and occasionally cause peripheral oedema.

9. NSAIDs can cause leucopenias, thrombocytopenias and other blood disorders.

10. NSAIDs antagonise the hypotensive effects of propranolol, possibly by inhibition of COX activity in the kidney.

11. α_2 receptor agonists provide little or no muscle relaxation but are good analgesics and sedatives.

12. Xylazine injection in the dog and cat produces analgesia over the head, neck and body but is minimal in extremities.

Short answers

1. List the signs of pain attributed to activation of the ANS.

2. What is nociception?

3. What substances released by damaged tissues stimulate nociceptive nerve endings?

4. Opioid analgesics have depressant and excitatory actions on the CNS – list the depressant actions.

5. How long after i.v. and i.m. injections of morphine are the peak analgesic effects seen?

6. List two contraindications of morphine use in dogs.

7. What effect on the heart does fentanyl have and what agent can be given to counteract this without compromising the analgesic effects?

8. Does ketamine have analgesic effects at sub-anaesthetic doses?

For answers go to page 246

Glossary

Acute of sudden onset, having a short course

Adenosine triphosphate (ATP) a molecule that stores energy for use in chemical reactions

Adhesion abnormal fibrous union of tissues, process of joining or sticking together

Adipose fat

Aerobic able to survive only in the presence of oxygen

Affinity attraction for – as between molecules, organisms or animals

Agar a derivative of marine seaweed used in some microbiology growth media

Albumin a major protein of blood plasma that is produced by the liver

Anabolism a chemical process involving the synthesis of organic compounds

Anaerobic organism one that grows in an atmosphere free of oxygen

Anaphylaxis a life-threatening allergic reaction in which a series of mediators cause contractions of smooth muscle throughout the body

Angiogenesis the formation of new blood vessels

Antibiotic a product of the metabolism of a micro-organism that is inhibitory to other micro-organisms

Antibody a highly specific protein molecule produced by plasma cells in response to a specific infection

Anticoagulant an agent that stops the clotting of blood

Antidote agent used to counteract poison

Anti-emetic agent that counteracts nausea and vomiting

Antifungal agent that inhibits or kills fungi

Antigen any chemical substance that elicits an immune response

Antihistamine agent that combats the effects of histamine

Anti-inflammatory agent that suppresses inflammation

Antipruritic agent that prevents or reduces itchiness

Antipyretic agent that reduces fever

Antitoxin antibody produced in response to exposure to a toxin produced by micro-organisms, insects or plants

Antitussive agent that combats coughing

Arrhythmia variation in the rhythm of the heart beat

Arthritis inflammation of a joint

Ascariasis infection by ascarids or roundworms of the genus *Ascaris*

Asepsis lack of infection or contamination by micro-organisms

Aseptic free of micro-organisms

Ataxia muscular incoordination, irregular muscular contraction

Attenuate to weaken, to decrease disease-producing capacity of a pathogenic organism

Azotaemia accumulation of nitrogenous urinary wastes in the blood, without apparent clinical signs

Bacillus, bacilli a rod-shaped bacterium

Bacterin vaccine made from bacteria

Bacteriology study of bacteria

Benign not malignant, with a favourable prognosis

Binary fission an asexual process by which a cell divides to form two new cells

Bradycardia abnormally slow heart beat

Bronchospasm spasmodic constriction of the bronchi

Budding an asexual process in fungi by which a new cell forms at the border of a parent cell

Capsid the surrounding layer of protein that encloses the genome of a virus

Capsule a layer of polysaccharides and small proteins that adheres to the surface of certain bacteria to protect the cell from the environment

Cardiopathy any disease of the heart

Catabolic promoting conversion of tissue or complex compounds into simple compounds, i.e. tissue breakdown

Cathartic causing evacuation of the bowel

Catecholamines epinephrine and norepinephrine

Chemoautotroph an organism that derives energy from chemical reactions and uses the energy to synthesise nutrients from carbon dioxide

Chemotherapy treatment of disease with chemical agents, especially cancer

Chromatin the readily stainable portion of the nucleus comprising the genetic material of the cell

Chromosome a structure in a cell nucleus that contains genetic information in the form of DNA

Cocci, coccus a spherical bacterium

Contraindication a circumstance, condition or disease that renders a particular treatment inappropriate or undesirable

Culture a growth of micro-organisms on living tissue cells or an artificial medium; to perpetuate micro-organisms

Decongestant agent that reduces swelling or congestion of tissues

Dermatophyte fungus that lives on skin

Diuresis increased production of urine

Drug a substance that can modify a biological activity

Ecchymosis small area of haemorrhage in the skin or mucous membranes (an ecchymosis is larger than a petechia)

Efficacy ability to produce the desired effect

Emesis act of vomiting

Endogenous growing or originating from within an organism

Erythrocytosis increased number of red blood cells

Eukaryote organisms whose cells contain organelles, a nucleus with multiple chromosomes, a nuclear membrane and undergo mitotic division

Euphoria sense of wellbeing, absence of pain or distress

Excretion act of removing or discharging products from the body, such as urine or perspiration; material that is excreted or discharged

Exogenous growing or originating from outside an organism

Expectorant agent that promotes ejection of mucus and other fluids from the lungs and trachea

Facultative organism one that grows in the presence or absence of oxygen

Fimbriae short hair-like structures used by bacteria for attachment

Flagellum long hair-like proteins used by bacteria and protozoa for motion

Functional group a group of atoms functioning as a unit

Fungi one of the five kingdoms of living things, composed of non-green eukaryotic micro-organisms

Gene a segment of DNA that provides the information for protein synthesis and inherited traits

Generic referring to a drug name not protected by a trademark

Genus category in classification of organisms

Glycolysis glycogen is broken down into energy molecules

Hepatitis inflammation of the liver

Heterotrophic an organism that feeds on preformed organic matter and obtains energy from this matter

Histamine naturally occurring substance found in all body tissues that causes dilation of capillaries, smooth muscle contraction, increased gastric secretions and increased heart rate

Homeostasis stability of the normal physiological state

Hormone substance produced by an organ causing a specific effect on other organs or tissues

Hyperalgesia increased response to a stimulation that is usually painful

Hyperplasia abnormally increased numbers of normal cells in a normal arrangement in tissues

Hypertension persistently high arterial blood pressure

Hypertrophy abnormal growth of an organ or tissue through increased size of its constituent cells

Hypha the basic unit of a fungus

Hypotension abnormally low blood pressure

Hypoxia reduced oxygen supply to tissues

Iatrogenic resulting from the actions of treatment

Icterus yellow discolouration of the skin and mucous membranes caused by deposition of bile pigments, jaundice

Idiopathic of unknown cause

Idiosyncratic pertaining to susceptibility to an adverse reaction from a drug or agent in an individual

Immune highly resistant to disease because of formation of antibodies

Immunoglobulin protein with antibody activity, synthesised by lymphocytes and plasma cells

Interferon an antiviral protein produced by the cells of the body in response to viral infection (inhibits viral replication)

Intermediary host the host in which the larval or other intermediary stage of a multicellular parasite is found

Infection invasion of the body by micro-organisms

Inflammation localised tissue response to injury, characterised by heat, swelling, redness, pain and loss of function

Integument the skin

Intercostal between the ribs

In vitro within a test tube, outside the body

In vivo inside the living body

Irrigate to wash out or flush, lavage

Isotonic having equal tone or equal osmotic pressure

-itis suffix denoting inflammation

Keratitis inflammation of the cornea

Labile chemically unstable

Lacrimal pertaining to tears

Lethal deadly or fatal

Leukaemia malignant disease characterised by proliferation of leucocyte precursors in the bone marrow and increased numbers of white blood cells in the peripheral blood

Leucocytosis increased numbers of circulating white blood cells

Leucopenia decreased numbers of circulating white blood cells

Lysis destruction of cells

Lysosome an organelle that contains digestive enzymes

Malignant tending to becoming progressively worse and result in death, often used to define potentially fatal tumours

Medicine any drug or remedy; the art of treating disease by non-surgical methods

Medullary inner portion of an organ or structure

Melanocyte cell that produces melanin

Metabolic the physiological process by which cells and tissues are produced and maintained

Metastasis transfer of disease from one organ or area of the body to another not linked to it

Micro-organism minute living organism, such as viruses, bacteria, fungi and protozoa

Miosis constriction of the pupil

Morphology study of form and structure of organisms

Mucosa membrane lining tubular organ such as alimentary tract

Mycology the study of fungi

Mydriasis dilatation of the pupil

Necrosis death of tissue and its component cells

Necrotoxin substance produced by certain *Staphylococcus* bacteria, which kills tissue cells

Neoplasm any new or abnormal growth, especially that which is progressive and uncontrolled; a tumour

Nephrosis any disease of the kidney, especially degenerative conditions of the renal tubules

Nociception reception, conduction, and central nervous processing of nerve signals from pain receptors

Nucleoid the chromosomal region of a bacterium

Organelle a membrane-enclosed compartment in a cell

Phagocytosis a process in which solid particles are taken into a cell – important in cell defence

Parasiticide agent that is destructive or lethal to parasites

Pathogen a parasite that causes disease in a host organism

Pathogenicity the ability of a parasite to gain entry into a cell and cause disease

Pediculosis infestation with lice

Permeable permitting passage of a substance

Pharmaceutical pertaining to drugs; a drug

Pharmacodynamics effects of the drug on the body, the mechanism of their action

Pharmacognosy branch of pharmacology dealing with the features of natural drugs

Pharmacokinetics the effect of the body on the drug, its absorption, distribution, metabolism and excretion

Pharmacology the study of the effect of drugs on the structure and metabolism of normal tissues

Photoautotroph an organism that uses light energy to synthesise nutrients from carbon dioxide

Polyuria increased quantities of urine

Postprandial after eating

Proprietary name trade or brand name of a drug

Protista one of the five kingdoms composed of protozoa and various other simple forms

Pure culture a culture or colony of micro-organisms of one type

Recrudescence recurrence of signs after temporary abatement

Remission diminution, lessening or abatement of signs of a disease; the period when signs of disease have abated or decreased

Resistance natural ability of the body to remain unaffected by poisonous substances and pathogenic micro-organisms; in microbiology, it refers to a lack of efficacy of a drug on a micro-organism

Retro- prefix meaning backward or behind

Sabouraud dextrose agar a growth medium for fungi

Saprophytic an organism that feeds on dead organic matter

Saturated unable to hold in solution any more of a given substance; describing a fatty acid with all single bonds between carbon atoms

Sedatives calm the patient and make them sleepy

Selective medium a growth medium that contains ingredients to inhibit the growth of some organisms whilst encouraging the growth of others

Sepsis presence of micro-organisms or their toxins in the blood

Septicaemia presence of micro-organisms or their toxins in the blood

Somatic pain pain from tissues other than viscera, i.e. skin, skeletal muscle and the peritoneum

Spore a highly resistant structure formed from several types of bacteria; also a reproductive structure formed by a fungus

Sterilisation the removal of all life forms, especially spores

Styptic an astringent or haemostatic agent

Subcutaneous beneath the skin

Susceptible not immune to the actions of a pathogenic organism or an antimicrobial drug

Systemic affecting the body as a whole

Teratogenic tending to produce birth defects

Therapeutics concerned with the application of drugs in the treatment of disease

Thrombolysis dissolution of a clot

Toxicology the study of poisons and the investigation of toxic side effects accompanying the use of drugs

Toxicosis any condition caused by poisoning

Toxin a poison

Toxoid a vaccine made of modified bacterial toxins

Tranquillisers relieve anxiety but do not cause drowsiness

Uraemia toxic condition, characterised by vomiting resulting from accumulation of nitrogenous urinary waste in the blood

Vaccine a suspension of killed or attenuated micro-organisms that, when introduced into the body, stimulates an immune response against that micro-organism

Vasoconstriction decrease in diameter of a blood vessel

Vector a living organism that transmits the agents of disease

Virulence the degree of pathogenicity of an organism

Virus a particle of nucleic acid (either DNA or RNA) surrounded by a protein sheath and sometimes an envelope

Yeast a type of fungus that resembles bacteria in culture

Zoonosis a disease of animals that can be transmitted to people under natural conditions

Appendix

Multiple Choice Questions

Multiple Choice Questions General

1. How many schedules are there for categorising controlled drugs?
   a. 3
   b. 4
   c. 5
   d. 6

2. Which of these drugs is an example of a Schedule 2 opioid?
   a. morphine
   b. carprofen (Rimadyl)
   c. ampicillin
   d. isoflurane

3. What act is in place to prevent the misuse of the drugs of abuse?
   a. The Dangerous Drugs Act 1971
   b. The Criminal Act 1971
   c. The Control of Substances Hazardous to Health Regulations 1994
   d. The Misuse of Drugs Act 1971

4. Which term describes a drug to relieve pain?
   a. analgesic
   b. anthelmintic
   c. antitussive
   d. analeptic

5. Which term describes a drug to reduce coughing?
   a. analgesic
   b. anthelmintic
   c. antitussive
   d. analeptic

6. Which term describes a drug used to treat parasite infestation?
   a. analgesic
   b. anthelmintic
   c. antitussive
   d. analeptic

7. What does an ecbolic drug do?
   a. cause the airways to dilate
   b. cause the uterus to contract
   c. cause the gut motility to increase
   d. kill ectoparasites

8. What is the definition of a diuretic drug?
   a. a drug to treat kidney infections
   b. a drug to increase urine production
   c. a drug to lower blood pressure by causing vasodilation
   d. a drug to treat heart failure by reducing coughing

9. Which is an example of an anticonvulsant?
   a. phenobarbital
   b. fenbendazole
   c. enrofloxacin
   d. enalapril

10. What does an expectorant do?
    a. increase the volume of respiratory secretions but make them less viscous
    b. decrease the volume of respiratory secretions

c. remove fluid from the lungs by increasing the volume of urine

d. decrease coughing by suppressing the cough reflex

11. Which of the following is a drug that induces vomiting?
    a. anti-emetic
    b. emetic
    c. ecbolic
    d. demulcent

12. What does a neuroleptanalgesic do?
    a. treat damaged spinal cords
    b. reduce inflammation
    c. increase blood supply to the brain
    d. produce pain relief and sedation

13. What does a tranquilliser do that a sedative does not?
    a. cause vomiting
    b. maintains alertness, i.e. does not cause drowsiness
    c. cause drowsiness
    d. dilates pupils

14. Which of these medications requires the handler to wear gloves?
    a. griseofulvin
    b. erythromycin
    c. fenbendazole
    d. glucosamine sulphate

15. Which of the following is a legal requirement to display on a drug label?
    a. dose/directions for use
    b. name and strength of product
    c. name of animal
    d. name and address of veterinary surgeon

16. What should be dispensed in a fluted or ridged bottle?
    a. liquids for internal use, i.e. cough medicines
    b. liquids for external use, i.e. shampoos
    c. semi-solid emulsions
    d. liquids for either internal or external use but not creams or emulsions

17. Which of the following means the same as 'to be given once a day'?
    a. q1h
    b. q.i.d.
    c. q24h
    d. q12h

18. How do you calculate the dose required of a drug?
    a. dose needed (mg) = dose rate (mg) × body weight (kg)
    b. dose needed (mg) = dose rate (mg) ÷ body weight (kg)
    c. dose needed (mg) = body weight (kg) ÷ dose rate (mg)
    d. dose needed (mg) = number of tablets × body weight (kg)

19. What is meant by the term parenteral administration?
    a. orally
    b. avoiding the digestive system, e.g. injected
    c. given with food
    d. only to be given on an empty stomach

20. Where is a suitable site for an i.m. injection?
    a. gluteals
    b. under the scruff
    c. into the cephalic vein
    d. triceps

Multiple Choice Questions for Level 2 SVNs

1. Which of the following drugs is legally required to be kept in a lockable cupboard?
   a. pentobarbitone
   b. diazepam
   c. buprenorphine
   d. phenobarbital

2. Which of the following drugs is a Schedule 3 partial agonist?
   a. pentobarbitone
   b. diazepam
   c. buprenorphine
   d. methadone

3. Which of the following drugs is light sensitive and requires storage in brown bottles?
   a. injectable amoxicillin
   b. injectable oxytetracycline
   c. oral amoxicillin with clavulanate
   d. injectable methylprednisolone

4. What storage requirements does injectable carprofen (Rimadyl) have?
   a. refrigerate until opened then store at room temperature
   b. room temperature until opened then store at 4–8°C
   c. always at room temperature
   d. always keep refrigerated

5. Which is a proprietary name for a NSAID?
   a. salicylic acid
   b. meloxicam
   c. phenylbutazone
   d. ketofen

6. How should preparations for external use be dispensed?
   a. coloured fluted bottles
   b. plain round-necked bottles
   c. plain fluted bottles with child-resistant closures
   d. coloured round-necked bottles with child-resistant closures

7. What does the abbreviation a.c. mean in prescription writing?
   a. after meals
   b. before meals
   c. with food
   d. once a day

8. What does the abbreviation o.m. mean in prescription writing?
   a. in the morning
   b. at night
   c. three times a day
   d. not orally

9. What does the abbreviation p.c. mean in prescription writing?
   a. at night
   b. correctly

c. after meals
d. at pleasure

10. Which correctly defines the half-life of a drug?
    a. the rate of elimination, i.e. the longer the half-life of a drug, the longer the duration of drug action for a given dose
    b. the rate of absorption
    c. the middle of the dose rate of a drug
    d. the margin of safety

11. Which of the following drugs has been proved to be teratogenic and should not be used in breeding animals?
    a. vitamin B
    b. penicillins
    c. griseofulvin
    d. carprofen

12. Which is an example of a drug interaction?
    a. displacement of protein binding
    b. bronchodilation
    c. vomiting
    d. skin changes

13. What is an example of a contraindication?
    a. an adverse effect
    b. a method of administration that is unsuitable, e.g. rapid i.v. injection of pethidine in dogs
    c. a reason for use of the drug
    d. how not to dispose of the drug

14. Which of the following is an example of an anthelmintic?
    a. fluconazole
    b. fenbendazole
    c. amphotericin B
    d. tetracycline

15. Which is an example of an antiepileptic drug?
    a. vincristine
    b. salazopyrin
    c. trilostane
    d. potassium bromide

16. Which is a property of the NSAIDs?
    a. antipyretic
    b. stimulate inflammatory mediators

c. increase prostaglandin production

d. stimulate local nerve endings

17. How quickly are peak plasma levels reached following an i.m. or s.c. injection of a drug given as an aqueous solution?
    a. 1–3 minutes
    b. within 30 minutes
    c. over 1 hour
    d. 6–12 hours

18. Which are the most common drugs to be given as sustained-release preparations?
    a. antiparasiticides
    b. diuretics
    c. anti-emetics
    d. antimicrobials

19. What does percutaneous absorption mean?
    a. can not be absorbed through the skin
    b. accidental skin contamination
    c. can be absorbed through the skin
    d. the drug is in a water emulsion base

20. Before entering the systemic circulation, what must a drug administered as an oral dose undergo?
    a. release from dosage form, diffusion across the GI mucosal barrier into the portal circulation, passage through the liver
    b. protection in dosage form until it reaches the alkaline intestines, direct absorption into the systemic circulation
    c. dissolution of the drug and biotransformation by the stomach acids
    d. dissolution of the drug, absorption in the colon and metabolism by the local tissues, liver and lungs

21. When are antibiotics contraindicated?
    a. if the causal agent is a fungus
    b. if the patient is immunosuppressed
    c. if the patient has renal failure
    d. with concurrent antiviral therapy

22. How quickly will an i.v. injection of furosemide work compared to an oral dose?
    a. 1 minute if injected i.v. and 10 minutes if given orally
    b. 5–30 minutes if injected i.v. and within 1 hour if given orally
    c. 60 minutes if given i.v. and up to 3 hours if given orally
    d. 2–3 hours if given i.v. and 12 hours if given orally

23. When are diuretics contraindicated?
    a. in congestive cardiac failure
    b. in renal failure
    c. in dehydrated patients
    d. in patients with systemic infections

24. What type of drug is the calcium sensitiser pimobendan?
    a. anthelmintic drug
    b. antimicrobial drug
    c. analgesic agent
    d. cardiovascular agent

25. Which category of drugs does the agent gentamicin come into?
    a. antibacterial
    b. antifungal
    c. antiparasitic
    d. antiprotozoal

Multiple Choice Questions for Level 3 SVNs

1. What affects the rate of induction of anaesthesia of the gaseous anaesthetics?
    a. blood solubility
    b. lipid solubility as most inhalational agents are insoluble in lipid
    c. metabolism site
    d. local tissue irritation

2. Which of the following drugs is a tranquilliser-sedative?
    a. pentobarbitone
    b. chloral hydrate
    c. acepromazine
    d. medetomidine

3. Which of the following premedicant agents is a parasympatholytic?
   a. midazolam
   b. diazepam
   c. butorphanol
   d. atropine

4. Which of these is a side effect of the α-2-adrenergic drugs?
   a. tachycardia
   b. hypoglycaemia
   c. increased urine volume
   d. mild arterial hypotension followed by prolonged hypertension

5. Which is an effect of the opioid drugs?
   a. increased intestinal motility
   b. stimulation of the medullary respiratory control centre
   c. CNS sedation in some species and CNS arousal (excitement) in others
   d. anti-emetic

6. Which is a dissociative drug that causes somatic analgesia?
   a. thiopental
   b. pentobarbitone
   c. ketamine
   d. propofol

7. Which of the following agents is an example of an opioid?
   a. benzodiazepines
   b. etomidate
   c. ketamine
   d. fentanyl

8. Which of the following is an undesirable effect of atropine?
   a. pupil constriction
   b. excessive respiratory tract secretions
   c. reduced gastrointestinal motility
   d. bradycardia

9. Which agent can be safely used i.v. in any species?
   a. barbiturates
   b. saffan
   c. opioids
   d. pethidine

10. Which is a property of the inhalational anaesthetics?
    a. they are not metabolised but excreted unchanged
    b. they cause a reversible depression of the CNS
    c. they stimulate alveolar ventilation
    d. some of the agents have no effect on the cardiovascular system

11. To avoid hypoxaemia, what is the highest amount of nitrous oxide that can be safely inspired by a healthy individual?
    a. 33%
    b. 50%
    c. 66%
    d. 75%

12. Which is a property of an ideal injectable anaesthetic agent?
    a. long duration of action
    b. cumulative effects
    c. slowly metabolised and/or excreted
    d. have a specific and complete reversal agent

13. Which agent does not belong to the barbiturate group?
    a. fentanyl
    b. methohexitone
    c. pentobarbitone
    d. thiopental

14. What effect on the respiratory system does sub-anaesthetic doses of barbiturates have?
    a. increases respiration rate
    b. decreases respiration rate
    c. has no effect on the pre-induction respiratory rate
    d. causes prolonged apnoea

15. Which intravenous agent is insoluble in water and so is available in an emulsion without preservatives and therefore supports bacterial growth?
    a. sevoflurane
    b. methohexitone
    c. propofol
    d. midazolam

16. Which agent stimulates the cardiovascular system and increases central venous pressure and heart rate?
    a. ketamine
    b. saffan
    c. thiopental
    d. morphine

17. What is codeine most commonly used for in veterinary medicine?
    a. analgesia
    b. premedicant sedative
    c. antitussive
    d. emetic

18. Which of the following is a partial agonist opioid?
    a. butorphanol
    b. morphine
    c. pethidine
    d. naloxone

19. Which of the following agents is suitable for topical anaesthesia?
    a. procaine
    b. lidocaine
    c. prilocaine
    d. bupivacaine

20. Which is the most commonly consumed NSAID in accidental poisoning?
    a. carprofen
    b. meloxicam
    c. piroxicam
    d. ibuprofen

21. Which is the most common and serious side effect of the NSAIDs?
    a. platelet impairment
    b. bone marrow dyscrasias
    c. nephropathy
    d. GI damage

22. Which of these would be a suitable treatment for hyperadrenocorticism?
    a. an agent that decreases glucocorticoid production
    b. an agent that increases glucocorticoid production
    c. an agent that increases mineralocorticoid production
    d. an agent that decreases mineralocorticoid production

23. What is a contraindication of steroid use?
    a. intra-articular
    b. topical ophthalmic use in the presence of a corneal ulceration
    c. intralesional
    d. systemic use

24. Which of the following is an antiviral agent?
    a. amphotericin B
    b. fenbendazole
    c. acyclovir
    d. griseofulvin

25. Which is an example of a chemo-therapeutic used in neoplastic disease?
    a. vincristine
    b. piperazine
    c. sulfadimidine
    d. phenylbutazone

Multiple Choice Questions for the Pharmacy Certificate

1. What is meant by bioavailability?
    a. the extent to which a drug administered as a particular dosage form enters the systemic circulation intact
    b. the method of metabolism
    c. the route of excretion
    d. the way the drug acts on the body

2. Why does the bioavailability of digoxin vary between the different administration routes: 100% i.v., tablets 60% and elixir 75%?
    a. due to the coating on the tablets and additives in the elixir
    b. due to the patient losing some drug through the action of salivary enzymes
    c. due to the acid in the stomach destroying some of the orally administered drugs
    d. due to the first-pass metabolism by the liver of oral digoxin

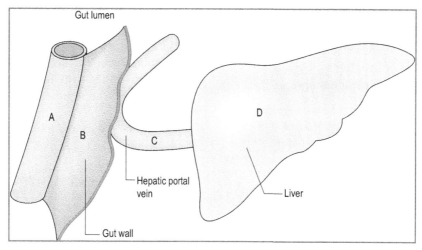

Gut lumen

A

B

C

Hepatic portal vein

Gut wall

D

Liver

Fig. A.1

3. Referring to Figure A.1, where does dissolution of solid drugs take place?
   a. A
   b. B
   c. C
   d. D

4. Referring to Figure A.1, where are the sites of metabolism of an orally administered drug?
   a. A
   b. A, B and D
   c. B and D
   d. D

5. How do drugs pass across cell membranes?
   a. active transport
   b. passive transport
   c. both active and passive transport
   d. drugs do not cross cell membranes but act in the plasma and extracellular fluid

6. What increases the penetration of a drug across the blood–brain barrier?
   a. enteric coating
   b. intravenous administration
   c. fever or inflammatory disease
   d. giving intravenous fluids at the time of drug administration

7. If the acidic urine of carnivores promotes the passive re-absorption of acidic drugs from the distal portion of the nephron, what will urinary alkalinisation do?
   a. increase their re-absorption
   b. promote their excretion by favouring ionisation of organic acids
   c. have no effect on the re-absorption or excretion unless the drug is completely metabolised first by the liver
   d. destroy the drug in the urine

8. The following drugs are basic (alkaline): narcotic analgesics, ketamine, diazepam, anti-arrhythmic agents. Where will they concentrate?
   a. in fluids that are more basic than them
   b. in fluids that are basic relative to plasma
   c. in fluids that are acidic relative to plasma, such as intracellular fluid
   d. they do not concentrate in a particular fluid, but are evenly distributed throughout the body

9. What constitutes parenteral administration?
   a. i.v., i.m. and s.c. injections only
   b. oral medications
   c. inhalational drugs only
   d. injections, inhaled drugs, tissue infiltration, intra-articular, subconjunctival and epidurals

10. What should never be injected i.v.?
    a. non-clear liquids
    b. drugs in an oily vehicle
    c. mixtures of two drugs
    d. non-steroidal anti-inflammatory drugs

11. Which of the following is the main factor affecting drug absorption from a site?
    a. vascularity of the injection site
    b. drug concentration in parenteral solution
    c. lipid solubility of the drug
    d. the area of the absorbing surface to which the drug is exposed

12. How does the epinephrine added to local anaesthetic agents procaine and lidocaine potentiate the drugs' effects?
    a. reduces the local tissue metabolism
    b. causes local vasodilation by acting on the β-adrenoceptors
    c. causes vasoconstriction by acting on the α-adrenoceptors
    d. competitively antagonises the agents at their nerve binding sites

13. How do sustained-release preparations give long durations of therapeutically effective plasma drug concentrations?
    a. they have a limited rate of absorption, which may be attributable to slow dissolution and/or absorption of the drug
    b. they are not metabolised before being excreted
    c. they are not excreted but remain in the circulation after metabolism
    d. they are not distributed around the body but remain at the site of injection

14. Why are surfactants added to topical drugs?
    a. to increase the metabolism of the drug in the lungs
    b. to prevent absorption systemically
    c. to potentiate the drug's effects on the skin surface
    d. to increase skin penetration of water-soluble substances

15. Why are drugs like griseofulvin and spironolactone micronised to decrease the particle size?
    a. it increases the dissolution of the drug (which is the rate-limiting step in release of the drug from its solid state)
    b. it makes it more stable in GI fluids
    c. it increases lipid solubility and therefore absorption
    d. it allows packaging in smaller capsules/tablets

16. Which antibiotics, because of their low solubility in lipid, are poorly absorbed from the GI tract and can not be taken orally?
    a. penicillins
    b. tetracyclines
    c. aminoglycosides
    d. sulphonamides

17. Which drug shows a considerable amount of first-pass metabolism by the liver when taken orally?
    a. diazepam
    b. amoxicillin
    c. neomercazole
    d. meloxicam

18. Which of these drugs is not extensively bound to plasma proteins?
    a. phenylbutazone
    b. furosemide
    c. diazepam
    d. morphine

19. Which of these is not a method of drug elimination?
    a. biotransformation
    b. hepatic metabolism
    c. renal excretion
    d. widespread extravascular distribution

20. Which of these is the principal method of excretion of drugs?
    a. bile
    b. kidneys
    c. lungs
    d. salivary, mammary glands and sweat

21. Which are the most potent and most commonly prescribed diuretics?
    a. osmotic diuretics
    b. inhibitors of carbonic anhydrase
    c. drugs acting on the collecting duct
    d. inhibitors of the sodium-potassium-chloride pump acting on the thick ascending limb of the loop of Henle

22. What is the method of action of the interferons?
    a. promote viral binding, penetration and uncoating
    b. affect RNA and DNA viral replication at many stages of the viral reproductive cycle
    c. stimulate viral protein synthesis
    d. promote synthesis of messenger RNA

23. If a drug, such as ketoconazole, inhibits the hepatic enzyme P-450, what effect on other drugs might it have?
    a. increase metabolism of other drugs
    b. decrease metabolism of other drugs
    c. increase protein binding of other drugs
    d. decrease protein binding of other drugs

24. Which of the following antibiotics has antifungal properties?
    a. penicillin
    b. tetracycline
    c. amphotericin B
    d. sulfadimidine

25. How does the avermectin selamectin kill ectoparasites?
    a. prevents larval growth
    b. inhibits DNA replication
    c. induces muscular paralysis by modulating movement of chloride ions through channels
    d. prevents cross-linking in cell walls and therefore causes cell lysis

Calculations

1. A solution contains furosemide at 10 mg/ml. How many mg are in 1.5 ml of the solution?
   a. 1.5
   b. 5
   c. 15
   d. 20

2. A suspension contains phenytoin 125 mg/5 ml. How many mg of drug are there in 20 ml of the suspension?
   a. 50
   b. 75
   c. 150
   d. 500

3. A suspension contains erythromycin 250 mg/5 ml. How many mg in 1 ml?
   a. 25
   b. 50
   c. 100
   d. 250

4. A patient requires cimetidine, which is available in 200 mg tablets. The dose required is 30 mg/kg and the dog weighs 10 kg. How many tablets does he need for a single dose?
   a. 0.66
   b. 1
   c. 1.5
   d. 6

5. How many 30 mg tablets of morphine are needed for a dose of 0.06 g?
   a. 0.5
   b. 1
   c. 2
   d. 2.5

6. A dog needs 450 mg of aspirin which is available in 300 mg tablets. How many tablets are required for a single dose?
   a. 0.5
   b. 1
   c. 1.5
   d. 2

7. Diazepam comes in 5 mg tablets. How many of these are to be administered to a 12.5 kg dog if the dose rate is 1 mg/kg?
   a. 1.5
   b. 2
   c. 2.5
   d. 3

8. Digoxin is required at a dose rate of 10 µg/kg for the above patient. Tablets available are 0.25 mg. How many tablets should be given?
   a. 0.5
   b. 1
   c. 1.5
   d. 2

9. Calculate the volume to be given of a penicillin solution containing 125 mg/5 ml if the dose required is 500 mg.
   a. 5 ml
   b. 10 ml
   c. 15 ml
   d. 20 ml

10. What volume of buprenorphine is required if the solution contains 10 mg/2 ml and the dose rate is 1 mg/kg to a 5 kg cat?
    a. 0.5 ml
    b. 1 ml
    c. 1.5 ml
    d 2 ml

11. What volume of morphine hydrochloride is required if the solution is 40 mg/ml and the dose required is 10 mg/kg to a 10 kg dog?
    a. 1.5 ml
    b. 2 ml
    c. 2.5 ml
    d. 3 ml

12. What volume of erythromycin is required for a 7.5 kg dog if the dose rate is 100 mg/kg and the mixture is 125 mg/5 ml?
    a. 3 ml
    b. 10 ml
    c. 25 ml
    d. 30 ml

13. Stock heparin has a strength of 5000 units per ml. What volume must be drawn up to give 6500 units?
    a. 1.1 ml
    b. 1.2 ml
    c. 1.3 ml
    d. 1.4 ml

14. 75 mg of pethidine is required to be injected i.m. Stock ampoules contain pethidine 100 mg in 2 ml. Calculate the volume of stock required.
    a. 1.1 ml
    b. 1.5 ml
    c. 1.75 ml
    d. 1.85 ml

15. A patient requires 60 mg gentamicin by i.m. injection. Ampoules contain 80 mg/2 ml. Calculate the volume required.
    a. 1.5 ml
    b. 1.75 ml
    c. 1.85 ml
    d. 1.95 ml

16. Stock ampoules of ranitidine contain 50 mg/2 ml. A 4 kg patient requires a single i.v. injection. The dose rate is 10 mg/kg. What volume should be injected?
    a. 1.1 ml
    b. 1.5 ml
    c. 1.6 ml
    d. 1.8 ml

17. Morphine 5.5 mg is prescribed. Stock ampoules contain 10 mg/ml. What volume should be drawn up for injection?
    a. 0.45 ml
    b. 0.55 ml
    c. 0.65 ml
    d. 0.75 ml

18. Penicillin 450 mg is ordered for a 14 kg dog. Stock ampoules contain 600 mg in 5 ml. Calculate the volume to be injected.
    a. 1.75 ml
    b. 2 ml
    c. 2.75 ml
    d. 3.75 ml

19. Digoxin ampoules contain 500 µg in 2 ml. A single 0.15 mg injection of digoxin is required. What volume should be drawn up?
    a. 0.6 ml
    b. 1.1 ml
    c. 6 ml
    d. 6.1 ml

20. The drawings in Figure A.2 represent syringes without needles. Which contains the correct volume of liquid to administer a 2% solution to a 5 kg dog if the dose rate is 1.5 mg/kg.
    a. syringe A
    b. syringe B
    c. syringe C
    d. syringe D

21. A dog is to receive 500 ml normal saline. The drip rate is adjusted to deliver 25 ml/h. How long will the infusion take?
    a. 12 hours
    b. 20 hours
    c. 25 hours
    d. 50 hours

22. A 2.5 kg cat requires shock rate (90 ml/kg) fluids i.v. If the infusion pump is set to deliver 150 ml/h, how long will the infusion take?
    a. 1 hour
    b. 1.5 hours
    c. 2 hours
    d. 2.5 hours

23. If a 20 kg dog requires penicillin V at 50 mg/kg/day in four equal doses, how much will a single dose be?
    a. 250 mg
    b. 100 mg
    c. 200 mg
    d. 1000 mg

24. If a 3 kg cat needs amoxicillin at a dose rate of 45 mg/kg/day in 3 equal doses, how much will a single dose be?
    a. 3 mg
    b. 35 mg
    c. 45 mg
    d. 135 mg

25. How many 0.25 mg tablets of digoxin are needed for a 7-day course if the dose rate is 11 µg/kg q 12 h and the dog weighs 11.3 kg?
    a. 4
    b. 5
    c. 6
    d. 7

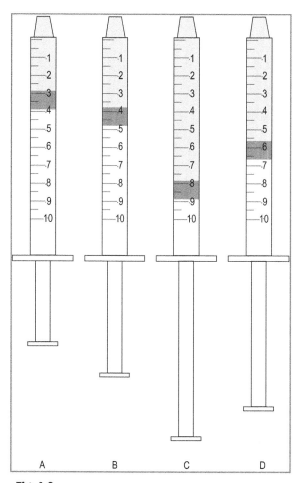

A   B   C   D

Fig. A.2

Answers for General MCQs

1. c	8. b	15. d
2. a	9. a	16. b
3. d	10. a	17. c
4. a	11. b	18. a
5. c	12. d	19. b
6. b	13. b	20. a
7. b	14. a	

Answers to SVN Level 2 MCQs

1. c	10. a	19. c
2. c	11. c	20. a
3. b	12. a	21. a
4. a	13. b	22. b
5. d	14. b	23. d
6. a	15. d	24. d
7. b	16. a	25. a
8. a	17. b	
9. c	18. d	

Answers to SVN Level 3 MCQs

1. a	10. b	19. b
2. c	11. d	20. d
3. d	12. d	21. d
4. c	13. a	22. a
5. c	14. a	23. b
6. c	15. c	24. c
7. d	16. a	25. a
8. c	17. c	
9. a	18. a	

Answers to Pharmacy Certificate MCQs

1. a	10. b	19. d
2. d	11. a	20. b
3. a	12. c	21. d
4. b	13. a	22. b
5. c	14. d	23. b
6. c	15. a	24. c
7. b	16. c	25. c
8. c	17. a	
9. d	18. d	

Answers to Calculations

1. c
2. d
3. b
4. c
5. c
6. c
7. c
8. a
9. d
10. b
11. c
12. d
13. c
14. b
15. a
16. c
17. b
18. d
19. a
20. b
21. b
22. b
23. a
24. c
25. d

Answers for Chapter 1

1. Place the drug, in its original packaging, in two external containers of different colours. Alternatively, write a warning in large letters on the outside of the packets

2. Right drug, right dose, right patient, right route, right time

3. A side effect is an expected, but unwanted effect of normal drug therapy, usually related to its actions in parts of the body other than the area being treated. An adverse reaction is an unexpected, harmful effect of drug therapy. It can be due to the drug, its administration or the patient

4. To the veterinary surgeon in charge of the case and the Veterinary Medicines Directorate (SARSS)

5. Checking patient alertness, body strength and ability to interact with nurse, temperature, pulse and respiratory rate measurement, monitoring 'special precautions' patients, nutritional intake, elimination patterns, checking the skin and mucous membranes, urinalysis, faecal examination and blood sampling, monitoring therapeutic effect

6. Written materials such as pamphlets, video recordings, models, slides, audiocassettes, photographs, charts, verbal, computer demonstrations, practical demonstrations, sign language

7. Avoid creating a mirror image, teach the correct methods only, demonstrate a skill first then describe it, teach each in stages and reiterate points of importance, demonstrate other skills required, make use of 'props', once you have demonstrated, ask the client to repeat the demonstration

8. Educate the client, demonstrate how to give medication and encourage the owner to repeat the dosing technique, offer medication aids, use written instructions and take advantage of commercially produced literature, call the client one or two days following commencement of treatment, assure the client they can return to check progress, offer nurse consultations for patients diagnosed with long-term conditions, consider a system of named nurses for chronically ill patients, check repeat prescriptions are being ordered at the correct time intervals, ask the client if they are able to manage the treatment programme easily when they call for a repeat prescription, ensure clients bring their pets back for routine blood testing if applicable, make sure the client is competent to collect a urine sample and understands storage requirements, check the drug is having the desired therapeutic effect

Answers for Chapter 2

1. S4
2. S3
3. S2
4. S3
5. S2

Answers for Chapter 3

1. 2400 g
2. 1020 mg
3. 600 µg
4. 7100 ng
5. 0.25 l
6. 100 ml
7. 0.9 mg
8. 0.002 kg
9. 3000 µg
10. 0.0024 g
11. 20/100 × 100% = 20%
    20% × 10 = 200 mg/ml
12. 25/100 × 100% = 6.25%
    6.25% × 10 = 62.5 mg/ml
13. 30/100 × 100% = 3%
    3% × 10 = 30 mg/ml
14.
    Volume of solution administered
    = 2 × 15 ml = 30 ml
    Solution contains 2.5% × 10 =
    25 mg/ml
    25 × 30 = 750 mg administered per day
    750 mg/dog/day – but we want the
    dose in mg/kg/d
    750/7.5 = 100 mg/kg/d
    Amount given in weight was 750 mg a
    day (which = 0.75 g)
    0.75 × 5 = 3.75 g in 5 days
15. 25, 1, 12.5, 180, 333, 0.1, 0.01, 1, 10,
    0.3

16.
    – Solution A (25/750) × 100 = 3.33%
    – Solution B (253/1750) × 100 =
      14.46%
    – Solution C (2.56/78) × 100 = 3.28%
    Therefore B is the most concentrated
17. Weight of drug required = 8 kg × 6 mg
    = 48 mg every 8 hours
    There are 40 mg/ml
    48 mg/40 mg/ml = 1.2 ml per injection
18.
    once daily
    to be taken once daily
    every day (used to mean once a day)
    repeat as required
    before food
    after food
    every morning
    every night
    a sufficient quantity
    contraindicated
    dosing interval
19. a
20. d
21. b
22. a

Answers for Chapter 4

1. Alfaxalone/Alfadolone (Saffan)
2. Only isoflurane. All of the others
   increase or decrease plasma levels,
   increase the risk of dysrhythmias or
   increase the incidence of seizures
3. Tetracyclines are bacteriostatic and
   therefore should not be given with
   bacteriocidal antibiotics such as
   Synulox as they work in opposition
4. Sedatives, as drowsiness is a
   potential side effect of antihistamines
5. Antirobe
6. Steroids and female hormones such as
   megestrol acetate (Ovarid)

7. Hypokalaemia (low blood potassium)
8. Ivermectin
9. Azathioprine, cyclophosphamide, oestrogens, chloramphenicol, cisplatin, doxorubicin, metronidazole, phenytoin, progesterone

10. ACE inhibitors e.g. Fortekor, trimethoprim (Trimacare), antifungals, some antineoplastic drugs, e.g. vincristine, anti-thyroid drugs, e.g. carbimazole, Vitamin A, phenytoin

Multiple choice answers

1. b
2. a
3. c
4. a
5. c
6. d
7. c
8. a
9. c
10. d
11. c

Answers for Chapter 5

Short answers

1. A protease is an enzyme that catalyses the hydrolysis of peptide bonds of target proteins
2. Trypsin and chymotrypsin
3. Blood plasma is about 5% of body weight and combined with interstitial fluid makes up the extracellular fluid (15% of body weight). Limits of the ECF volume are ill defined and lymph cannot be separated from the ECF and is measured with it. It includes joint fluid, aqueous humor and the fluid in relatively avascular tissues such as dense connective tissue, cartilage and bone. The intracellular fluid volume makes up about 40% of body weight and although the water content of lean body tissue is constant, fat is relatively free of water and therefore the IFV varies depending on the amount of fat present. The amount of fluid decreases with age
4. Osmosis encourages the uptake of water
5. Integral proteins pass through the membrane and peripheral proteins stud the inside and outside of the membrane. There are 7 different functions, structural, pumps, carriers, ion channels, receptors, enzymes and antigens
6. Ligands bind to cell membranes in special coated pits and form endosomes. It is responsible for internalisation of low-density lipoproteins, an important part of the metabolism of cholesterol

Multiple choice answers

1. c
2. e
3. b
4. e
5. G
6. L
7. S
8. G
9. G
10. L

True/false

1. F	23. F	45. F
2. T	24. F	46. F
3. F	25. F	47. F
4. T	26. T	48. T
5. T	27. F	49. T
6. T	28. T	50. F
7. F	29. F	51. T
8. F	30. T	52. T
9. F	31. F	53. F
10. F	32. F	54. F
11. T	33. T	55. F
12. T	34. F	56. F
13. T	35. F	57. T
14. F	36. T	58. T
15. T	37. F	59. T
16. F	38. F	60. F
17. F	39. T	61. F
18. T	40. T	62. T
19. T	41. F	63. T
20. T	42. F	64. T
21. F	43. T	65. T
22. T	44. F	

Answers for Chapter 6

1. Unlike Universal Indicator, litmus solution does not measure the pH as litmus only changes colour when going from acidic to basic solutions

2. Neutralisation should occur, giving a green colour

3.

$$C + O_2 \rightarrow CO_2$$
$$CaCO_3 + H_2SO_4 \rightarrow CaSO_4 + H_2O + CO_2$$
$$KOH + HCl \rightarrow KCl + H_2O$$

4.

$$CaCO_3 \rightarrow CaO + CO_2$$
$$MgO + 2HCl \rightarrow MgCl_2 + H_2O$$
$$2SO_2 + O_2 \rightarrow 2SO_3$$
$$Na_2CO_3 + 2HNO_3 \rightarrow 2NaNO_3 + H_2O + CO_2$$
$$N_2 + 3H_2 \rightarrow 2NH_3$$

5. 24 g

6. 2 moles

7. They are basically the same – just different terms for the same value

8. Two or more atoms

9. Chemical bonding

10. 1 or more pairs of electrons

11. Both atoms can effectively have a full shell

12. Noble gasses

13. moles = mass/RMM

14. Hydrocarbon – saturated

15. Unsaturated

16. Methane, ethane, propane

17. Ethene, propene, butene

18. Burn exothermically, make good fuels

19. The most reactive group on a compound. The part which gives its name to the compound

20. $MgOH_2 + 2HCl \rightarrow 2H_2O + MgCl_2$
21. Dock leaves contain alkali, which neutralises the acidic sting of nettles
22. Bee stings are acidic and therefore bicarbonate of soda neutralises the sting. Wasp stings are alkaline and vinegar is a suitable neutralising agent

Answers for Chapter 7

1. Bacteria and viruses
2. a and b exist as unicellular fungi and c and d form mould colonies
3. Strongly
4. An organism able to grow in the presence of atmospheric oxygen
5. Water leaves the organism by osmosis and the organism dehydrates, becomes inactive and may die
6. 20–45°C
7. The viral protein coat is broken and the viral genetic material is released into the host cell
8. Organisms that spread disease from one host to another such as ticks
9. An inanimate object that spreads disease from one animal to another such as a feeding bowl
10. Outside the cell wall

Answers for Chapter 8

1. All of the listed agents
2. Cestodes and trematodes do not use GABA as a neurotransmitter and the drugs work by affecting the nervous impulse transmission at the synapse of parasites that use GABA
3.
   – Benzimidazoles – bind to nematode tubulin
   – Imidazothiazoles, e.g. levamisole – a direct cholinergic (stimulates ganglia) and paralyses nematodes by sustained muscle contraction
   – Tetrahydropyrimidines, e.g. pyrantel – a depolarising neuromuscular blocker

– Organophosphates – inhibition of AChE leading to paralysis of the parasite
– Macrocyclic lactones, e.g. selamectin. Bind to and potentiate GABA-gated chloride channels
– Heterocyclic compounds, e.g. piperazine. Hyperpolarises nerve membranes at the neuromuscular junction and induces paralysis in the parasite

4. Tubular damage occurs because amphotericin B binds to cholesterol in the tubular cells which results in electrolyte leakage from the cells and renal tubular acidosis. Induced renal vasoconstriction and impaired acid excretion contribute to the toxicity

Answers for Chapter 9

1. T
2. F – it is a form of active immunity as the body has to actively respond to the product and formulate an immune response
3. F – it is the administration of an antigen or organism
4. T
5. T
6. F – they can still replicate but have been altered so they do not cause infection
7. F – FeLV is a viral vaccine
8. T
9. F – there are vaccines available for both of these infectious agents
10. F – polyvalent vaccines fit this definition
11. T – 31 infectious organisms have been identified as causes of kennel cough, including 12 different viruses and bacteria. Currently vaccines are available for three of the known components: parainfluenza, adenovirus type 2 and *Bordetella bronchiseptica*. Vaccination for these three organisms prevents 90% of the cases of kennel cough

12. **T** – by doing this, the virus will adapt to its new host environment and lose its virulence for the original host

13. **T**

14. **F** – there is no evidence to support anti-inflammatory doses of steroids prevent a response to vaccination, but it is wise to use a killed vaccine or monovalents to reduce the challenge to the immune system

15. **T** – this condition prevents the adrenal gland from secreting steroids in response to stress, including that from vaccination. The deficiency can result in lethargy, loss of appetite, weakness, vomiting, seizures, shock and death in severe cases

16. **T**

17. **F** – the speed of protection varies depending on the type of vaccine given. Consult the datasheets for advice. Live intranasal vaccines, for example, can be used in the face of an outbreak due to their rapid response and the kennel cough vaccine confers immunity within 72 hours

18. **F** – in one study, 20% of dogs were found to have circulating maternal antibody as late as 18 weeks of age and therefore susceptible dogs may benefit from a final booster at 20 and 22 weeks of age

Answers for Chapter 10

1. b
2. b
3. b
4. a
5. c

Answers for Chapter 11

1. Increasing the strength of contraction and therefore increasing cardiac output

2. Oxygen demand is dependent on the cardiac workload. It is therefore affected by heart rate, the strength of contraction, afterload (aortic blood pressure) and the size of the heart (how much the myocardial fibres stretch)

3. The term glycoside in general refers to a compound linked by an oxygen atom to a sugar molecule(s)

4. Increased myocardial contractility, increased cardiac output, diuresis, reduction of oedema, control of arrhythmias, reductions in venous pressures, heart size and heart rate

5. Decrease all variables

6. The decrease in calcium entering the heart cells results in a reduction in myocardial contractility, vasodilation in peripheral and coronary arterial beds, reduced pressure against left ventricular outflow, reduced myocardial oxygen demand, slowed AV node impulse conduction

7. A reduction in blood volume leads to a decreased venous return, a reduction in filling of the heart and so a reduction in cardiac output unless positive inotropic drugs are used concurrently

Answers for Chapter 12

1. The abbreviation E denotes an emetic and AE denotes anti-emetic
   a. E
   b. AE
   c. E
   d. E
   e. AE
   f. E
   g. AE
   h. E
   i. E
   j. AE
   k. AE

2.
   a. HA
   b. DP
   c. A
   d. HA

3. Misoprostol
4. They are intestinal motility modifiers that increase segmental intestinal contractions and decrease peristaltic contractions, thereby slowing gastrointestinal transit time
5. Antibiotics may destroy the normal protective microflora and allow colonisation of the mucosa by potential pathogens. They should therefore be reserved for cases showing bloody diarrhoea, pyrexia, leucopaenia, and leucocytosis

Answers for Chapter 13

1. F – hyperventilation secondary to stress is the most common cause
2. F
3. T
4. T
5. F – it can be bought without prescription at pharmacies
6. F – amlodipine, a second-generation dihydropyridine calcium channel blocker whose main effects are in the peripheral vessels, is the first-choice agent to manage systemic hypertension in cats
7. F – even at the higher dose rate, there have been no adverse effects reported to date
8. F – the partial agonist opioids can be given orally as a suspension. For example, 2 ml of butorphanol mixed in 30 ml of metatone syrup to disguise the taste is a useful way to provide analgesia at home
9. F – antibiotics should not be given unless absolutely necessary as this is likely to generate drug-resistant bacteria. It is better to start antibiotic therapy on removal of the catheter, with the agent selected according to culture of the catheter tip
10. T

Answers for Chapter 14

1. F – transmission is usually in one direction as fibres are either motor or sensory
2. F – over 40 different substances have been found and many are active in the CNS
3. T
4. F – it has an inhibitory action
5. T
6. T

Answers for Chapter 15

1. The test is used to diagnose hyperadrenocorticism and for the definitive diagnosis of primary adrenal hypofunction. ACTH is well absorbed following i.m. injection and can be given by this route or by i.v. injection. A basal cortisol level reading is taken before the aqueous synthetic ACTH is administered. Plasma cortisol levels peak at 30–90 minutes due to the short half-life of ACTH, therefore most sampling protocols advise sampling at 1 hour post-injection. Administration of 250 µg of synthetic ACTH to dogs results in similar cortisol levels regardless of whether it was given i.m. or i.v. This is not, however, the case in cats
2. The TRH stimulation test is designed to evaluate the pituitary's responsiveness to TRH as manifested by the change in serum TSH concentration. In primary thyroid gland failure the pituitary response to TRH is increased; in hyperthyroidism it is decreased
3. It is the most definitive non-invasive test for the diagnosis of primary hypothyroidism. The administration of exogenous bovine TSH followed by the measurement of serum T_4 tests the secretory reserve of the thyroid gland
4. Aqueous ADH or ADH analogues are currently the only formulations

available for the treatment of total and partial central diabetes insipidus. The synthetic analogue DDAVP (desmopressin acetate) is the most commonly used and has also been used for bleeding disorders

5. The sources of progesterone include the corpora lutea (CL) in animals undergoing oestrus cycles and the placenta in some species. Progesterone and its synthetic analogues (the progestins) mimic the effects of a CL and thereby inhibit oestrus during the period of administration

6. A variety of drugs may impair plasma or tissue binding of the thyroid hormones or alter thyroid hormone metabolism. Drugs include the glucocorticoids, anticonvulsants, salicylates, phenylbutazone and radiocontrast agents. The mechanism by which they exert their effects varies. Salicylates and furosemide directly displace thyroid hormone from plasma binding sites. Phenylbutazone has a direct antithyroid effect. Exogenous glucocorticoids have a profound effect on thyroid function tests in the dog but less so in the cat. The anticonvulsant drugs, including phenobarbital, decrease serum T_4 levels by enhancing its rate of metabolism and excretion. Trimethoprim/sulfamethoxazole (commonly used to treat bacterial skin infections) interferes with iodine metabolism by the thyroid gland and therefore decreases serum T_4

7. Fifteen percent of cats show mild side effects of anorexia, vomiting and lethargy. In most cats these are transient and resolve despite continued treatment. Severe gastrointestinal signs do persist in some cats and treatment should be stopped. Renal values should be monitored due to the possibility of developing renal failure because of reduced renal blood flow. Remember to check if the owner is pregnant, warn them of the teratogenicity of the drug and advise the use of gloves for handling the drug and especially when cleaning out the litter tray

8. Whether the shock is toxic, haemorrhagic and/or traumatic, the body's response is similar. Catecholamines are released which cause vasoconstriction in selected areas of the body. As the peripheral circulation is affected by the shock process, there is an increase in peripheral resistance, venous return of blood to the heart is decreased and there is a decrease in cardiac output. Tissue perfusion decreases and cells become hypoxic. The first organs affected are the kidneys, bowel, liver, lung and skin. As shock progresses, there is continued vasoconstriction, greater increase in peripheral resistance, decreased venous return, tissue anoxia, acidosis, oedema and eventually there is so much tissue damage that the animal will die.

High doses of glucocorticoids cause vasodilation. This causes the blood to start flowing again, lowers peripheral resistance, increases venous return, improves cardiac output and increases tissue perfusion.

Methylprednisolone at high doses has the additional effect of protection of capillary membranes, preventing leakage of fluid into surrounding tissues and preventing pulmonary oedema. There is also protection of cell membranes, preventing cells disrupting and dying, and protection of lysosomal membranes, preventing release of enzymes which cause further cell death

9. Feline hyperadrenocorticism poses problems both in terms of diagnosis and management as the cat is less responsive to the ACTH stimulation test. The interpretation of results is further complicated by

the effects of non-adrenal illness, particularly diabetes mellitus, on the hypothalamic–pituitary–adrenal axis. Cats show a variable response to mitotane and an unpredictable response to ketoconazole with unwanted side effects. Trilostane has been used to treat cats and may prove to be a useful alternative, but at present the treatment of choice is bilateral adrenalectomy. Unilateral adrenalectomy is indicated in cats with a unilateral cortisol-secreting adrenocortical tumour. Bilateral adrenalectomy is indicated in cats with pituitary-dependent bilateral adrenocortical hyperplasia

Answers for Chapter 16

1. c
2. b
3. c
4. b

Answers for Chapter 17

1. a
2. b
3. a
4. a, b and c are correct
5. d
6. d
7. a – DMSO enhances absorption of a variety of agents including water, hydrocortisone, antibiotics and oestradiol by an unknown action
8. d
9. b
10. c

Answers for Chapter 18

1. c
2. c
3. a
4. d
5. b

Answers for Chapter 19

1. b
2. c
3. b
4. d

Answers for Chapter 20

1. d
2. d
3. a
4. d

Answers for Chapter 21

1. D, D, D, D, D, D
2. D, I, D, D, D, D
3. I, D, D, I, I
4. I, D, D, I, I, I
5. Recovery of consciousness from thiopental depends on redistribution from the brain to the muscles and then to adipose tissue (fat). The drug then slowly redistributes from the fat back into the circulation over many hours to be excreted. As sighthounds possess reduced amounts of body fat, the drug remains in the circulation for longer and recovery is prolonged. It may also be that sighthounds do not possess the liver enzymes needed for the breakdown of the drug
6. Isoflurane is stable in light and contains no additives. It has a higher MAC value, implying a higher vaporiser setting is required. There is a lower blood solubility resulting in faster induction and recovery. Halothane reduces cardiac output through its effects on myocardial contractility and heart rate, but has relatively little effect on the peripheral vasculature, while isoflurane causes little change in cardiac output but leads to marked peripheral vasodilation. Isoflurane does not sensitise the heart to catecholamine-induced arrhythmias,

and a more stable cardiac rhythm is usually observed. Isoflurane causes a greater dose-dependent depression of respiration, is a more potent muscle relaxant and there is some evidence to suggest it provides more analgesia

7. Liver disease, malnutrition, chronic anaemia, burns, certain malignancies, cytotoxic drugs, pregnancy

8. Inspired concentration, potency, alveolar ventilation, blood/gas solubility, cardiac output and alveolar to systemic venous anaesthetic partial pressure difference

9. Sevoflurane has a lower blood/gas partition coefficient (0.69) than isoflurane (1.46). This means it will provide a more rapid induction of and recovery from anaesthesia and allow for greater control of anaesthetic depth during the maintenance phase. Mask induction is 80% faster than with isoflurane. Sevoflurane is less pungent and causes less irritation to airway mucosa than isoflurane

Answers for Chapter 22

True or false

1. T
2. T
3. F – they increase the sphincter tone by this mechanism
4. T – they bind to receptors in the medullary vomiting centre and though emesis often occurs initially, opioid analgesics such as fentanyl can prevent vomiting due to other narcotics
5. F – opiates and several of their derivatives are potent inhibitors of the medullary cough centre at sub-analgesic doses and are therefore classed as centrally acting antitussives
6. T
7. F – inhibition of COX-2 in the large bowel can worsen inflammatory bowel disease and they are therefore contraindicated in ulcerative colitis, although salicylic acid is used specifically to treat inflammatory bowel disease when ulceration is not present
8. T
9. T
10. T
11. F – they provide good muscle relaxation
12. T

Short answers

1. Dilated pupils, altered pulse and respiration rate, panting, sweating, piloerection, vomiting
2. Initial physiological perception of the painful stimulus
3. Prostaglandins, histamine
4. Analgesia, sedation, respiratory depression, cough suppression, constipation
5. 20 and 90 minutes respectively
6. Respiratory distress and head injuries as it causes a rise in intracranial pressure
7. Bradycardia; atropine
8. Yes

Index

In the case of entries referring to drug groups/types, readers should also see specific drugs.

A

abortifacients, 139
accidents, 31, 42
    see also hazardous drugs; health and safety
ACE inhibitors *see* angiotensin converting enzyme (ACE) inhibitors
acepromazine, 99, 200, 201–202, 207
    combinations, 203
    dog breeds sensitive to, *202*
acepromazine maleate, *201*
acetazolamide, 161
acetylcholine (ACh), 141–143, *142, 143*
acetylcholinesterase (AChE), 99, *142,* 142–143
acetylcysteine, 112, 185
acetyl L carnitine choline, *194*
aciclovir (Zovirax), 95, 161
acid(s), 76–78
acid-base indicators, 78, *78*
acid-base reactions, 77
acid citrate-dextrose (ACD), 197
activated charcoal, 132, 184, 187, 188
activated prothrombin time (APTT), 197
acute disseminated encephalomyelitis, 105
acute respiratory distress, 113
adenine, 53–54, *54*
adenosine, 149–150
adenosine triphosphate (ATP), 50, 52, 54, 59
adenosylmethionine, 195
adenovirus-1 (CAV-1) vaccination, 104, 106
adrenal corticosteroids, 178
    see also corticosteroids

adrenal glands, 150–154
adrenaline, 204
adrenergic drugs, *138*
α-adrenergic receptor agonists, 162, 219
α-adrenergic receptor antagonists, 120
adrenolytic drugs, 153–154
adsorbents, 132, 187
    see also specific substances
adverse reactions
    classification, *6*
    definition, 5
    hypersensitivity *see* hypersensitivity reactions
    suspected, 5, 32
    toxicity, 16, 36–39, *38,* 94, 142–143
    see also specific drugs/substances
aerobic glycolysis, 54
aerosolisation (of drugs), *114,* 114–115
agar plates, *85*
    see also cultures, micro-organisms
α₂ agonists, 202–204
agonists, definition, 37
albendazole, 98
albumin, 196
albuterol, 113
alcohols, 79
aldosterone, 150
alendronate, 179
alfentanil, 216
alkanes, *78,* 78–79
alkenes, 79, *79*
alkylating agents, 177
allergic reactions *see* hypersensitivity reactions
allergic rhinitis, 162
allopurinol (Zyloric), 99

alopecia, chemotherapy-induced, 175–176
alphadolone (Saffan), 200, 207
alphaxalone, 200, 207
Aludex (amitraz), 97, 170
aluminium silicate (kaolin), 39, 131, 132
alveoli, 65
amantadine, 95
amiloride, 120
amino acids, 49–50, *50*
aminoglycoside antibiotics, *39,* 90, 91
5-aminolaevulinic acid, 179–180
aminophylline, 113, 124
amitraz (Aludex), 97, 170
amitriptyline, 10
    feline idiopathic cystitis, 137
    indications, *43,* 145
amlodipine, 122, 136
amoxicillin, 10, 89, 136
    brand names, 4
ampakines, 145
amphotericin B, 94
AMTRA training courses, 14
anabolic steroids, 40, 147
anaerobic glycolysis, 54
anaesthetics, 203–210
    dissociative, 207
    drug interactions, 124
    exotic patients, 28
    inhalational, *208,* 208–210, *209*
    injectable, 206–208
    local, *204,* 204–206, *206*
    metabolism, factors affecting, 36
    minimum alveolar concentration, 209
    topical, 160, 203
analeptics, 145
anal furunculosis, 180

blood pressure control, 61–62, 123, *124*
blood vessels *see* circulatory system
blood volume restoration, 124
'blue eye,' 104
body secretions/excretions, disposal, 29
botulism, 142
bovine cartilage, 194
BR-16A, *194*
bradyarrhythmias, 118
bradycardia, 122, 207
breast cancer, 139
British Veterinary Association (BVA) Code of Practice on Medicines (2000), 32
brodifacoum, *186*
bromadiolone, *186*
bromhexine, 112
bronchi, 64–65
bronchioles, 65
bronchodilators, 113
budesonide, 132
buffer solutions, 78
bupivacaine, 205
buprenorphine
    feline idiopathic cystitis, 137
    pharmacological action, 217
    storage, 17, *22*
butane, structure, 79, *79*
N-butanol, 198
butorphanol, 112, 156, 163
    combinations, 203
    pharmacological action, 217
butyrophenone fluanisone, 203
butyrophenones, *201*, 201–202
BVA Code of Practice on Medicines (2000), 32

C

cabergoline (Galastop), 139, 154
caffeine, 113
calcineurin inhibitors, 168
calcium borogluconate, 193
calcium carbonate, 193
calcium channel blockers, 121–122, *122*, 124
calcium gluconate, 135
Campylobacter, 83
cancer, 173–180
    antineoplastic drugs *see* antineoplastic drugs
    development, 173–174
    photodynamic therapy, 179–180
    tumour development, 173–174

canine adenovirus-1 (CAV-1) vaccination, 104, 106
canine atopy, 167–168
canine cognitive dysfunction, 145
    see also dogs
canine distemper virus vaccination, 105, 106, *106*
canine hypothyroidism, 155
canine parvovirus vaccination, 103, 106
canine pyoderma, 89
capillaries, 63
Capoten (captopril), *120, 121*
captopril (Capoten), *120, 121*
carbamates, 96
    poisoning antidotes, *184*
carbamazepine, 145
carbimazole, 124, *154*
carbohydrates, 52–53
carbonic anhydrase inhibitors, 161
carboplatin, *177*, 179
carcinogenesis, 173–174
    see also cancer
cardiac arrhythmias, 117–118
cardiac failure, 118, 119
cardiac glycosides, *39*
cardiac muscle, 61, *61*
cardiovascular disorders, 117–125
    management
        β-blocking agents, *123*, 123–124, *124*
        blood volume restoration, 124
        calcium channel blockers, 121–122, *122*, 124
        diuresis, *119*, 119–120
        goals, 118
        systolic force strengthening, 118–119
        vasodilators, *120*, 120–121
    see also specific disorders
cardiovascular system, 61–63, *62*, 215
    see also circulatory system
carprofen (Rimadyl), 30, 217, 218
cascade system, 15, 27
castor oil, 128
cathartics, 128
cats
    chronic renal failure, 136
    drug metabolism issues, 36
    eosinophilic skin lesions, 169
    idiopathic cystitis, 136–137
    oral drug administration, 20
    steroid anaesthetics, 207
    vomiting reflex, 128
    see also under feline

cell(s), 53–61, *56*
    classification, *55*
    dimensions, *50*
    division, 66
    metabolism, 54
    structure and function, 55–56, *57*
    transport, 56
cell cycle, *175*, 175–176
cell membranes, 56, *57*
    calcium channels, *122*
cellulitis, 168
central nervous system (CNS), 141–148
    blood-brain barrier, 36, 141
    neuromuscular drugs, 147–148
    neuromuscular junction, 141–143, *142*
    opiate analgesics, effects, 215
    sensitisation, 214
    stimulants, 145
charcoal *see* activated charcoal
chelonia, 26
chemical reactions, 76
chemistry, 73–80
chemoreceptor trigger zone (CRTZ), 128, 129, *129*
chemotherapeutic agents *see* antineoplastic drugs
chemotherapy drug spill kits, 42
Cheyletiella infestation, 96, 97
chitosanide, 166
chlorambucil, 132, *177*, 180
chloramphenicol, 92
    drug interactions, *39*, 144
    mode of action, 90
    ophthalmic use, 161
    otitis interna, 162
chlorazepate, 144–145
chlorhexidine, 163, 166
    shampoos, 166, *169*
chloroform, 208
chlorothiazide (Saluric), 120
chlorphacinone, *186*
chlorpheniramine (Piriton), 10, 162
chlorpromazine, *201*
chlortetracycline, 91
cholecalciferol, 157, *184*
cholinesterase inhibiting insecticides, poisoning, 184–185
chondroitin, 192, 195
chromatin, 65
chyle, 63
ciclosporin, 132, 168, 180
    eosinophilic skin lesions, 169
    ophthalmic use, 160

toxicity, 16, 36–39, *38*, 94, 142–143
    see also specific drugs/substances
toxoplasmosis, ocular, 161
trachea, 64–65
training courses, AMTRA, 14
tranquilisers, *201*
transition metals, 75
triamcinolone acetonide, 168
triamterene, 120
triazoles, 94
tricaine methanesulfonate (MS222), 28
trichomoniasis, 132
tricyclic antidepressants, 10, 137, 145
trifluridine, 95
triglycerides, *51*, 51–52
trilazad mesylate, 146
trilostane, 153–154
trimeprazine, *201*
trimethobenzamide hydrochloride, 130
trimethoprim, 91
trimethoprim-sulphadiazine, 161, 162
tropicamide, 161
Trusopt (dorzolamide), 161
trypsin, 50
tumours *see* cancer
turmeric, 192
tylosin, 92

U

ulcerative keratitis, 161
urethral spasm, 137, *137*
urinary acidifiers, 137
urinary alkalinisers, 137
urinary incontinence, 137–138
urinary retention, 138
urinary tract, 60, 135–139, 215
    infections, 10, 136

V

vaccination, 101–109
    administration routes, 105–106

adverse effects/contra-
    indications, 104–106, *106*
efficacy, factors affecting, *103*, 103–104
flea bite hypersensitivity, 168
homeopathic, 106
types, *102*, 102–103, 106–108
viral-induced diseases, 94
    see also specific diseases
vaccine interference, 104
Valium *see* diazepam
valproic acid, 145
vasculitis, vaccine-induced, 105
vasoconstrictors, 204
vasodilators, *120*, 120–121
Vasotop (ramipril), *121*
vectors, 84
vecuronium, 147
ventilatory muscles, strengthening, 124
verapamil (Cordilox), 121, 122
Veterinary Medicinal Products
    definition, *14*
    retail supplies, RCVS advice, 16
    see also drug(s)
The Veterinary Medicines Directorate
    (VMD), 5, 38
Veterinary Medicines Guidance
    Notes, 16
Veterinary Medicines Regulations
    2005, 13, 14
    see also pharmacy law
Vetmedin (pimobendan), 122
Vetoquinol (ipakitine), 136
vidarabine, 95
vinblastine, *177*, 178
vinca alkaloids, 178, *179*
vincristine, 177, 178, 180
    administration, *42*
    drug interactions, 122
    mode of action, *177*
Virbac (gentamicin), 27, 90, 91, 161
viruses, 49, 54, 94
    replication, 84, *84*
vitamin(s), 194

vitamin A, 27
vitamin C, 19, 137
vitamin D, 157, *184*
vitamin K, 186
Vivitonin (propentofylline), 145, *146*
VMD (Veterinary Medicines
    Directorate), 5, 38
vomiting, 128–130, *129*

W

warfarin, 39, *184*, 186
waste disposal, 30–31
    contaminated body secretions/
        excretions, 29
    pharmaceutical
        DOOP bins, 29, 31
        drug administration
            equipment, 29
water
    function, 55
    structure, 55, 75–76, *76*
whole blood, 197
whole bowel irrigation, 188

X

xylazine
    combinations, 203
    emesis, 128, *129*
    indications, 187
    pharmacological action, 219
xylazine stimulation test, 41, *41*

Y

yeasts, *82*, 83–84
yohimbine hydrochloride, 203

Z

Zantac (ranitidine), 130–131, *131*
zidovudine (AZT), 95
zinc poisoning, antidotes, *184*
zinc sulphate, 193
zolazepam, *201*
zoonoses, 84
Zovirax (aciclovir), 95, 161
Zyloric (allopurinol), 99

Printed and bound by CPI Group (UK) Ltd, Croydon, CR0 4YY

08/06/2025

01896874-0006